Practical Approach to
Cosmetic & Regenerative Gynecology

Dr. Garima Srivastav (MD, MRCOG) &
Dr. Fahad Usman (MD)

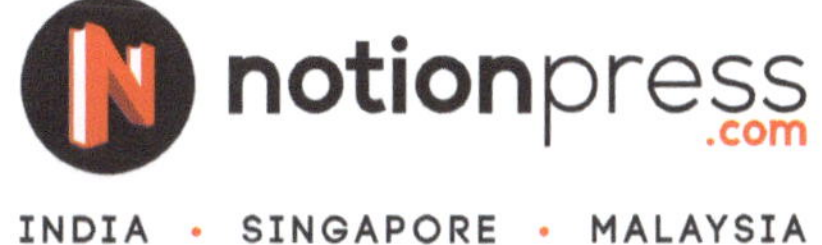

Copyright © Dr. Garima Srivastav & Dr. Fahad Usman 2024
All Rights Reserved.

ISBN
Paperback 979-8-89322-854-0
Hardcase 979-8-89415-043-7

This book has been published with all efforts taken to make the material error-free after the consent of the author. However, the author and the publisher do not assume and hereby disclaim any liability to any party for any loss, damage, or disruption caused by errors or omissions, whether such errors or omissions result from negligence, accident, or any other cause.

While every effort has been made to avoid any mistake or omission, this publication is being sold on the condition and understanding that neither the author nor the publishers or printers would be liable in any manner to any person by reason of any mistake or omission in this publication or for any action taken or omitted to be taken or advice rendered or accepted on the basis of this work. For any defect in printing or binding the publishers will be liable only to replace the defective copy by another copy of this work then available.

**Dedicated to the Three pillars of my life…..
My Parents, Husband and Daughter**

ACKNOWLEDGEMENT

In the profound journey of exploring the nuances of cosmetic gynecology, this book stands as a collective effort of unwavering dedication, tireless research, and the relentless pursuit of excellence. To the authors whose expertise and passion have woven together the fabric of knowledge within these pages, your invaluable contributions have illuminated pathways for understanding and advancement in this specialized realm.

We extend our heartfelt appreciation to the practitioners, researchers, and professionals whose insights and commitment have shaped the very essence of this evolving field. Your continuous efforts in pushing the boundaries of cosmetic gynecology have not only expanded the horizons of medical understanding but also empowered countless individuals to embrace holistic well-being.

To the editors, designers, and all those behind the scenes who worked tirelessly to bring this endeavor to fruition, your dedication and meticulous attention to detail have ensured the delivery of a comprehensive and enlightening source.

Last, but certainly not least, we express our gratitude to the readers and enthusiasts who with an insatiable thirst for knowledge, seek to further their understanding of cosmetic gynecology. It is your curiosity and eagerness that propel the perpetuation of discovery and innovation in this field.

May this book serve as both a guiding light and a testament to the collaborative spirit that defines the realm of cosmetic gynecology!

Dr. Garima Srivastav

CONTRIBUTORS

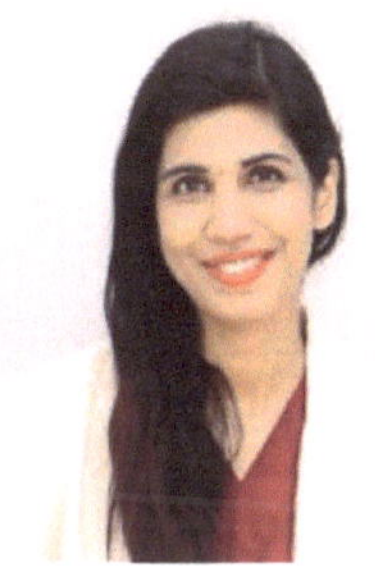

Dr. Garima Srivastav (M.D., D.N.B., M.R.C.O.G.)
- Consultant Gynecologist, Board Certified Cosmetic Gynecologist, International Trainer, Speaker, Influencer, Entrepreneur, Author, Mother.
- Faculty: American Board Aesthetic Association
- President: Indian Association of Cosmetic Gynecology
- Co-Founder: Orange Klinic & Dr. Snug
- Social Media Influencer & Educator
- Fellowship in Laparoscopy, SHIMIST
- Fellowship in ART & Reproductive Medicine (Kiel School, Germany)
- Fellowship in Cosmetic Gynecology (Dubai)
- Fellowship in Ultrasound (USA)

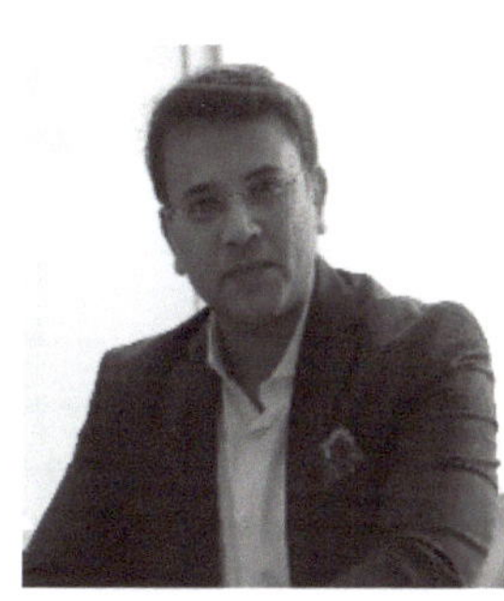

Dr. Fahad Usman M.D.
- Stem Cell Consultant, Dermatologist & Board- Certified Aesthetic Physician International Trainer, Researcher & Speaker
- Dip.Derm (UK) - 2015
- Certificate In Aesthetic Medicine (AAAM - USA 2016
- Diploma in Aesthetic Medicine (AAAM-USA) 2016
- Fellowship in Aesthetic Medicine -American Board Of Aesthetic Medicine & Surgery USA 2016
- Fellowship In Cutaneous & Laser Surgery -Institute Of Dermatology Bangkok Thailand 2017
- Fellowship In Cosmetic Gynaecology 2018
- Board Certified in Aesthetic Medicine - American Board Of Aesthetic Medicine & Surgery USA 2018
- Certification In Regenerative Medicine - ISSCA Global Stem Cells Group USA - 2018

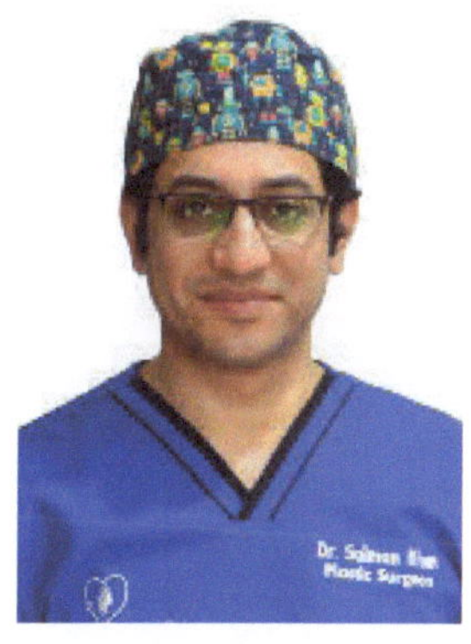

Dr. M. Salman Khan, M.D.
- Fellowship in Plastic Surgery, Consultant Plastic Surgeon
- Senior Faculty ARM - US,
- Master Trainer for Liposuction, Hair Transplant, and Cosmetic Gynecology, Dubai.

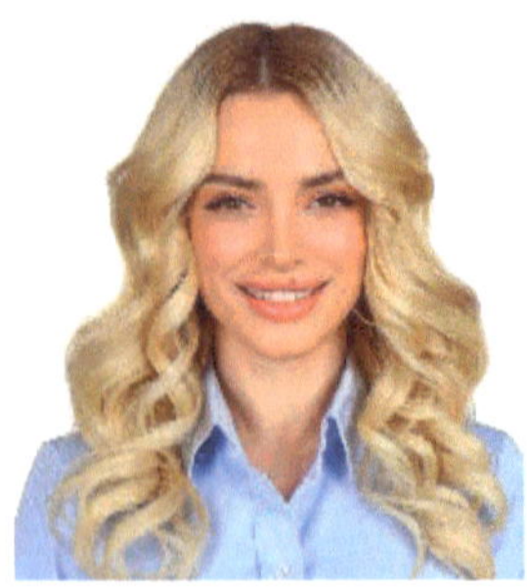

Dr. Sibel Ustunel M.D.
- Consultant gynecologist
- Assistant Professor Altınbaş MedicalPark University Hospital
- Faculty – American Board of Aesthetic Gynecology

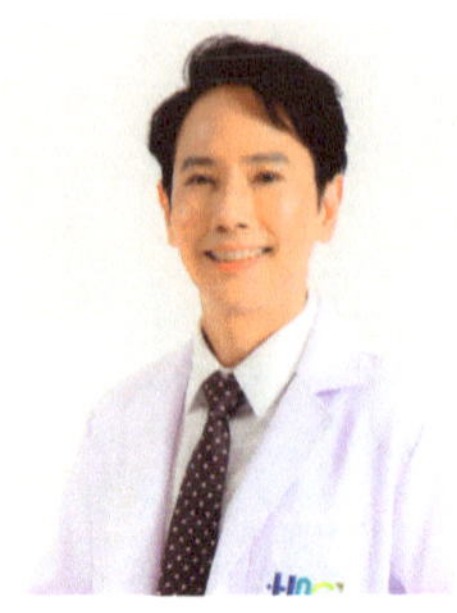

Dr. ATIWUT KAMUDHAMAS M.D., DHS, Ph.D.,
- Present administrative position: Head of the Department of Obstetrics and Gynecology, Faculty of Medicine, Thammasat University
- Special fields at work: 1. Obstetrics and Gynecology 2. Clinical sexology and Sexual medicine
- Division of Clinical Sexology and Sexual Medicine,
- Department of Obstetrics and Gynecology,
- Faculty of Medicine, Thammasat University, Klong-Luang, Pathumthani, 12120, THAILAND.

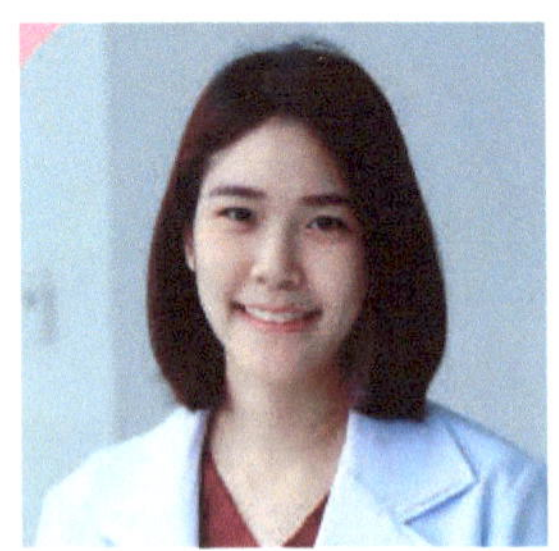

Dr. Nopwaree Chantawong
- Fellowship in Cosmetic Gynecology 2023
- American Board of Aesthetic Gynecology,
- American Academy of Aesthetic and Regenerative Medicine
- Fellowship in Cosmetic Gynecology 2023
- International Society of Aesthetic Genital Surgery and Sexology
- Certificate in Gynaecological Endoscopy 2023
- Faculty of Medicine, Ramathibodi Hospital, Bangkok, Thailand
- Diploma in Sexual Medicine 2021
- Faculty of Medicine, Thammasat University, Pathumthani, Thailand
- Diploma, Thai Sub-Board of Gynecologic Oncology 2019
- Faculty of Medicine, Chiang Mai University, Chiang Mai, Thailand
- Diploma, Thai Board of Obstetrics and Gynecology 2017
- Faculty of Medicine, Chiang Mai University, Chiang Mai, Thailand
- Doctor of Medicine 2012
- Faculty of Medicine, Thammasart University, Bangkok, Thailand

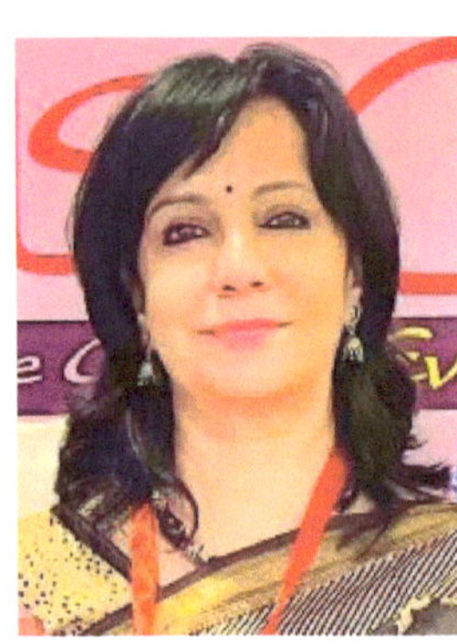

Dr. Minie Anand M.S.
- Consultant Obstetrician and Gynecologist
- Cosmetic laser & Gyne Surgeon, Sun Hospital, Patna, Bihar
- Professor Madhubani Medical College, Madhubani, Bihar, India.
- Fellowship in Cosmetic Gynecology

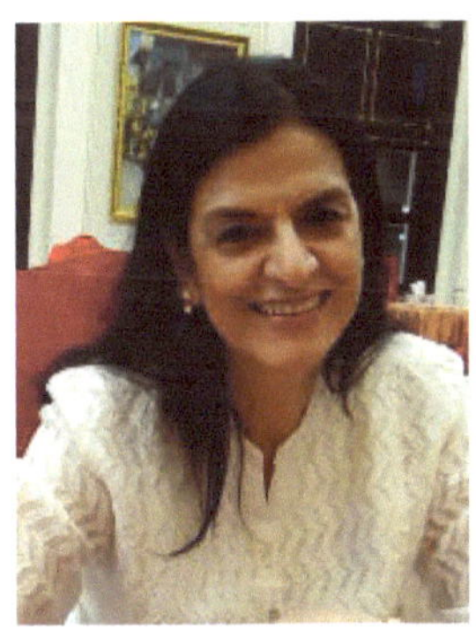

Dr. Chitra Jha MBBS, DGO, FRCOG
- Senior Consultant Obstetrics and Gynaecology
- Graduated from the Armed Forces Medical College Pune, India, and subsequently served in the Indian Army for 5 years.
- Was head of the Maternal Medicine and High-Risk Pregnancy and Gynaecology unit at the Royal Hospital, Oman. Currently employed at Muscat Private Hospital Oman.
- Completed her membership and has been a Fellow of the Royal College of Obstetricians and Gynecologists, UK since 2014
- Has a special interest in Aesthetic Gynecology and is passionate about patient safety and Risk Management.
- Being actively involved in teaching and research has presented several papers at National and International conferences.

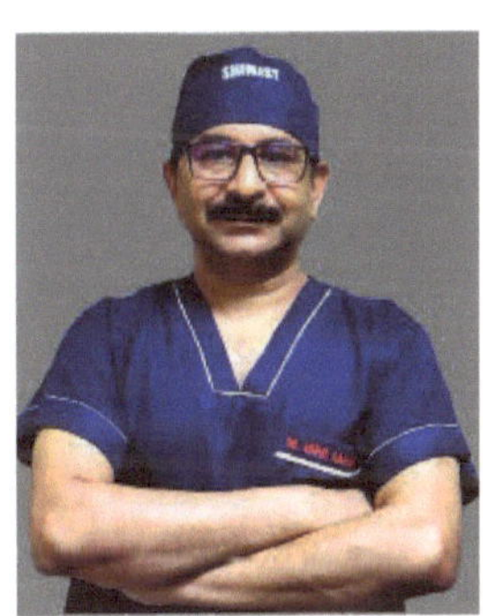

Dr. Akhil Saxena M.S.
- HOD Consultant Surgeon (Minimal Access Surgery), SHIMIST, India
- Director – SMH & SHIMIST – Training Centre for Minimal Access Surgery, Gynecology, Urology & Urogynecology Course Director:
- Diploma in Gynecological Laparoscopy, Hysteroscopy & Urogynecology by UKSH, Germany in India & UAE
- SHIMIST-SAARC German Course on MIS in Gynecology & Urogynecology in India, UAE & Germany
- MAS training programs at Kathmandu- Nepal
- MAS training program at BIMAS & OGSB Hospital - Dhaka

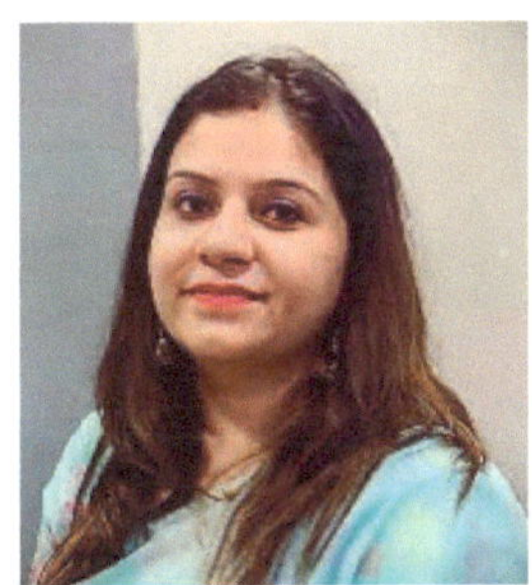

Dr. Sandhya Deora M.D.
- MRCOG (London)
- Laparoscopic surgeon
- Laser and cosmetic gynecologist, India

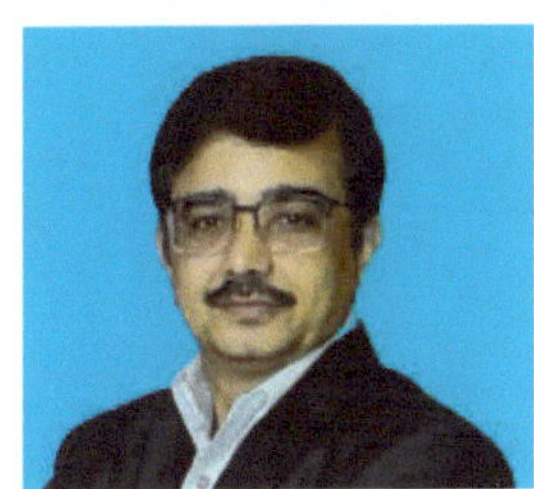

Dr. Jignesh Vaghasia
- MBBS DGO
- Fellowship in Cosmetic Gynecology
- Vaghasia Hospital, Talala, Gujarat, India

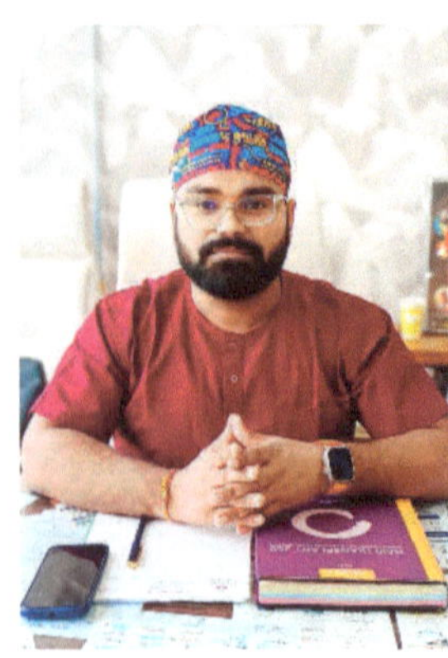

Dr. Nitesh Prajapati
- Cosmetic Sexologist & Cosmetic Gynecologist
- MBBS From MGM MC Indore MP.
- DVD (SKIN & VD) From VIMS Mumbai
- FCG-fellowship in cosmetic gynecology
- Diploma in male cosmetic andrology
- (Expert in shock wave, botox filler, PRP & PRF)
- Director of
  1- Manmantha Mens Clinic
  2- All India Institute of Aesthetic & Cosmetic Surgery- Academy
  (Branches- Lucknow, Indore, Dehradoon, Ahmedabad, Surat, Allahabad)

CONTENTS

Module 3

ADJUVANT THERAPIES

Module 4

SURGICAL ASPECT

Module 5

RECENT ADVANCES

MODULE 1

UNDERSTANDING THE BASICS OF COSMETIC GYNECOLOGY

INTRODUCTION TO COSMETIC & REGENERATIVE GYNAECOLOGY

Garima Srivastav

DEFINITION & SCOPE

- Cosmetic & Regenerative Gynecology is the fastest-growing branch in women's healthcare. Cosmetic gynecology aka Aesthetic gynecology aka Female Genital Plastic / Cosmetic surgery (FGPS) aka Regenerative gynecology has caught the attention of all in current times. Together with its promise of improving female sexual health, it is THE branch in the field of Cosmesis.

- The various names have mirrored the semantic direction of their individuals/authors. For example, the various terminologies given are Female Cosmetic Genital Surgery (FCGS), Vulvovaginal Aesthetic Surgery (VVAS), Aesthetic Vulvovaginal Surgery (AVS), Cosmetic Plastic Gynecology (CPG). In the current book, we will use the term Aesthetic or Cosmetic gynecology.

- It is a futuristic branch that spans gynecology, dermatology, urogynecology, urology & and plastic surgery. It covers not only women's genitalia but complete female aesthetics from head to toe.

- As the popularity of our practice rises, we have mounting data on published clinical experience, operative methods, and scientific data, we have sufficient data for patient selection, procedures, minimal complication rates as well as published evidence on psychological benefits.

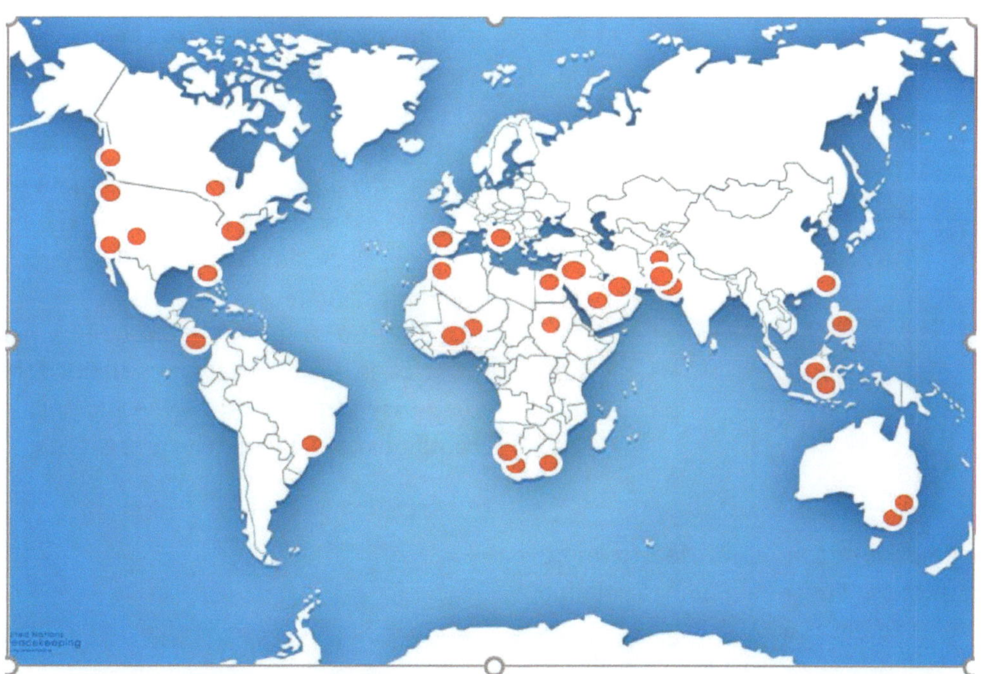

Regions with increasing demand for Cosmetic Gynecology

WHAT IS COSMETIC GYNAECOLOGY?

- It covers a variety of procedures that includes both cosmetic procedures to enhance the aesthetic appearance of the vulva/vaginal region as well as functional vaginal repairs to enhance or help restore sexual function following the changes that may occur following childbirth or aging.
- The author feels that Cosmetic or aesthetic gynecology is the first step toward women being unapologetic and forthcoming about their sexual health concerns beyond the scope of reproduction. The discussion of female arousal issues, orgasmic disorders, or reduced sensitivity never caught the eye of researchers unlike that of male sexual dysfunction. The separate subspecialty not only helps us as health care providers to talk about these issues with our women but also helps spread the concerns and treatment around these issues more effectively.
- The branch is here to revolutionize the sexual health of women at all phases of their lives.

PREVALENCE OF SEXUAL PROBLEMS

Age (y)	Lacked interest in sex	Unable to achieve orgasm	Experienced pain during sex	Sex not pleasurable	Anxious about performance	Trouble lubricating
57-64	45.4 (37.9-52.9)	35.0 (28.9-41.2)	18.2 (13.8-22.7)	23.4 (17.6-29.2)	10.7 (6.5-14.9)	36.1 (29.7-42.6)
65-74	37.6 (28.3-46.9)	33.4 (25.4-41.3)	18.9 (11.0-26.8)	22.4 (15.3-29.4)	12.7 (6.4-19.1)	43.7 (35.3-52.1)
75-85	49.3 (36.8-61.9)	38.2 (23.7-52.8)	11.8 (4.3-19.4)	24.9 (14.8-35.0)	9.9 (1.7-18.2)	43.6 (27.8-59.3)

Note: Statistics provided in this table are the prevalence and the 95% confidence interval.

HISTORICAL PERSPECTIVE

Since time immemorial people have tried to improve beauty and aesthetics. Sushruta Samhita mentions labioplasty written as early as 600 BC.

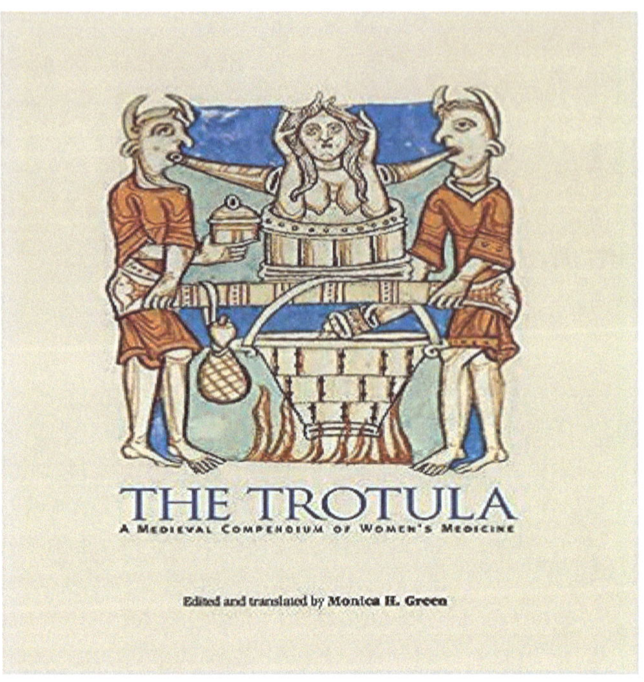

The work of female physician, TROTULA de RUGGIERO is believed to have first described vaginoplasty.

The history of cosmetic gynecology is a testament to the ever-evolving landscape of women's healthcare and societal perceptions of beauty and body image.

While the roots of cosmetic gynecology can be traced back to the late 20th century, its development gained momentum in the early 2000s making a significant shift in the field of gynecology.

Pioneering surgeons like Dr. Gary Alter, David Matlock, and Michael P. Goodman played pivotal roles in the early promotion and refinement of labioplasty.

The other noted physicians in the field are Dr. Red Allinsod, Dr. Adam Ostrzenski Dr. Marco Pelosi 11, and Dr. Charles Runnels.

The use of laser, radiofrequency, and HIFU which have been used in face aesthetics for a long found their way into cosmetic gynecology as well. The field continues to evolve till the present day.

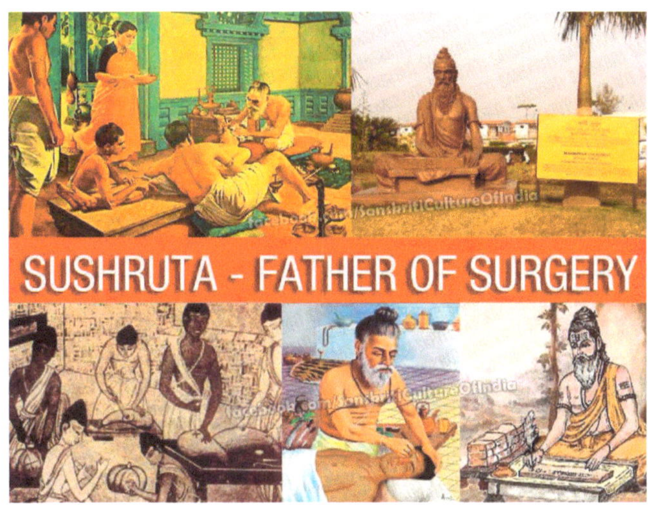

- Influence of social media on perceptions of beauty and aesthetics.
- Distorted view of normal genitalia as shown in porn sites and adult videos.
- Social media like Instagram Snapchat or Pinterest.

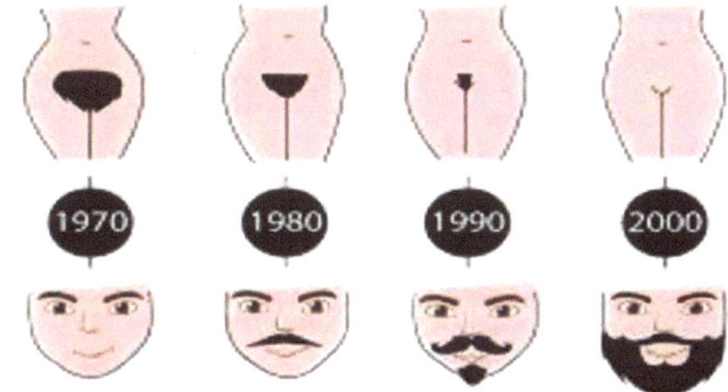

GAINING POPULARITY

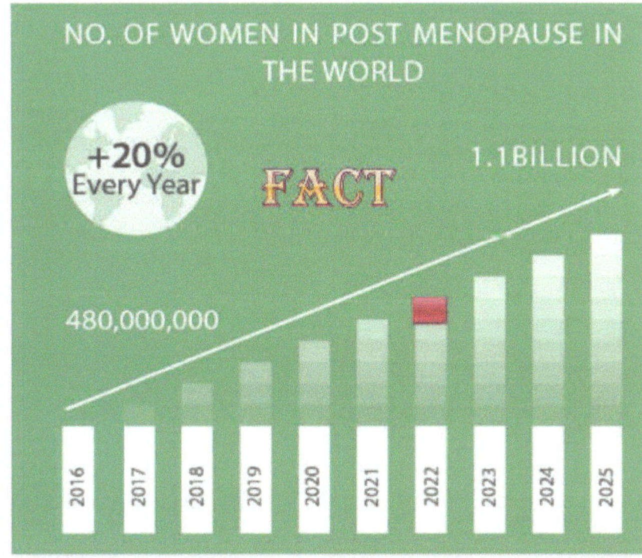

- Studies have shown with increasing awareness & and susceptibility to the internet: Women are becoming more aware of their beauty and sexuality.
- 30% of all visitors to porn sites are women: Desire for a perfect body and to mimic the appearances of such models is becoming common.
- Increase in the longevity of life: The average woman spends 1/3rd of her life in the post-menopausal phase.
- Financial-independence and women empowerment.
- Changes in grooming practices and more focus on aesthetics by women.

WHY GYNECOLOGISTS MUST KNOW ABOUT THIS FIELD??

It is the fastest-growing subspecialty of gynecology. Not knowing about this field is like living under a rock.

Unlike other counterparts like ART and Endoscopy, which require a long learning curve and investments, this branch has a much easier learning curve and is easy to master.

It does not require a hospital setting unlike other branches but can be started in a clinic set up as well.

In countries like India, usually, women's first point of contact is a gynecologist for most of their needs. Earlier gynecologists used to refer most of these patients to other specialties. Understanding this speciality makes you an overall healthcare provider including sexual health problems.

Almost all our obstetrics and gynecology patients are good candidates for this branch, yet as doctors we never realized that we can offer a simpler treatment for all these issues due to the lack of training and knowledge among doctors.

Patients with these issues cannot locate a provider for some of these sexual health issues and go to a sexologist because they feel their doctor does not address these issues.

In the end just want to emphasize the huge demand and potential in the market which is left for us doctors to address.

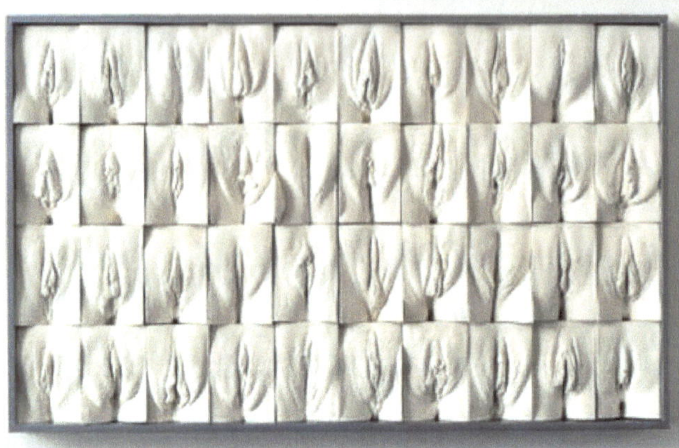

The great wall of Vagina; McCartney

COMMON PROCEDURES IN COSMETIC GYNECOLOGY

Energy-based devices (EBD) like Lasers, Radio-frequency, Highly Focused Ultrasound (HIFU), and Carboxytherapy have made it possible to treat conditions previously considered untreatable or difficult to treat, without hospitalization, no downtime, early recovery, and reduced cost. Patients have a high degree of satisfaction provided we select our patients well. The various modalities that are discussed in subsequent chapters are:

- Lasers (CO_2, Erbium, Diode, LLLT)
- Radiofrequency
- HIFU
- Electromagnetic Field Therapy
- Carboxytherapy
- Chemical treatments for lightening
- PRP
- Labial Fillers
- BOTOX
- Plasma Therapy
- Fat Grafting
- G spot augmentation

Surgical Procedures
- Labioplasty
- Labia majora reduction / augmentation
- Vaginoplasty
- Vaginal intraorbital repairs
- G spot amplification
- Clitoral hood reduction
- Hymenoplasty
- PerineoplastY

Regenerative gynecology
- Fat graft
- Platelet-rich plasma
- Stem cells
- Amniotic fluid
- Amniotic membrane

FACTORS AFFECTING TISSUE REMODELING
- Ageing
- Delivery
- Genetic predisposition
- Radiation
- Diet
- Exercise
- Smoking
- Surgery
- Pollution

Is Cosmetic Gynecology effective?

The majority of studies regarding patient satisfaction and sexual function after vaginal aesthetic and functional plastic procedures report beneficial results, with overall patient satisfaction in the 90–95% range, and sexual satisfaction over 80–85%. These data are supported by outcome data from non-elective vaginal support procedures. Complications appear minor and acceptable to patients.

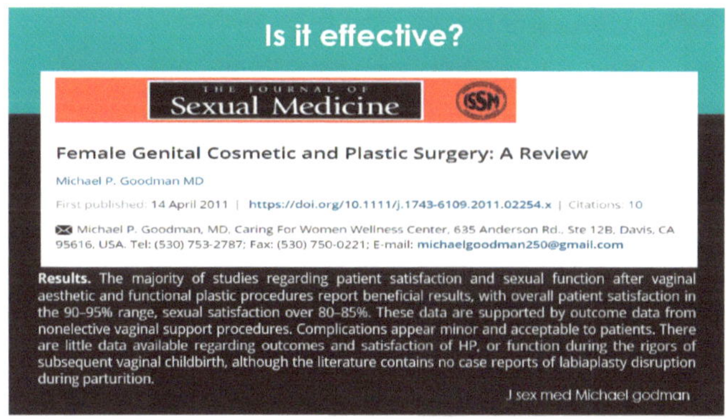

As this field is relatively new, we are at that point in history where major advancements may continue to happen and we will be able to offer evidence-based medicine in this field as well.

More and more studies are citing the benefits of energy-based devices with little side effects, it is speculated that it is only a matter of time before these devices may get recognized by various organizations. HIFEM technology is FDA-approved for male and female non-invasive urinary incontinence treatment.

FDA has not approved other devices for "vaginal rejuvenation" till the date of writing of this chapter.

CHALLENGES TO THE FIELD
- Knowledge and awareness are deficient in both patients as well as doctors.
- Aware patients often find it difficult to identify a qualified surgeon.
- Lack of long-term prospective studies.
- Historically a taboo subject often enables shyness in patients and their inability to seek treatment.
- Most traditional gynecologists may not address such issues.
- Lack of training in doctors.
- Lack of aesthetic wound closure skills in gynecologists.

COMMERCIAL NOMENCLATURES
- Vaginal rejuvenation
- Designer laser vaginoplasty
- Revirgination
- Barbie vulva
- Designer vulva

The target consumers often mistakenly believe such official-sounding terms to medically recognized procedures. Remember these are not medically recognized words and should not be used in your documentation for legal safety.

COMMON FEMININE CONCERNS ADDRESSED
- Vaginal dryness, burning, itching.
- Loss of elasticity and tone. (VRS)
- Urinary incontinence.
- Vaginal atrophy.
- Symptoms of menopause.
- Thrush and bladder infections.
- Painful intercourse.
- Vagina/vulva pain.
- Mild prolapse.
- Reduced sensitivity & sexual arousal.
- Lichen sclerosis.
- Vulval skin resurfacing for scars, and tissue laxity.

EVIDENCE-BASED MEDICINE
The existing scientific literature on cosmetic gynecology has been steadily growing. Some key aspects covered in the literature include:

Studies have confirmed the rising trend of cosmetic gynecological procedures due to various factors and cultural factors affecting women's decisions.

A lot of research continues to show improved patient satisfaction, better psychological well-being, and quality of life after undergoing these procedures.

Various studies are confirming the safety aspects of these procedures including potential complications, and short-term and long-term risks which will be covered in each section of the subsequent chapters.

Literature has also shown the positive psychological impact of cosmetic gynecological procedures including their influence on body image, self-esteem, and sexual satisfaction.

Some literature has also started to investigate the long-term effects and potential complications of these procedures to provide a more comprehensive understanding of safety and efficacy.

CAUTION
American College of Obstetrics and Gynecology (ACOG) recommends that patients should be made aware that procedures to change sexual function and appearance (except done for clinical indications like female sexual dysfunction, pain during intercourse, vaginal prolapse, or incontinence) are not medically indicated, pose a substantial risk and their safety and effectiveness has not been established.

Further, US Food and Drug Administration (FDA) warns against the use of Energy -based devices to perform "vaginal rejuvenation" of vaginal cosmetic procedures as the safety and effectiveness of these devices have not been established. (30th July, 2018)

FDA issued a warning to women, healthcare providers, and industry: Energy-based vaginal rejuvenation procedures marketed for the treatment of vaginal symptoms related to menopause, urinary incontinence, or sexual function are not proven safe and effective and are dangerous to women.

- FDA-approved laser to be used on face and vagina for surgical procedures.
- Approved for Destruction of abnormal or pre-cancerous cervical, and vaginal tissues, condylomas, and warts.

The author believes it is only a matter of time before we have enough citations and studies that all major guidelines approve energy-based devices for their various aforementioned indications.

The thickness of vaginal mucosa is 4mm while the penetration of lasers and other EBDs is much less, therefore theoretically they are safe options to be used in the vaginal mucosa. In the last few years, we have witnessed more and more studies citing the benefits of these procedures.

One of the early indicators of the direction where we may be heading is the fact that the HIFEM technology has been approved by the US FDA for male and female non-invasive urinary incontinence treatment.

CONCLUSION

In conclusion, cosmetic gynecology represents a growing and significant aspect within the broader field of gynecology. As societal norms and cultural influences continue to evolve, women's perception of their bodies has taken center stage, giving rise to increasing demand for cosmetic procedures tailored to intimate and aesthetic concerns of female anatomy.

While cosmetic gynecology offers promising opportunities for enhancing self-esteem and quality of life, it must prioritize patient–centered care and ethical considerations. Thorough per-operative counseling, informed consent, understanding patient's concerns, and setting realistic patient expectations are integral to fostering a positive influence.

Safety remains of paramount importance. As the literature highlights potential risks and complications, it is imperative that practitioners employ evidence-based approaches, adhere to best practices, and continuously prioritize patient well-being.

ACOG recommends proper counseling of patients including risks and limitations of procedures and informed consent should be taken before undertaking any cosmetic procedure.

In experienced hands, these procedures are quite safe with a high degree of patient satisfaction and life-changing benefits. However, it should preferably be advised for managing clinical conditions rather than purely cosmetic reasons.

REFERENCES

1. Fisher LL Sex, Romance and Relationships: AARP survey of midlife and older Adults April 2010.

2. Shindel AW,Parish SJ. Sexuality education in North American Medical Schools: current status and future directions. J Sex Med 2013; 10(1):3;17.

3. Maes CA, Louis M Nurse practitioners sexual history taking practices with adults 50 and older. J Nurse Pract 2011; 7(3);216-222.

4. Got M Hinchliff S, Galena E. General Practitioner Attitudes to discussing sexual health issues with older people. SCI Med 2004; 58(11)2093-2103.

5. Kleinplatz PJ sexuality and older people. BMJ. 2008; 337:a239.

6. Layman EO Glasser DB, Neves RC, Moreira ED Jr; GSSAB Investigators groupA population-based survey of sexual activity, sexual problems, and associated help-seeking behavior patterns in mature adults in the United States of America. Int J Impost Res.2009, 21(3):171-178.

7. Moore A, Arthur R, Hull A, Faught B, Glass C. Sexual Health Issues in the aging population. In: cash JC, Glass CA, Ed's Adult-Gerontology Practice Guidelines. New York, NY: Springer Publishing Co;2016:516-535.

8. Laumann EO Waite LJ sexual Dysfunction among older adults: prevalence and risk factors from a nationality representative. J Sex Med 2008; 5 (10): 2300-2311.

9. Dailymail.com, Erica Tempestafor. Women reveal the biggest mistakes that men make in the bedroom. 13 November 2020.

10. Bhagyashri S, Lalitkumar. V concept of cosmetology in ancient India concerning Sushruta Samhita. Int. A Med J. 2018;6(4):893-4.

11. Pelosi M. The history of cosmetic vaginal surgery: part 1, 2 Oct, 2013.

12. Aximmrc.com cosmetic gynecology market Trend analysis report.

13. Vaginal Laxity. The frequent problem that is infrequently addressed. Medresults Network (cited 2020, August 24.

14. Millheiser L Kingsberg S Paul's R. A cross-section of the survey to assess the prevalence and symptoms associated with laxity of vaginal introitus. Neurourol urodyn 2010.

15. Lindau ST Gavrilova N Sex health and years of sexually active life gained due to good health: evidence from 2 US-based population-based cross-sectional surveys of aging. BMJ. 2010; 340 (7746):580.

16. Luber KM: Risk factors for stress urinary incontinence. Rev Urol 2004; 6(3):3-9.

17. Kontula O: sex life challenges: the Finnish case. International encyclopedia Sov Behav sci second edition 2015 March, 26:665-71.

18. Data M cosmetic surgery National Data bank statistics. Aesthetic Surgery Journal J.2018; 38:1-24.

19. Committee on gynecological practice. ACOG COMMITTEE OPINION no 795: elective female genital cosmetic surgery. Vol 107, ACOG. 2006.pg 213.

20. FDA warns against use of energy-based devices to perform rejuvenation or vaginal cosmetic procedures: FDA Safety communication 2018.

MEDICO-LEGAL ASPECTS IN AESTHETIC AND REGENERATIVE GYNECOLOGY

CHAPTER 02

Garima Srivastav

Medico-legally these procedures are different from other treatments that gynecologists have performed traditionally.

In many cases there may not be any medical indications but they are done on demand of the patients. The purpose of the treatment may be purely cosmetic.

We as gynecologists have yet to face any of the procedures done only for cosmetic purposes and hence, we must understand the legal implications of the same and understand the purpose of documentation.

WHO CAN DO COSMETIC SURGERIES?

Any Registered Medical practitioner with experience and training in the field of cosmetology can do a cosmetic treatment.

But we must remember that one cannot write cosmetologist or specialist or cosmetic gynecologist unless they have a postgraduate or super specialty recognized by MCI in India. The rules are different for each country and one must abide by the medical regulations of their own country.

Many diplomas in the market have no validity in the court of law, except they can be considered as training obtained. With an original degree, you can write "Special Interest In Cosmetic Gynecology" in India.

PROCEDURES

- Laser hair reduction
- PRP for hair loss
- Non-Surgical vaginal resurfacing for vaginal relaxation syndrome
- Body contouring & weight loss
- Laser vaginal tightening
- Mommy makeover
- Treatment of pigmentation and stretch marks
- Sexual dysfunction
- Vaginismus
- Nonsurgical treatment of menopause, ui, prolapse
- Hymenoplasty, labioplasty, clitoral hood reduction, vaginoplasty, perineoplasty
- Fat grafting

What is FGM?

- WHO defines FGM as "All procedures involving partial or total removal of external female genitalia or another injury to female genital organs whether for cultural, religious or nontherapeutic reasons."
- WHO has classified FGM into various categories.
  - Type 1: Partial or total removal of the prepuce or clitoris (clitoridectomy)
  - Type 2: Partial or total removal of the clitoris and the labia minora, with or without excision of labia majora.
  - Type 3: Narrowing of the vaginal orifice with the creation of a covering seal by cutting and positioning the labia minora and /or labia majora with or without excision of the clitoris (infibulation).
  - Type 4: All other harmful procedures to the female genitalia for nonmedical purposes, for example, picking, piercing, incising, scraping, and cauterization.
- UNICEF claims that worldwide over 125 million women and girls have undergone FGM.
- It is a traditional cultural practice in 29 African countries. FGM is practiced in Yemen, Iraq, Indonesia, and Malaysia. Smaller numbers are also recorded in India, Pakistan, Sri Lanka, UAE, Oman, Peru, and Columbia.
- FGM in most countries is illegal. It is illegal to arrange or assist in any of these procedures and offense for those with parental responsibility to fail to protect a girl from FGM.

HOW ARE SURGICAL COSMETIC PROCEDURES DIFFERENT FROM FGM?

There are 4 principles of Ethics which help us differentiate between the two procedures:

- Principle of Non-maleficence: (Not harm) One should not have the intention to harm others.
- Principle of Autonomy of the patient: Every person has the right to decide what she wants to undergo or not. We have to respect the autonomy of the patient.
- Principle of Beneficence: (to do good) We must do whatever is good for the patient and positively impacts her physical and mental health.
- Principle of Justice: There should be equality and impartiality in treatment. The procedure should not be performed at the expense of others and surgeons should do it ethically and should be able to justify it.

These 4 principles of ethics prevent female genital cosmetic surgery from falling under the category of FGM.

These situations are common in aesthetic practice If the procedure is not harmful to the patient, then we can proceed with the same respecting the autonomy of the patient but when something is harmful to the patient, then it becomes our duty to inform the patient about the possibility of harm in detail before proceeding for the same.

If everything is normal physiologically yet the patient demands these procedures, proper counseling is a must. If the patient still wants to undergo treatment, then we have to respect the autonomy of the patient but if the procedure is harmful then it is best avoided. To refuse to treat the patient is the right of the doctor but in this case, it is advisable to document the reason for refusal.

INFORMED CONSENT

Obtaining informed consent is a critical medico-legal requirement for any procedure more so with cosmetic procedures. Patients must be adequately informed about the nature of the procedure, potential risks and complications, expected outcomes, and alternative options. Written consent must be documented, ensuring patients fully understand and consent to the treatment.

Informed consent consists of these 6 parameters.
- Purpose of the treatment
- Procedure in detail
- Alternatives available.
- Success/ failure rates
- Risks/ side effects
- Risks of not undergoing treatment

PATIENT SELECTION AND COUNSELING:

Medical professionals must carefully assess patient candidacy for cosmetic gynecological procedures. Patients should be evaluated physically and psychologically to ensure they have realistic expectations and are mentally prepared for the procedure. Proper patient counseling is essential to address concerns, potential limitations, and postoperative expectations.

A detailed explanation is mentioned in the subsequent chapter.

PROFESSIONAL COMPETENCE

Cosmetic gynecological procedures require specialized skills and training. Surgeons performing these procedures should have qualifications as discussed earlier and training /experience in the field.

Maintaining professional competence and staying updated with best practices is essential to minimize the risk of complications and ensure patient safety.

RISK DISCLOSURE AND MANAGEMENT

Medical professionals have a legal obligation to disclose potential risks associated with these procedures. Patients should be informed about the possible risks of the surgery and any specific complications that may arise. Adequate risk management protocols should be in place to handle adverse- events, should they occur.

PATIENT PRIVACY AND CONFIDENTIALITY

Given the intimate nature of these procedures, ensuring patient privacy and confidentiality is paramount. Medical practices should have robust data protection measures in place to safeguard patient information, complying with relevant privacy laws and regulations.

ADVERTISING AND MARKETING

Medical professionals offering cosmetic gynecological services must adhere to ethical advertising and marketing practices. Claims about procedure outcomes and benefits should be accurate, and the use of before and after images must comply with relevant advertising guidelines.

CULTURAL SENSITIVITY

Cosmetic gynecologists should be culturally sensitive and considerate of patient backgrounds and beliefs. Procedures like hymenoplasty should be approached with cultural sensitivity and consideration.

MALPRACTICE INSURANCE

Medical practitioners should carry adequate malpractice insurance to protect themselves in case of legal claims arising from these procedures.

DOCUMENTATION

Documentation is the only evidence in the court of law to prove your case. Good documentation is good defense, poor documentation is poor evidence and no documentation is no evidence.

Complications are not negligence. If complications are explained in detail before starting the treatment, then it becomes more acceptable.

Any complications should be treated according to medical norms.

Full confidentiality has to be maintained for these procedures, exceptions about the court of law, notifiable diseases, and serious risks to the person or community.

In some procedures as in orgasmic shots, patients should be informed that the improvement cannot be guaranteed and there is no measure to know the fact your claim of no improvement will not be entertained.

In minor it is better to avoid cosmetic procedures, consent if required, may have to be taken from the legal guardian.

Most insurance does not cover cosmetic procedures, yet every procedure is under the Consumer Protection Act.

CONCLUSION

- To address aesthetic, functional, and sexual concerns cosmetology is emerging as an upcoming field.
- Potentially beneficial in chronic debilitating conditions like Lichen Sclerosis, SUI, Sexual Dysfunction, scars, vulvodynia, and side effects of chemotherapy.
- ACOG recommends proper counseling including risks & and limitations and takes informed consent.
- Cosmetic surgery has its place in the modern-day scenario. However, since its inception, teething problems have arisen and one such issue is medicolegal issues.
- It is always better to consult a medico-legal consultant in such issues.

REFERENCES

1. Indian Medical Council (Professional Conduct, Etiquette and Ethics) Regulation 2002. Section – 3.7.2 and section 3.7.3
2. Indian Medical Council (Professional Conduct, Etiquette and Ethics) Regulation, 2002- section 2.2
3. Ministry of Health and Family Welfare (Department of Health and Family Welfare) by Notification – New Delhi 11th March 2020- The Drug And Cosmetics Rule, 1945.
4. Samira Kohli vs Dr. Prabha Manchanda & Anr on 16th January 2008.

PATIENT SELECTION & CONSULTATION

Garima Srivastav

CONSULTATION RULES IN COSMETIC GYNAECOLOGY

- A patient seeks aesthetic gynecological procedures to improve her comfort with her genitalia and her perception of her body. This is directly related to her sexual function and performance.
- The surgeon who has mastered cosmetic procedures involving the genital area can educate her patients on the best alternatives for their sexual well-being.
- An effective aesthetic gynecologic consultation remains one of the major challenges for doctors.
- As doctors, we are not trained to sell our services, only to perform them.
- Converting consults into actual procedures is a crucial step to maintaining a financially thriving practice.
- Look professional. Do not use casual clothing or scrubs when you conduct a consult.
- Manners: Knock on the door gently, greet the patient by her name, and introduce yourself while looking her in the eye and shaking hands.
- Build rapport: Spend a few minutes learning about the patient as a person. Comment on their occupation or perhaps the person who referred them (you can get that information from your patient information sheet).
- Listen while they talk. Look the patient in the eye, nod, and take notes to let them know you are listening and understanding.
- Now, ask more open-ended questions to determine if the patient's expectations are reasonable and within the scope of your expertise and abilities.
- If it is not, ask yourself: Should you refer this customer to another colleague? Confirm that the results they are seeking can be reached safely and they are rational about the entire process.
- Use a mirror to the patient to show you her concerns.
- Ask an open-ended question such as
  - "How can I help you today?" and "What brings you into our practice?"
  - "Have you had other consultations? if so, what information did I tell you that you didn't already know?"
- Do not interrupt the patient. Resist the temptation to interrupt with your recommendations. Be sure the patient has completely and thoroughly relayed their concerns to you before responding to them.
- Use layperson terms. Be concise and keep it simple while explaining how you would address their concerns.
- Never offer too many choices, a confused patient will decide to do nothing.
- Sell yourself, and show your expertise. Inform patients what makes you the best aesthetic gynecologist in comparison to the competition. Mention your board certification, training, talks, or written articles.
- Sell your skills. Patients must be informed you have performed many of these procedures or treatments with excellent results and you will do the same for them.
- Explain all the possible side effects of a treatment. Go over the items in your procedure consent forms. Make sure you tell the patient how many complications you had, and that you can manage them if they occur.
- Never spend more than 20-30 minutes in a consultation. Some patients think too much time spent in a consult is a sign of a non-busy practitioner. They wonder why you are not busier.
- Never bad-mouth your colleagues. Always remember, it puts you in a bad position and makes you look worse than your competition.
- Prepare and rehearse a closing statement that sounds natural. Tell the patient you look forward to working with her to help them and you hope to see them again soon.
- Do not use these phrases:

- I will make it disappear completely.
- It will be perfect.
- I am going to erase that line (soften).
- I will give you a touch They will all come for it oops.
- I promise it will go away in (3) times.

EXPLORE THE REASONS FOR THE PROCEDURE

- Discomfort with tight clothing.
- Information on digital media.
- Physical discomfort like pain, dyspareunia, difficulty in maintaining hygiene, and vaginal laxity.
- Limited genital education.
- Comments directed by others at them or otherwise.
- Intimate partner abuse or sexual abuse.
- Grooming practices for pubic hair like waxing, epilation, shaving, or laser.
- Decreased sexual satisfaction by self or partner (feeling of looseness or laxity).
- Decreased lubrication.
- Dribbling of urine on sneezing or coughing.
- Hypertrophied or dark labia.

ASSESS THE DEGREE OF CONCERN AND ANXIETY

- Is her concern affecting her intimate relationship, self-esteem, confidence, and ability to function happily?
- Feeling unpleasant during sexual activity and how she addresses the issue.
- Smoking and alcohol may lead to compromised results.
- Pregnancy, active local infection, sexually transmitted infection, and untreated genital malignancies are contraindications.

ASSESSMENT OF MENTAL HEALTH AND SEXUAL ABUSE ISSUES

- Existing issues of depression, anxiety, PTSD, addictions, low self-esteem, and stress are likely to give poor results.

- Body dysmorphic disorder and marital discord should be ruled out.
- A sexual history and function evaluation are advisable and may include a variety of established questionnaires such as the Arizona Sexual Experience Questionnaire or the Female Sexual Function Index

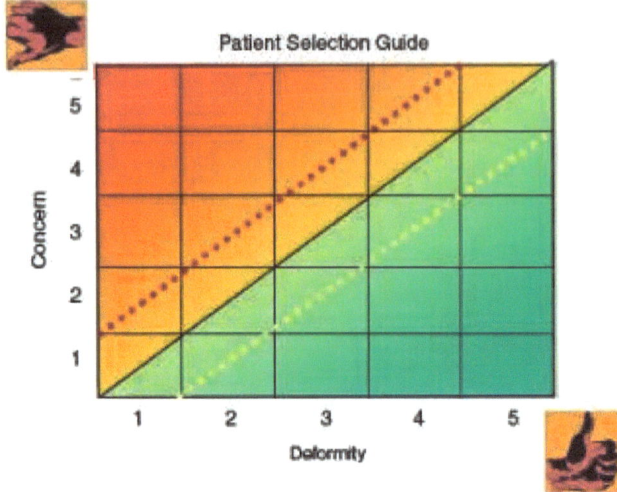

"Gorneygram" shows higher risks in treating patients with minimal deformities. Prospective patients with greater deformity and less concern (represented in the right lower side of the chart) tend to do much better than patients perceiving their minimal deformity as huge (represented in the upper left area of the chart). Caution is suggested when caring for patients whose balance of deformity and concern lies in this upper left area.

FEMALE SEXUAL FUNCTION INDEX SCORING

Appendix 1.   Female Sexual Function Index Scoring

Question	Response Options
1. Over the past 4 weeks, how **often** did you feel sexual desire or interest?	5 = Almost always or always 4 = Most times (more than half the time) 3 = Sometimes (about half the time) 2 = A few times (less than half the time) 1 = Almost never or never
2. Over the past 4 weeks, how would you rate your **level** (degree) of sexual desire or interest?	5 = Very high 4 = High 3 = Moderate 2 = Low 1 = Very low or none at all
3. Over the past 4 weeks, how **often** did you feel sexually aroused ("turned on") during sexual activity or intercourse?	0 = No sexual activity 5 = Almost always or always 4 = Most times (more than half the time) 3 = Sometimes (about half the time) 2 = A few times (less than half the time) 1 = Almost never or never
4. Over the past 4 weeks, how would you rate your **level** of sexual arousal ("turn on") during sexual activity or intercourse?	0 = No sexual activity 5 = Very high 4 = High 3 = Moderate 2 = Low 1 = Very low or none at all
5. Over the past 4 weeks, how **confident** were you about becoming sexually aroused during sexual activity or intercourse?	0 = No sexual activity 5 = Very high confidence 4 = High confidence 3 = Moderate confidence 2 = Low confidence 1 = Very low or no confidence
6. Over the past 4 weeks, how **often** have you been satisfied with your arousal (excitement) during sexual activity or intercourse?	0 = No sexual activity 5 = Almost always or always 4 = Most times (more than half the time) 3 = Sometimes (about half the time) 2 = A few times (less than half the time) 1 = Almost never or never

Reed SD, Mitchell CM, Joffe H, Cohen L, Shifren JL, Newton KM, et al. Sexual function in women on estradiol or venlafaxine for hot flushes: a randomized controlled trial. Obstet Gynecol 2014;124.
The authors provided this information as a supplement to their article.
© Copyright 2014 American College of Obstetricians and Gynecologists.   Page 1 of 4

7. Over the past 4 weeks, how **often** did you become lubricated ("wet") during sexual activity or intercourse?

0 = No sexual activity
5 = Almost always or always
4 = Most times (more than half the time)
3 = Sometimes (about half the time)
2 = A few times (less than half the time)
1 = Almost never or never

8. Over the past 4 weeks, how **difficult** was it to become lubricated ("wet") during sexual activity or intercourse?

0 = No sexual activity
1 = Extremely difficult or impossible
2 = Very difficult
3 = Difficult
4 = Slightly difficult
5 = Not difficult

9. Over the past 4 weeks, how often did you **maintain** your lubrication ("wetness") until completion of sexual activity or intercourse?

0 = No sexual activity
5 = Almost always or always
4 = Most times (more than half the time)
3 = Sometimes (about half the time)
2 = A few times (less than half the time)
1 = Almost never or never

10. Over the past 4 weeks, how **difficult** was it to maintain your lubrication ("wetness") until completion of sexual activity or intercourse?

0 = No sexual activity
1 = Extremely difficult or impossible
2 = Very difficult
3 = Difficult
4 = Slightly difficult
5 = Not difficult

11. Over the past 4 weeks, when you had sexual stimulation or intercourse, how **often** did you reach orgasm (climax)?

0 = No sexual activity
5 = Almost always or always
4 = Most times (more than half the time)
3 = Sometimes (about half the time)
2 = A few times (less than half the time)
1 = Almost never or never

12. Over the past 4 weeks, when you had sexual stimulation or intercourse, how **difficult** was it for you to reach orgasm (climax)?

0 = No sexual activity
1 = Extremely difficult or impossible
2 = Very difficult
3 = Difficult
4 = Slightly difficult
5 = Not difficult

Reed SD, Mitchell CM, Joffe H, Cohen L, Shifren JL, Newton KM, et al. Sexual function in women on estradiol or venlafaxine for hot flushes: a randomized controlled trial. Obstet Gynecol 2014;124.
The authors provided this information as a supplement to their article.

© Copyright 2014 American College of Obstetricians and Gynecologists.

13. Over the past 4 weeks, how **satisfied** were you with your ability to reach orgasm (climax) during sexual activity or intercourse?

0 = No sexual activity
5 = Very satisfied
4 = Moderately satisfied
3 = About equally satisfied and dissatisfied
2 = Moderately dissatisfied
1 = Very dissatisfied

14. Over the past 4 weeks, how **satisfied** have you been with the amount of emotional closeness during sexual activity between you and your partner?

0 = No sexual activity
5 = Very satisfied
4 = Moderately satisfied
3 = About equally satisfied and dissatisfied
2 = Moderately dissatisfied
1 = Very dissatisfied

15. Over the past 4 weeks, how **satisfied** have you been with your sexual relationship with your partner?

5 = Very satisfied
4 = Moderately satisfied
3 = About equally satisfied and dissatisfied
2 = Moderately dissatisfied
1 = Very dissatisfied

16. Over the past 4 weeks, how **satisfied** have you been with your overall sexual life?

5 = Very satisfied
4 = Moderately satisfied
3 = About equally satisfied and dissatisfied
2 = Moderately dissatisfied
1 = Very dissatisfied

17. Over the past 4 weeks, how **often** did you experience discomfort or pain during vaginal penetration?

0 = Did not attempt intercourse
1 = Almost always or always
2 = Most times (more than half the time)
3 = Sometimes (about half the time)
4 = A few times (less than half the time)
5 = Almost never or never

18. Over the past 4 weeks, how **often** did you experience discomfort or pain following vaginal penetration?

0 = Did not attempt intercourse
1 = Almost always or always
2 = Most times (more than half the time)
3 = Sometimes (about half the time)
4 = A few times (less than half the time)
5 = Almost never or never

19. Over the past 4 weeks, how would you rate your **level** (degree) of discomfort or pain during or following vaginal penetration?

0 = Did not attempt intercourse
1 = Very high
2 = High
3 = Moderate
4 = Low
5 = Very low or none at all

Reed SD, Mitchell CM, Joffe H, Cohen L, Shifren JL, Newton KM, et al. Sexual function in women on estradiol or venlafaxine for hot flushes: a randomized controlled trial. Obstet Gynecol 2014;124.

The authors provided this information as a supplement to their article.

© Copyright 2014 American College of Obstetricians and Gynecologists.

TIPS FOR CONSULTATION

- Answer all questions to give the patient realistic expectations.
- Take good before pictures, and study them with the patient before and after treatment.
- Discuss the procedure details.
- Discuss the pre and post-operative instructions.
- Discuss possible complications.

RELATIVE CONTRAINDICATIONS

- Less than well-controlled diabetics
- STDs
- Smoking
- BDD (2%)
- Unrealistic expectations
- History of sexual abuse
- Psychologically unstable individuals
- If the doctor has ethical or principle objections

There are no absolute contraindications.

EXAMINATION

- Evaluate morphology
- Evaluate skin elasticity
- Evaluate muscle weakness

MEDICAL PHOTOGRAPHY

- Make sure pictures are taken from the same distance every time.
- Before and after pictures should always be consistent.
- Take consent for using pictures in marketing or education.
- A proportion of medical photography is for publication and presentation and is not essential to the care of any individual patient.
- Medical photography may have significant effects on the patient and their family.
- This is particularly true of aesthetic gynecology but is likely to apply to other patients.
- Patients undergoing medical photography must be fully informed as to the purpose of the photograph and full consent for each use must be sought.
- Pictures taken by other than photographic staff should be subject to the same storage and use regulations as those taken by the professional photographic staff.
- Whole-body naked photographs cause serious psychological sequelae and should not be taken. They do not educate or inform and should no longer be used for teaching and publication.

REASSURE THE PATIENT

- Reassurance regarding all her concerns.
- Explain why the procedure has been selected for her.
- Consent to be taken for both surgical and nonsurgical treatment.
- Consent should provide adequate information.
- Patient's consent is a must.
- Consent is considered informed when all of the below points are mentioned
- Purpose of the treatment
- Procedure in detail
- Alternatives available.
- Success/ failure rates
- Risks/ side effects
- Risks of not undergoing treatment.
- The unintended complications of the surgery should be properly mentioned in the consent like
- Bleeding
- Wound infection
- Altered sensation
- Dyspareunia
- Scarring
- Unknown delayed complications.

COUNSELING ALONE MAY BE BENEFICIAL

- Body image distress.
- Low self-esteem
- Social anxiety
- Sexual difficulties that are due to undue sexual expectations by the partner or from the partner
- Counselling of both partners may be considered.
  MINOR PATIENTS
- Girls requesting genital cosmetic procedures below age 18 should be counseled against them, irrespective of their consent.
- Genital maturation is not reached before the age of 18
- Hence unlikely to give long-term best results.

CAN WE DO SURGERY WHEN NOT MEDICALLY INDICATED???

- If the procedure is not harmful then we can proceed with the same respecting the autonomy of the patient.
- But when something is harmful to the patient, then we must inform the patient.
- To refuse to treat the patient is the right of the doctor but it is advisable to document the reason for refusal.

- Documentation is most important
- Courts are not courts of justices but courts of evidence.

CONCLUSION

- A loose vagina post-childbirth is the most subjective and commonly self-reported complaint for which treatment may be sought.
- More than 1/3 rd women have sex related issues which were told only when specifically asked for.
- Almost 50% of women have felt a decreased interest in sexual activity and were concerned about laxity post-childbirth.
- Prevalence of UI is almost 25-30%.
- Hence the problem is widespread but patients are hesitant to bring up these issues with the doctor for the fear of being dismissed, considering these normal aging signs, or simply due to shyness.

- It is our duty as clinicians and health care providers to hear their issues, be empathetic, and provide the best possible solution to their intimate-area issues.

SUMMARY

These procedures are no longer for rich and famous models or celebrities. It has now become readily accessible to the general public. Cosmetic procedures can benefit if patient expectations are realistic, which can be achieved by proper pre-procedure counseling.

Genital procedures should not be done before the age of 18 years. Always make sure the patient understands these procedures well and has given informed consent.

SAMPLE CONSENT FORMS

CHEMICAL PEEL CONSENT FORM

I………………………………………………………………………consent Dr. ….. or any of his staff associates or aestheticians to perform the treatment known as a chemical peel. The treatment has been explained to me by Dr. ……, and I have had the opportunity to ask questions.

I understand that the procedure may cause swelling redness, scabbing, or puffiness of my face or (body site treated that may be uncomfortable. The procedure may cause my skin to appear red and peel like sunburn. During and after the procedure the following may be experienced- stinging, itching, burning, mild pain, tightness, peeling, and scabbing of the superficial layers of the skin. These sensations will gradually diminish over the week as the skin returns to its normal appearance. However, some patients may react differently. For example, in severe cases, the skin may look like very bad sunburn. The peeling usually lasts about three to seven days although it may last longer.

I understand that there is a possible risk of developing a temporary or permanent pigment (color) change in the skin There is a small incidence of the reactivation of cold sores (herpes infections) in patients with a prior history of herpes. There is also a small incidence of a flare of acne-like lesions after the peel. I understand that that on rare occasions this peel can penetrate deeper in certain areas, causing crusting or a scab to form. There is a rare incidence of infection. I have been given a copy of the post-peel instructions and have reviewed them.

I understand that photographs may be taken and agree to waive ownership of these photographs and allow the physician or agents of the physician to copyright publish or use these photographs in conjunction with presenting case stuffy results.

I am aware that the practice of surgery is not an exact science and acknowledge that no guarantees have been made to me as to the results of the procedure nor are there any guarantees against an unfavorable result. I acknowledge that you will do your best for me but I also recognize that you lack infallibility and that mistakes and accidents can occur in medicine they can in any discipline.

In the absence of a deliberate premeditated act of negligence, I will not sue you

Patient (or Guardian)   Signature Patient Name

Date

Witness Signature

Date

PLATELET-RICH PLASMA

Platelet-rich plasma, also known as "PRP" is an injection treatment whereby a person's blood is used. A fraction of blood (20cc-55cc) is drawn up from the individual patient into a syringe. This is a relatively small amount compared to blood donation which removes 500cc. The blood is spun down in a special centrifuge (according to standard Harvest Techniques) to separate its components (Red Blood Cells, platelet-rich plasma, and Plasma). The platelet-rich plasma is first separated and then activated with a small amount of calcium to allow the release of growth factors from the platelets which in turn amplifies the healing process. PRP is then injected into the area to be treated. Platelets are very small cells in your blood that are involved in the clotting process. When PRP is injected into the damaged area it causes a mild inflammation that triggers the healing cascade. As the platelets organize in the clot they release several enzymes to promote healing and tissue responses including attracting stem cells to repair the damaged area As a result new collagen begins to develop. As the collagen matures it begins to shrink causing the tightening and strengthening of the damaged area. When treating injured or sun and time-damaged tissue they can induce a remodeling of the tissue to a healthier and younger state. The full procedure takes approximately 45 minutes- 1 hr. Generally, 2-3 treatments are advised, however, more may be indicated for some individuals. Touch-up treatment may be done once a year after the initial group of treatments to boost and maintain the results.

BENEFITS of PRP: Along with the benefit of using your tissue, therefore, eliminating allergies there is the added intrigue of mobilizing your stem cells for your benefit. PRP has been shown to have overall rejuvenating effects on the skin as improving skin texture, fine lines, and wrinkles, increasing volume via the increased production of collagen and elastin, and diminishing and improving the appearance of scars. Other benefits: minimal downtime, safety with minimal risk, short recovery time, natural-looking results, and no general anesthesia is required.

CONTRAINDICATIONS: PRP used for aesthetic procedures is safe for most individuals between the ages of 25 and 80. There are very few contraindications, however, patients with the following conditions are not candidates:

1. Acute and Chronic Infections
2. Skin diseases (i.e. SLE, porphyria, allergies)
3. Cancer 3) Chemotherapy
4. Severe metabolic and systemic disorders
5. Abnormal platelet function (blood disorders, e Haemodynamic Instability, Hypofibrinogenemia, Critical Thrombocytopenia)
6. Chronic Liver Pathology
7. Anti-coagulation therapy,
8. Underlying Sepsis,
9. Systemic use of corticosteroids within two weeks of the procedure, and
10. pregnant or breastfeeding.

RISKS & COMPLICATIONS: I have been informed that some of the Side Effects of platelet-rich plasma include: 1) Pain or itching at the injection site 2) Bleeding, and Bruising. Swelling and/or Infection 3) Short-lasting pinkness/redness (flushing) of the skin 4) Allergic reaction to the solution 51 Injury to a nerve and/or muscle 6) Nausea/Vomiting 71 Dizziness or fainting 8) Temporary blood sugar increase

RESULTS: Results are generally visible at 3 weeks and continue to improve gradually over the next 3-6 months with improvement in texture and tone. Advanced wrinkling cannot be reversed and only a minimal improvement is predictable in persons with drug, alcohol, and tobacco usage. Severe scarring may not respond. Current data shows results may last 18-24 months. Of course, all individuals are different so there will be variations from one person to the next.

PHOTOGRAPHS: I authorize the taking of clinical photographs for historical, training, and/or promotional purposes. I understand confidentiality will be maintained.

CONSENT: My consent and authorization for this elective procedure is strictly voluntary. By signing this informed consent form, I hereby grant authority to the physician/practitioner to perform Platelet Rich Plasma "aka" PRP Injections to the area (s) discussed during our consultation, for aesthetic enhancement and skin rejuvenation. I have read this informed consent and certify and understand its contents in full. All of my questions have been answered to my satisfaction and consent to the terms of this agreement. I agree to adhere to all safety precautions and instructions after the treatment. I have been instructed in and understand post-treatment instructions and have been given a written copy of them. I understand that medicine is not an exact science and acknowledge that no guarantee has been given or implied by anyone as to the results that may be obtained by this treatment. I also understand this procedure is "elective" and not covered by insurance and that payment is my responsibility. Any expenses which may be incurred for medical care elect to receive outside of this office, such as, but not limited to dissatisfaction with my treatment outcome will be my sole financial responsibility. Payment in full for all treatments is required at the time of service and is non-refundable.

I hereby give my voluntary consent to this PRP procedure and release ....medical staff, and specific technicians from liability associated with the procedure. I certify that I am a competent adult of at least 18 years of age and am not under the influence of alcohol or drugs. This consent form shall be binding upon my spouse, relatives, legal representatives, heirs, administrators, successors, and assigns. I agree, that if should have any questions or concerns regarding my treatment/results will notify this office immediately so that timely follow-up and intervention can be provided.

Patient Name (print)   Patient Signature   Date

Witness Name (print)   Witness Signature   Date

Physician Signature (print)   Physician Signature   Date

LASER CONSENT FORM

I (we) voluntarily request laser/light assisted treatment for vaginal remodeling/treatment of stress urinary incontinence...........................

1 (we) voluntarily consent and authorize that this laser/light-assisted treatment be performed by the staff of this clinic, including physicians, technicians, associates, technical assistants, and other health care providers as deemed necessary by the staff of this clinic.

I (we) hereby release this clinic, its staff, and any other participating healthcare providers from any liability for any adverse effects that may result from this treatment and related procedures.

For accurate record keeping in connection with the care and treatment that I am receiving and will subsequently receive from this clinic, I (we), the undersigned, consent to have this clinic's staff take before, during, and after treatment close-up photographs of the involved area(s) and the anatomical region surrounding the involved area(s). These photographs shall be used for medical records and shall be treated with the same confidentiality as the remainder of my record at this clinic.

I (we) recognize that this laser/light-assisted treatment is not an exact science and I (we) acknowledge that no guarantees or assurances have been made to me (us) as to the result or cure. There are risks related to the performance of these procedures. I (we) understand and acknowledge that the risks that may occur in connection with this particular procedure may include the following:

1. Infection - Albeit rare, skin infection is a possibility any time a skin procedure is performed. I acknowledge and understand that although rare, a skin infection can become a blood-borne widespread infection.
2. Blood clots in veins and lungs -Albeit extremely rare, it may be possible to develop a blood clot associated with this treatment that goes (embolizes) to the heart and/or lungs.
3. Allergic reactions - Although uncommon, I could develop an allergic reaction to medicines applied to the treated area and I could develop an allergic reaction to any medications that may be prescribed to me.
4. Haemorrhage and bruising - Bruising in the treated area is possible, especially if, within the last ten (10) days, I (we) have taken aspirin or aspirin-containing products, or other medications that "thin" the blood.
5. Recurrence of the lesion - I may not experience permanent results even with multiple treatments.
6. Painful or unattractive scarring - Scarring is a rare complication of laser-assisted treatment, but scarring is possible because the skin surface is disrupted by the laser. To minimize the chances of scarring, it is most important that I follow all postoperative instructions carefully.
7. Discomfort and pain - Some discomfort will be experienced during and after the laser treatment. I give my permission for the administration of topical and/or local injection of anesthesia when and if deemed appropriate.
8. Pigment changes (skin color) - During the healing process, the treated area may become either lighter or darker in color than the surrounding skin. This is usually temporary, but on a rare occasion, it may be permanent.
9. Poor The resultant open wound may require more than the usual one to three weeks to heal.
10. Blindness and even damage - The laser, without protective eyewear, may cause visual loss including blindness. It is important to keep these shields on at all times during the procedure and I should keep my eyes closed to protect my eyes from accidental laser exposure.

1 (we) understand and acknowledge that I have been informed using visual aids, as well as individual discussion, that multiple treatments are often required to cause long-term results and that some patients have no results even with multiple treatments. The usual number of treatments required is two to three, but more treatments may be required.

I (we) have been allowed to ask questions about my condition, alternate forms of anesthesia and treatment, the procedure to be used, and the risks and hazards involved, and I (we) believe that I (we) have sufficient information to give the informed consent. By signing below, I (we) certify that I (we) have read and fully understand the contents of this document and that (we) have received and understand all of the disclosures referred to herein. I certify that am a competent adult of at least 18 years of age, or that if I am a minor under the age of 18, understand that the consent of my parent/legal guardian having legal custody will also be required before treatment.

Signature of Patient

Signature of Person Authorized to Consent for Patient

Print Name of Patient

Print Name

Relationship

Date

Witness

POST LASER/LIGHT TREATMENT CARE –

1.00 Be careful with hot water and do not bathe with very hot water until healed.

2. Keep the area moist with Aloe Vera gel, or Aquaphor Healing Ointment until inflammation resolves and the area is healed.

3. Keep clothing from rubbing the treated area and avoid other irritation to the area.

4. Notify the clinic should you have any prolonged redness, excessive puffiness, or other unusual side effects.

Important Facts to Remember

1. There will be redness, and occasionally, mild blistering of the treated areas lasting for several hours to 3-14 days.
2. The treated area might be "crust". "fake", or look like a "cat scratch". This should be resolved within 3-14 days.
3. Each area to be treated usually requires two or more treatments approximately 2-12 weeks apart.
4. It might be impossible to remove the lesion forever. Even though the lesion may be diminished or "disappear" for long periods of 3-6 months, it might return in the future. The fact that the lesion responded to treatment and was disabled for an extended period almost invariably means it will respond to future treatment.
5. Medications Dispensed:………………………………………………….
   use as directed.

Signature of Patient

Print Name of Patient

Signature of Person Authorized to Consent for Patient

Print Name

Relationship

Date…….

REFERENCES

1. Mowat H Mc Donald K, Dobson AS, Fisher J, Kirkman. The contribution of online content to the promotion and normalization of female genital cosmetic surgery: A systematic review of literature BMC Women's Health 2015; November 25;15:110

2. Yurteri-Kaplan LA, Antosh DD, Sokol AI, Park AJ, Interest in cosmetic vulvar surgery and perception of vulvar appearance.AmJ obstetric gynecology 2012;207:428

3. Braunsteiner N, Vickers ER, Shapberg et al psychological issues for patients undergoing stem cell therapy & Regenerative medicine. Open J Regen Med 2018;7:1-17

4. Mirzabeigi MN, Jandali S, Mettel RK, Alter GJ. The nomenclature of vaginal rejuvenation and elective vulva vaginal plastic surgery. Aesthetic surgery Journal 2011;31(6):723-4

5. Schnatz PF Boardman LA Committee on Gynecology Practice, American College of Obstetricians and Gynecologists. ACOG Committee Opinion No 795

6. Vojvodic M, Lista F, Vastis P-G, Ahmad J Luminal reduction Hymenoplasty: a Canadian experience with Hymen restoration. Aesthetic journal surgery J 2018;38(7):802-6

7. Goodman MP. Female genital cosmetic and plastic surgery review. J Sex Med 2011;8:1813-25

8. Goodman MP, Placik, OJ, Benson RH, Miklos JK et al. A large multi-center outcome study of female genital plastic surgery. J Sex Med 2010;7:1565-77

RELEVANT ANATOMY IN AESTHETIC GYNECOLOGY

Garima Srivastav

Aesthetic Gynecology is the fastest-growing offshoot in gynecology. The procedures performed are Labioplasty, Clitoral Hood Reduction, Hymenoplasty, Vaginoplasty, Perineoplasty, and G spot augmentation to name a few.

These procedures are classified as FCGS (Female Cosmetic Gynecological Surgery).

ANATOMY AND PHYSIOLOGY

The external genital organs are mons pubis, labia majora, labia minora, Bartholin and clitoris.

The internal organs are the vagina, cervix hymen, uterus tubes, skene glands, and G spot.

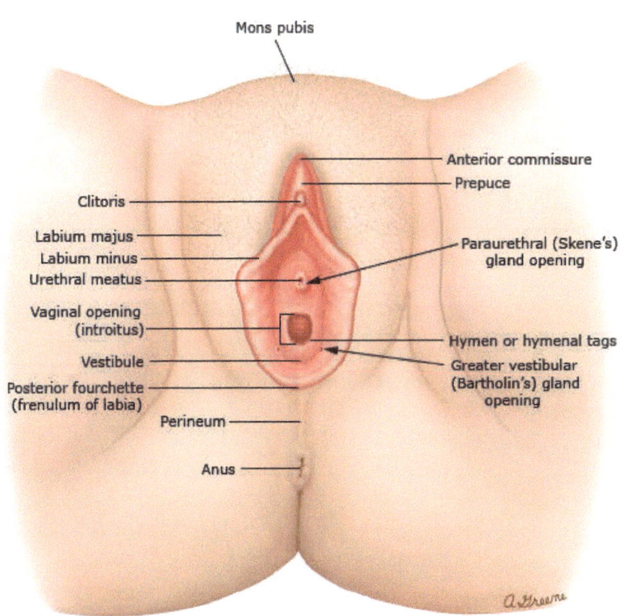

VULVA

Both urinary and reproductive structures form the female external genitalia, collectively called as vulva. It acts as sensory tissue during sexual intercourse, assists in micturition by directing the flow of urine, and protects the internal female reproductive tract from infection. It includes the following structures.

VULVAR COMPLEX

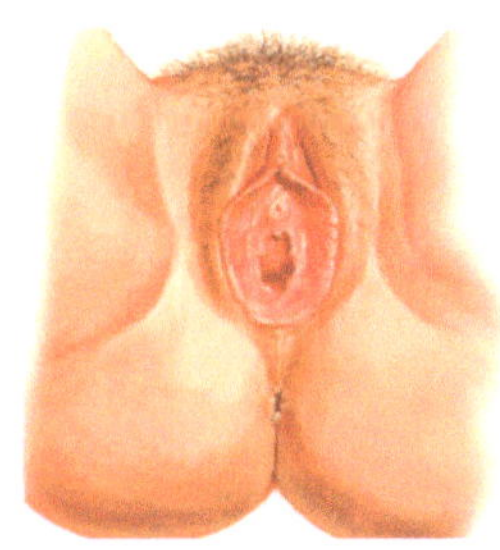

- Mons pubis
- Clitoris ve clitoral hood
- Labia majora
- Labia minora

MONS PUBIS

It provides a cushioning effect during sexual intercourse. Lack of fat in the mons may result in dyspareunia.

It contains sebaceous glands which produce pheromones that induce sexual attraction.

LABIA MAJORA

It covers and protects delicate and sensitive structures of the vulva. During aging, when fat atrophies, labial augmentation with fat, fillers, and PRP can be done.

LABIA MINORA

It protects the urethral and vaginal opening, directs the urine stream, and has sensory tissue.

The anatomic variation can be huge and depending on that, various classifications are proposed as discussed later in the chapter.

Labioplasty is one of the most commonly performed procedures in aesthetic gynecology. Documentation of the type of labia minora is hence, important for future purposes.

CLITORIS

It is analogous to the penis in males and hence the principal female erogenous organ. Superiorly it is located under a hood (prepuce) which is a part of labia minora anatomically that splits into frenulum on either side. Clitoral hood reduction surgery is offered in women with orgasmic dysfunction and thick clitoral fold to expose more of the clitoris anatomically.

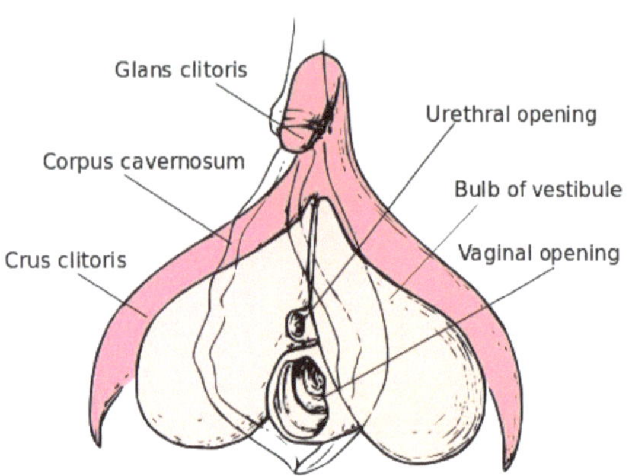

VESTIBULE

It is the almond-shaped area enclosed by the hart line laterally, the external surface of the hymen medially, the clitoral frenulum anteriorly, and the fourchette posteriorly.

BARTHOLIN'S GLAND

They are pea-sized glands located slightly posterior and on either side of the vaginal orifice.

It secretes mucus from ducts during sexual arousal. Bartholin gland cysts are common in sexually active women. It can be treated by co2 or diode laser similar to the procedure of marsipulization.

HYMEN

It is a thin membrane that surrounds the opening of the vagina. They come in various shapes and sizes.

Hymenoplasty is an office procedure that restores the structural integrity of the hymen. The reasons for the procedure are purely cultural and are banned in the Middle East.

Rarely imperforate hymen is seen leading to hematocolpos. it can be divided for free drainage of menstrual blood, secretion, and sexual intercourse.

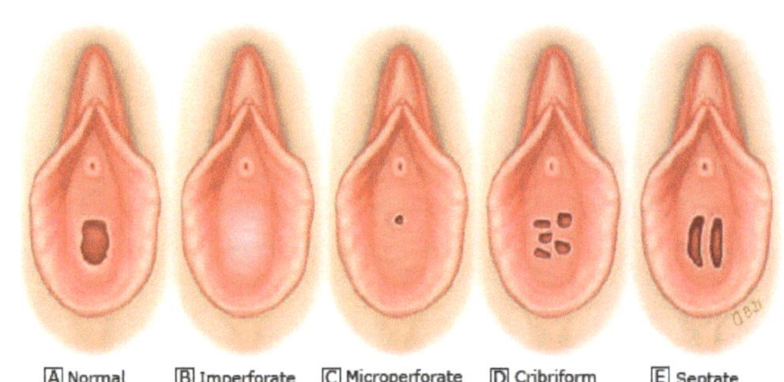

G SPOT

Also called the G zone / Grafenberg spot, it is believed to be a point 2-3 inches on the anterior vaginal wall, inside from the introitus. It is believed to be the confluence of several nerve endings and its stimulation is believed to lead to orgasm. The G spot can be augmented by fillers, PRP, or autologous fat transfer. It is often described as a sexual rejuvenation procedure, the details of which will be discussed in subsequent chapters.

G-SPOT

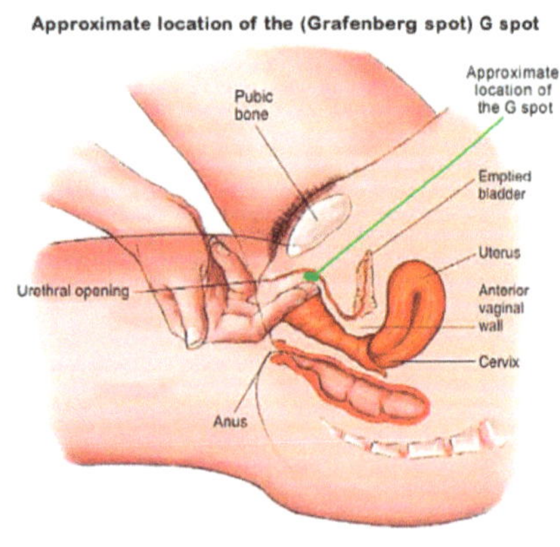

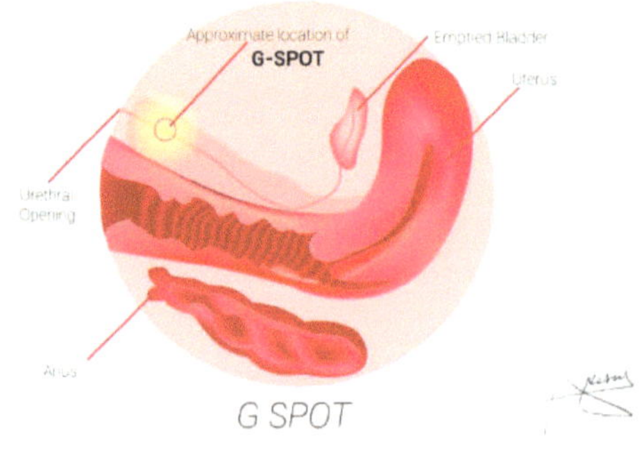

ANATOMIC VARIATION AND CLASSIFICATION

There are various anatomic classifications of Labia Minora given by various scholars.

Here we are mentioning the important few. These are important for understanding the diversity of labia minora and for documentation purposes in notes before undergoing any procedures.

The important ones discussed in the chapter are:

- Banwell classification
- Chang classification
- Felicio classification
- Motakef classification

Chang Classification of Labia Minora by Protrusion Beyond Labia Majora

Class	Protrusion Characteristics
1	<2 cm protrusion beyond the fourchette, without extension beyond the labia majora
2	>2 cm protrusion beyond the fourchette, with extension beyond the labia majora
3	Protrusion as in class 2, and beyond the clitoris anteriorly
4	Protrusion as in class 3, and beyond the vagina to the perineum or anus

Chang P, Salisbury M, Narsete T, et al. Vaginal Labiaplasty: Defense of the Simple "Clip and Snip" and a New Classification System, *Aesthetic Plast Surg*, 2013, vol. 375 (pg. 887-891)

Labia Minora Morphology

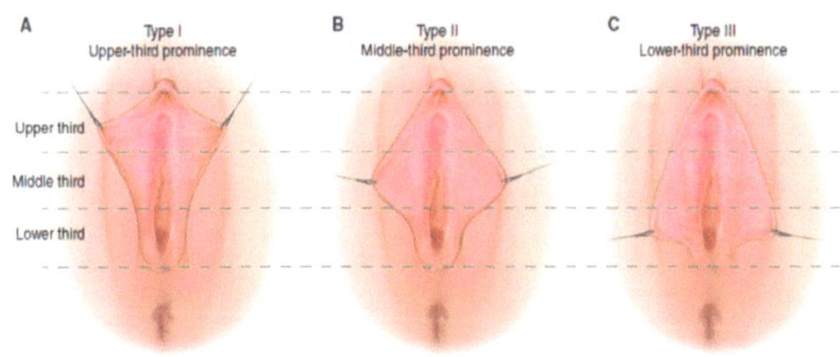

Banwell classification of labia minora morphology.
A, Type I: Upper-third enlargement (winging).
B, Type II: Middle-third enlargement.
C, Type III: Lower-third enlargement.

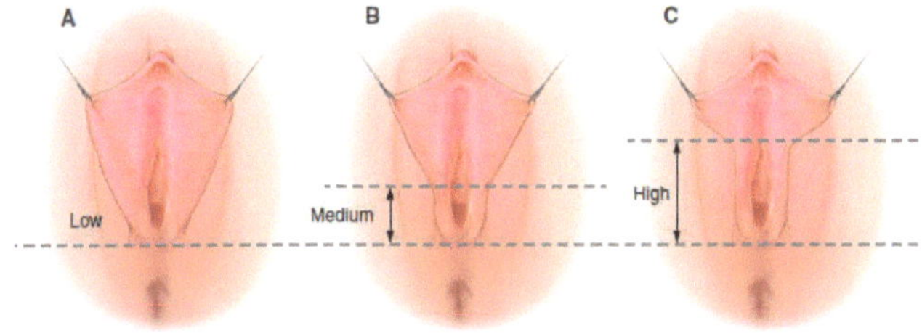

Felicio Classification of Labial Hypertrophy

Type	Length of Labium (cm)
I	<2
II	2-4
III	4-6
IV	>6

- Values represent the maximum length of each labium. Classification system developed by Felicio.

Felicio Y, Chirurgie Intime , *La Ver Chir Esth Lang ranc* , 1992, vol.677(pg. 37-43)

MOTAKEF CLASSIFICATION OF LABIAL HYPERTROPHY

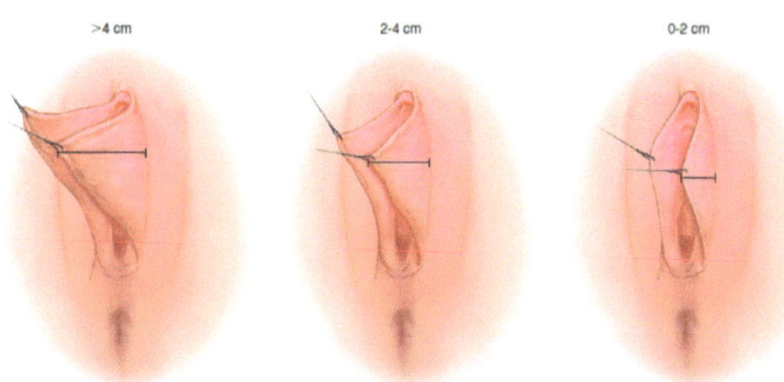

Fig. 1-12 Motakef classification for labial protrusion, which classifies the degree of protrusion of the labia minora past the labia majora. Class I (0 to 2 cm), class II (2 to 4 cm), and class III (more than 4 cm) may be amenable to different treatment paradigms. An "A" is added for asymmetry and a "C" for involvement of the clitoral hood.

MOTAKEF'S CLASSIFICATION

Fig. 1-12 Motakef classification for labial protrusion, which classifies the degree of protrusion of the labia minora past the labia majora. Class I (0 to 2 cm), class II (2 to 4 cm), and class III (more than 4 cm) may be amenable to different treatment paradigms. An 'A' is added for asymmetry and a 'C' for involvement of the clitoral hood.

BANWELL'S CLASSIFICATION

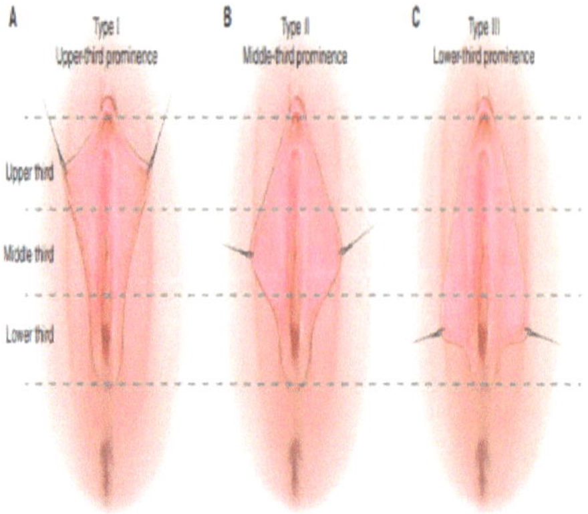

Banwell classification of labia minora morphology. A, Type I: Upper-third enlargement (winging). B, Type II: Middle-third enlargement. C, Type III: Lower-third enlargement.

BLOOD SUPPLY

Understanding the blood supply to the area is crucial to perform various surgeries.

Labioplasty is a common procedure. The main complication of this surgery is the dehiscence of the suture line. The dehiscence rate varies with different techniques and this might imply that that vascular anatomy is not respected.

Various studies have described a dominant central artery, 2 posterior arteries, and 1 small anterior artery. Furthermore, the connection between the anterior system of the external pudendal artery and the posterior system of the internal pudendal artery was confirmed.

This orients the surgeons to understand why the dehiscence rate is more common in the wedge technique in comparison to the edge or trim technique.

In wedge resection, the dominant central artery is cut at two specific points, hampering the blood supply and leading to more complications.

More precisely, when this wedge is placed at the more anterior part of the labia, the least perfused area is removed and a posterior flap is created that will preserve robust blood perfusion.

In edge resection the thinner aspect of the arteries is cut, respecting the vascular supply leading to fewer complications.

BLOOD VESSELS OF LABIA MINORA

A Cadaveric Study of the Arterial Blood Supply of the Labia Minora

Charalambos A. Georgiou, M.D.
Marc Benatar, M.D.
Pierre Dumas, M.D.
Bérengère Chignon-Sicard, M.D.
Thierry Balaguer, M.D.
Bernard Padovani, Ph.D.
Patrick Baqué, Ph.D.

Nice, France

Plastic and Reconstructive Surgery • July 2015

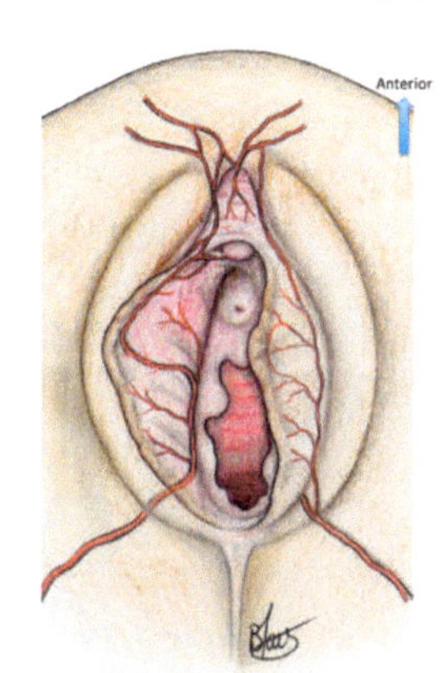

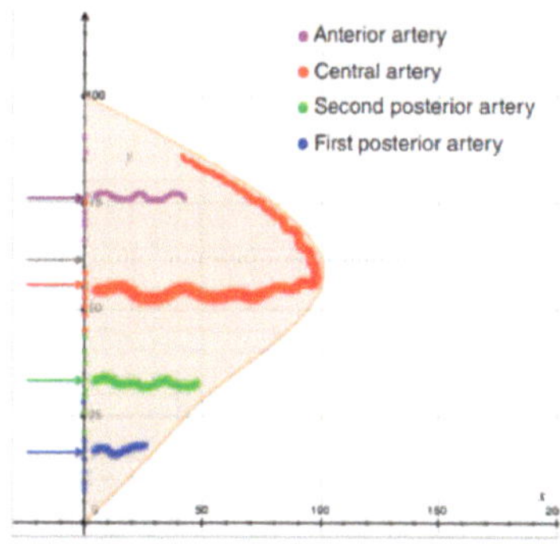

Arterial supply to the medial and lateral aspects of the labia minora, with contributions from the external pudendal artery anteriorly and the posterior system of the internal pudendal artery.

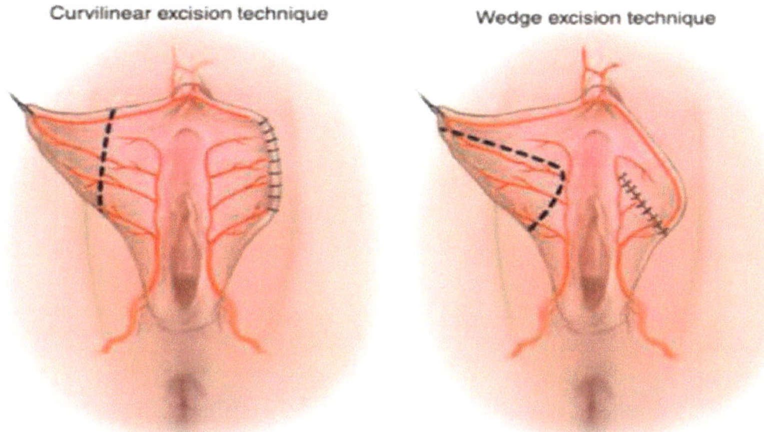

Fig. 1-9   The blood supply in relation to curvilinear and wedge excision techniques.

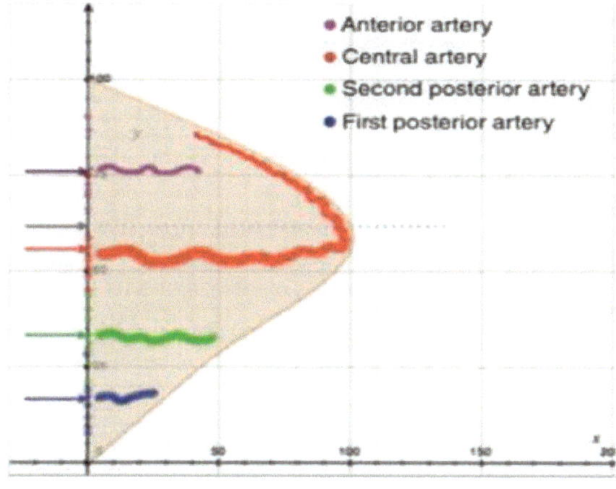

Fig. 1-10   Mapping of the labial arteries demonstrating the A, C, and P arteries.

REFERENCES

1. Goodman MP. Female cosmetic genital surgery 2009;113:154-9.
2. Journal of Plastic and Reconstructive Surgery: A cadaveric study of the arterial blood supply of Labia Minora 167-178, July 2015.
3. Hamori, Banwell, and Alinsod: Female Cosmetic Genital Surgery: 4-22.
4. Motakef S, Rodriguez- Feliz, Chung MT et al Vaginal labioplasty: current practices and simplified classification system for labial protrusion. plastic reconstructive surgery 135:774,2015.
5. Banwell PE. Classification and anatomical variation: implications for labioplasty surgery.
6. Banwell PE. labioplasty: anatomy, techniques, and new classification. clinical cosmetic and reconstructive expo, Olympia London, Oct 2013.
7. llyod J Crouch NS, Minto CL, et al: Female Genital Appearance: BJOJ 112:653, 2005
8. Franco T, Franco D. Hiperttrofia de ninfas J Bras Ginecol 103:163,1993.
9. Hamori CA discussion: Vaginal Labioplasty: Current practices and a simplified classification system for labial protrusion. Plastic Reconstructive Surgery 134:661,2014.
10. Placik OJ, Arkins JP Plastic Surgery Trends. Aesthetic Surgery 34:1083, 2014.

MODULE 2

ENERGY-BASED DEVICES

LASER PHYSICS AND HAIR REDUCTION

Fahad Usman

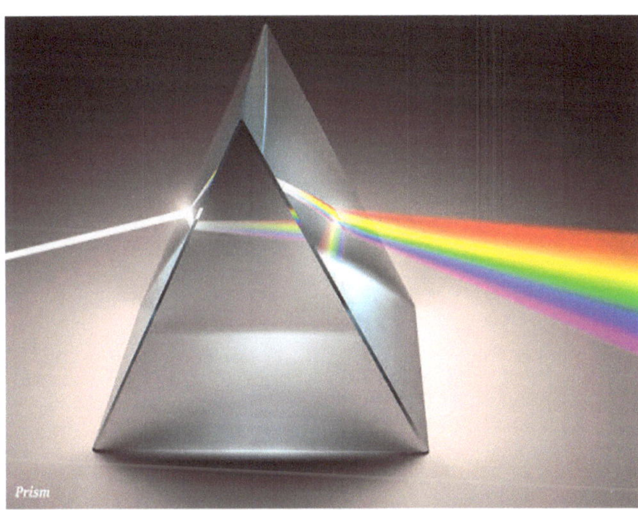

Figure 1: *Prism showing components of White Light*

Physics

Wave Length:

- Laser effect depends on its wavelength

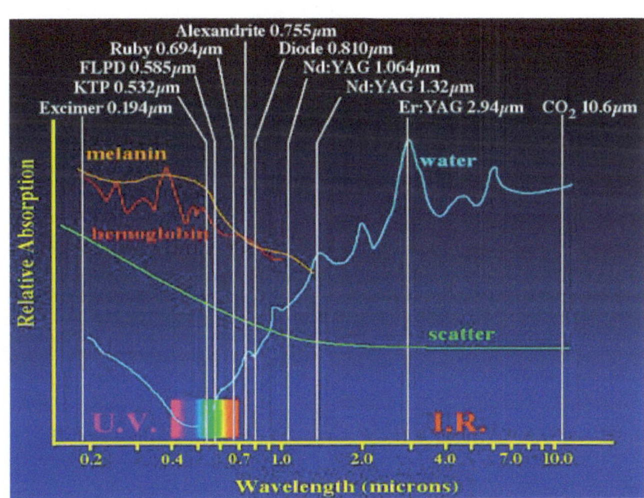

Figure 2: *Relative Absorption Vs. Wavelength*

Absorption Coefficient

- Absorption by a chromophore at a particular wavelength.
- The degree of absorption and effect on the skin varies with the *type* and *amount* of chromophores present in the recipient.

Hypertrichosis

Nonandrogen-dependent increase in hair growth at any body site out of normal range for sex age and race.

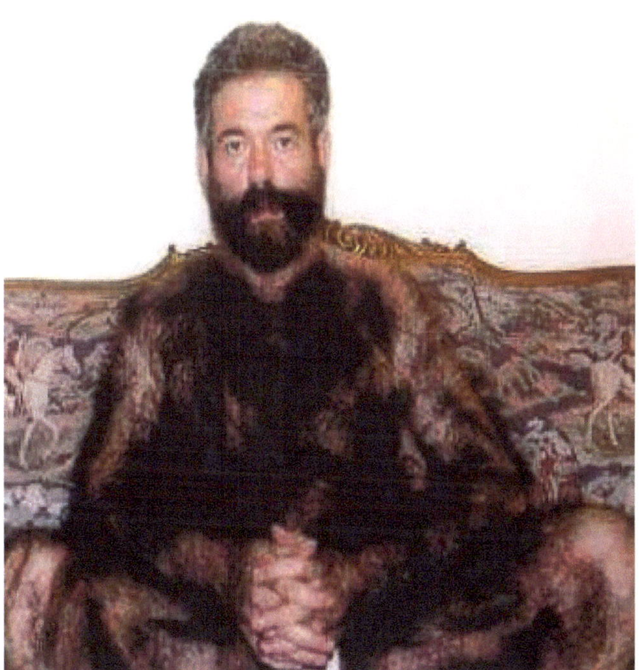

Figure 3: *Person with Hypertrichosis*

Hirsutism

- Abnormal growth of terminal androgen-dependent hair in women mimicking male pattern (chest and Face).

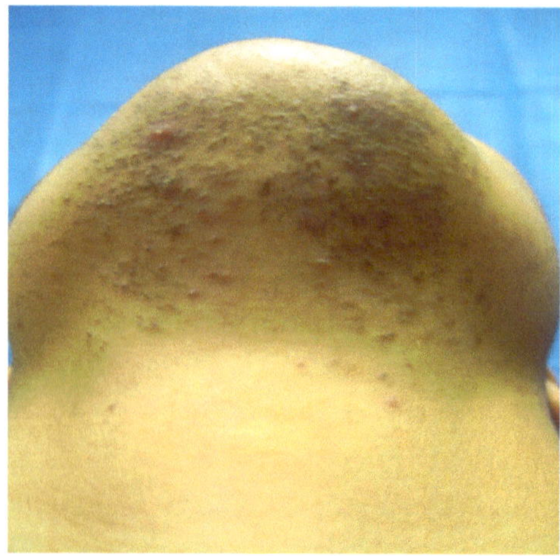

Figure 4: Excessive hair growth on chin

History

- **1963:** Goldman described ruby-laser injury to pigmented hair follicles.
- **1983:** Oshiro and Maruyama noted hair loss from nevi with a ruby laser. However, at fluences affecting hair follicles, the epidermis was severely damaged.
- **1996:** Grossman used a normal-mode ruby laser and reported the first application of Anderson and Parrish's theory for hair removal.
- **1998:** Dierickx published their report of a 2-year follow-up study demonstrating long-term, permanent hair removal with ruby laser.

Laser Hair Removal Mechanics

- Melanin is the chromophore.
- Number of sessions depends on various <u>parameters:</u>
- Location-Skin-type-Coarseness of hair-Reason for hirsutism-Gender

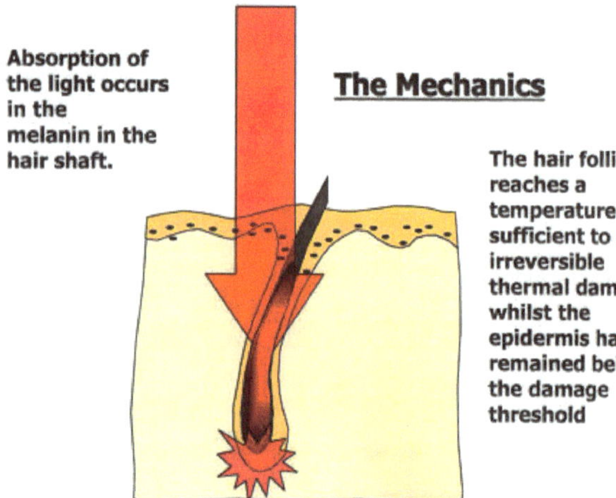

Figure 5: Laser Hair Removal Mechanics [1]

Hair Growth Cycle

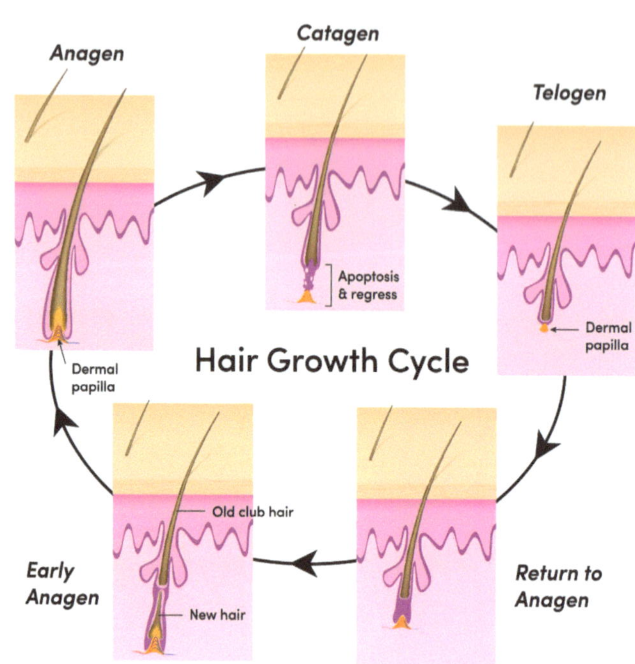

Figure 6: Hair Growth Cycle [2]

- Hair growth exhibits a cyclical pattern. The anagen phase is the growth phase, whereas the telogen phase is the resting state. The transition between anagen and telogen is termed the catagen phase.
- Phases vary in length according to anatomic location, and the length of the anagen phase is proportional to the length of the hair produced.
- At any one time at an anatomic location, follicles are found in all 3 phases of hair growth. This is extremely important for Laser hair removal, because follicles in the anagen phase are Susceptible to destruction, whereas resting follicles are more resistant.
- This explains why multiple treatments of an area may be necessary to ensure adequate hair removal.

LHR is a Melanin contest:
Follicular Vs. epidermal melanin

Ideal patient	Dark coarse hair, fair skin
Challenging patient	Dark coarse hair, dark skin
More Challenging patient	Light hair, dark skin
Very Challenging patient	Light thin hair
Impossible (so far)	White hair

LASER HAIR REMOVAL DEVICES

LASER	WL (nm)	PD (ms)	REMARKS
Ruby (epiLaser)	694	3-10	Oldest
Alexandrite (Photogenica)	755	3-20	Spray Cooling
Diode (Lightshear)	810	5-300	Versatile
Nd: YAG	1064	3-100	Safe for dark skin
IPL	600-1100	3-100	Versatile, can be dangerous
IPL+RF	600-1100		
Cooling	Cryogen > Cold Window Gel >Air		

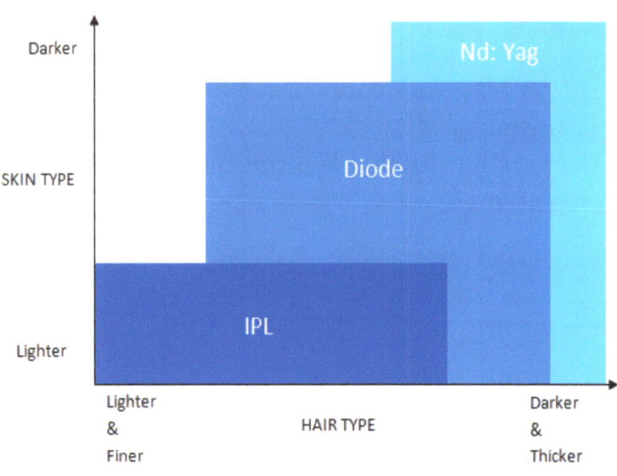

Figure 7: Laser for Different Skin & Hair Types

Most patients need a minimum of 7 treatments.

Wait 3-8 weeks between sessions depending on the area.

Certain areas (men's faces) require more treatments.

REFERENCES

1. https://bareuk.co.uk/laser-hair-removal-can-change-life/
2. https://hairlossmedicalsolutions.com.au/hair-replacement-cycle/

LASERS IN COSMETIC GYNAECOLOGY

Minie Anand

CHAPTER
06

Abstract:

Physiological changes in a woman's life, such as childbirth, weight fluctuations, and hormonal changes due to aging and menopause, may alter the laxity of the vaginal canal, damage the pelvic floor, and devitalize the mucosal tone of the vaginal walls, leading to stress urinary incontinence, vulvovaginal atrophy, and dryness affecting a women's quality of life, self-confidence, and sexuality. Vaginal rejuvenation has shown importance in recent times as women seek out these procedures to gain back their self-esteem, reduce functional discomfort and difficulties, and improve sexual pleasure. Various technologies are available now to address these issues in the form of energy-based devices which are the latest developments in this sector and are showing promising results in the alleviation of these concerns. The EBDs apply thermal or non-thermal energy to the skin tissue which stimulates collagen formation, contraction of elastin fibers, and neovascularization and induces tissue remodeling thus improving lubrication, the proliferation of vaginal epithelium, and increasing vascular and neural regeneration. Lasers have widely and successfully been used for treatments in aesthetic medicine and their application in the vaginal canal for feminine rejuvenation represents their wide expansion of therapeutic indications.

Introduction:

Laser is an acronym that stands for Light Amplification by the Stimulated Emission of Radiation. The use of laser technology in gynecology has become widespread since CO_2 laser was initially used by Kaplan and colleagues in 1973 for the treatment of cervical erosions. Since then, many advancements in laser technology have been made, and several types of lasers are now available, the common ones in use being Erbium:Yttrium-aluminum-garnet (Er: YAG) and diode lasers along with carbon dioxide (CO_2) lasers to treat the vulvovaginal area.

Laser Physics:

A simple way to understand how light is emitted in lasers is to look at an atom with its surrounding electrons (Fig. 1). The electrons occupy discrete orbits that shift to higher orbits when they absorb energy (Fig 2). Whenever the medium is activated, electrons are displaced to higher energy orbits. The electrons that are displaced quickly return to their resting orbits, releasing a package of energy in the process referred to as a photon (Fig. 3). This process of light generation is known as spontaneous emission. In the laser, however, these photons can further stimulate an already excited atom in its path to release an identical photon. This is called stimulated emission (Fig. 4).

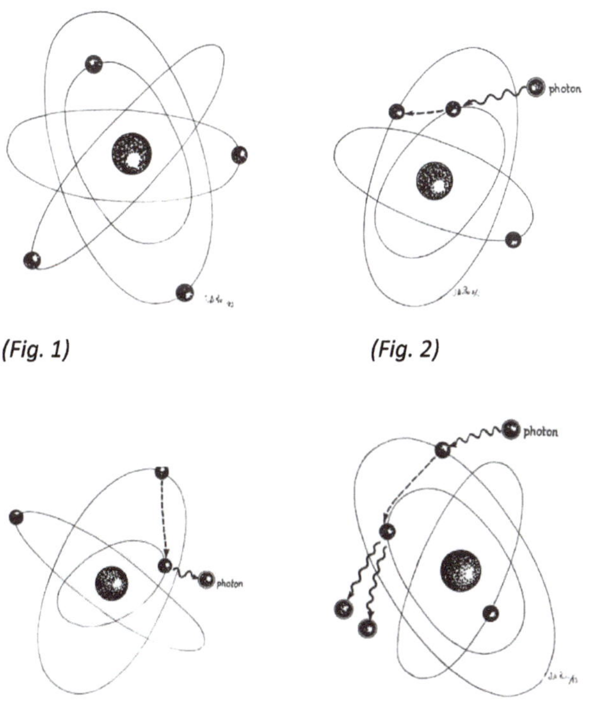

(Fig. 1)   *(Fig. 2)*

(Fig. 3)   *(Fig. 4)*

Basic Components of Lasers

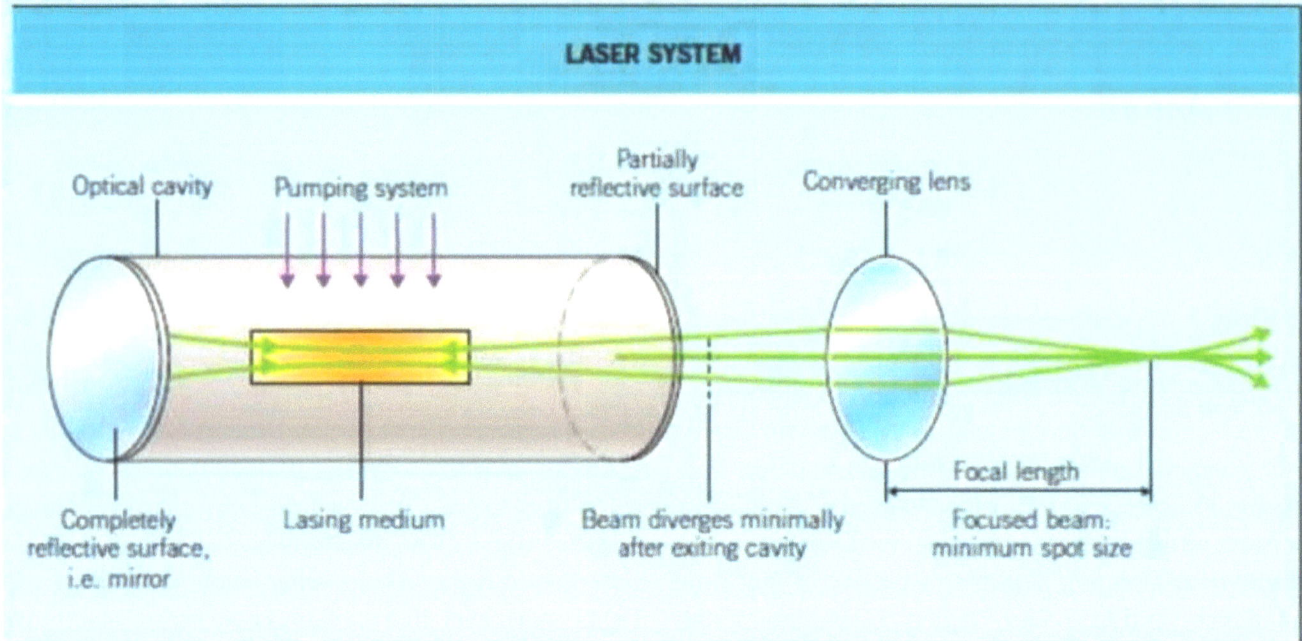

Properties:-

Laser light has three unique properties: –

- **Monochromatic:** - The luminous waves emitted come out with the same wavelength and energy thus allowing precise targeting within tissue while sparing adjacent structures.
- **Coherent:** - All the photons emitted vibrate in phase agreement both in space and time. Highly coherent beams can be more precisely focused.
- **Collimated:** - The light waves are parallel and not divergent and this directionality allows the laser beam to be focused on a very small spot size.

Laser Characteristics: -

- Wavelength (in nanometers)
- Spot size (in centimeters)
- Pulse duration (energy delivered per unit time in Watt)
- Fluence (energy delivered per unit area) joule/cm2
- Irradiance (power delivered per unit area) watt/cm2

Classification of Lasers according to the nature of the amplifying medium

TYPES OF LASER MEDIA		
Gas	**Liquid**	**Solid**
Argon	Rhodamine dye	Crystal
Carbon dioxide	dissolved in organic	• Alexandrite
Copper vapor	solvent†	• Erbium-doped yttrium aluminum garnet (YAG)
Helium–neon		• Holmium-doped YAG
Krypton		• Neodymium-doped YAG
Xenon chloride*		• Potassium titanyl phosphate
		• Ruby
		Semiconductor
		• Diode (e.g. aluminum gallium arsenide)

Penetration of Lasers: -

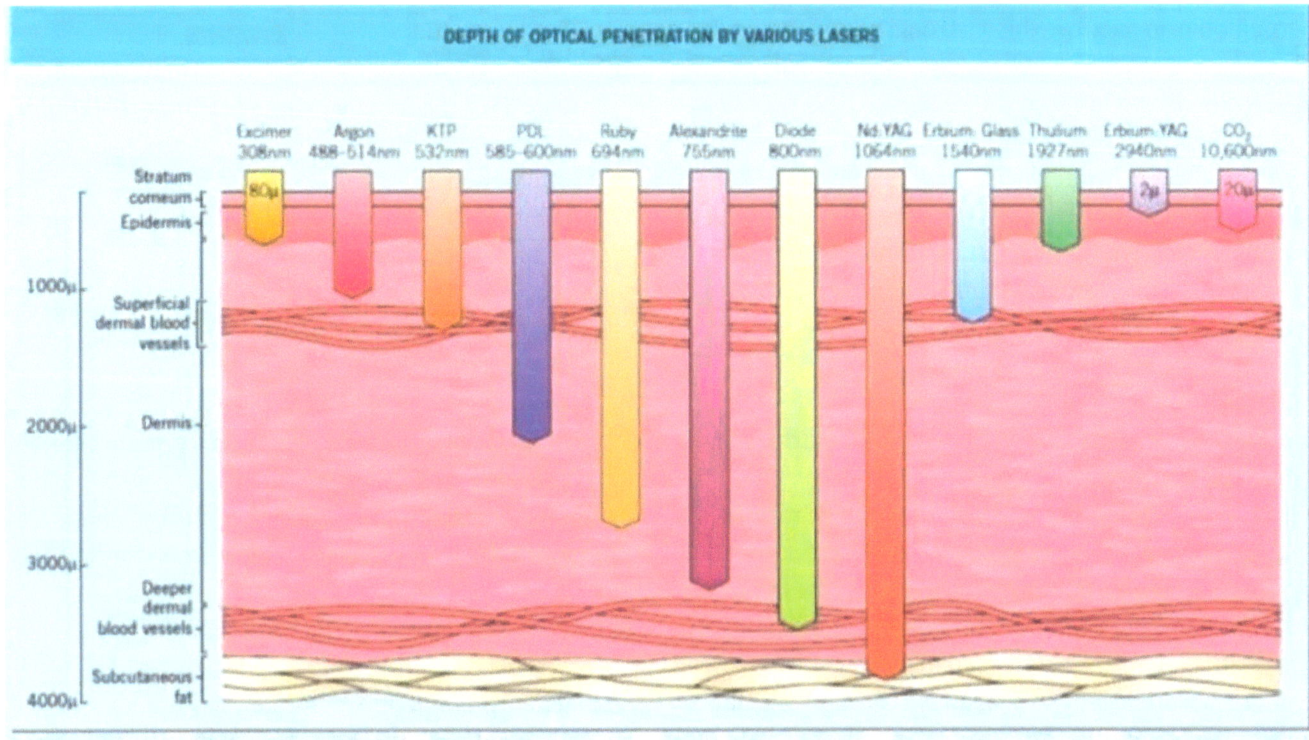

Ablative laser treatments work mainly on the epidermis. Non-ablative laser treatments work solely on dermal collagen. Fractional laser treatment works at both the epidermal and dermal layers of the skin.

The laser light interacts with tissue in unique ways
- Photoacoustic – A sound wave explodes the tissue.
- Photoablative – High energy vaporizes or cuts the tissue
- Photothermal – Heat coagulates/cuts the tissue
- Photochemical – Energy causes chemical and/or cellular changes

Thermal relaxation time (TRT) is defined as the time required for a particular heated tissue to cool halfway towards its initial temperature. Most of the absorbed energy is converted to heat which diffuses in the surrounding tissue. This diffusion via conduction is also called thermal relaxation. The key to clean ablation of tissue is to ablate it quickly before much heat is conducted into the surrounding tissue.

Identification of different types of medical lasers

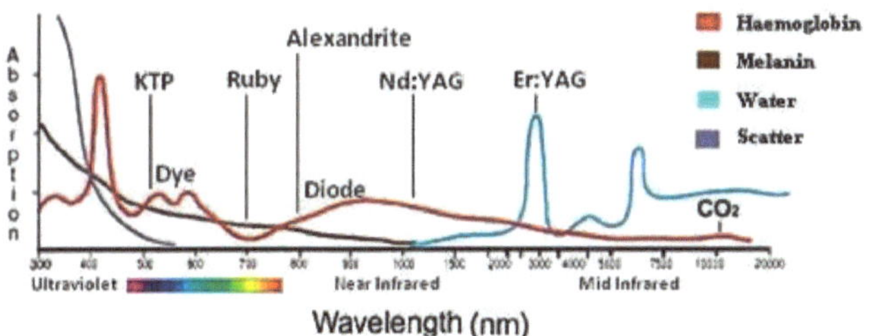

Chromophores (Absorbing Molecules)
Chromophores exhibit characteristic bands of absorption at certain wavelengths when absorption occurs, the photon surrenders its energy to chromophores. Once absorbed, the photon ceases to exist and the chromophore becomes excited. It is this fact that allows for the delineation of specific targets for laser activity.

Three primary skin chromophores are: -
- Water
- Hemoglobin
- melanin

Melanin absorbs broadly across the visible and ultraviolet (UV) spectrum. Oxyhemoglobin and reduced hemoglobin in blood exhibit strong bands in the UV, blue, green, and yellow regions. Water has strong absorption in the infrared (IR) region.

Lasers have recently been used for several urological and gynecological conditions like lichen sclerosis, condylomata acuminate, vaginal laxity, vulva vaginal dryness, mild to moderate urinary incontinence, mild pelvic organ prolapse, vulval diseases like lichen sclerosis and condylomata acuminate.

COMPARISON OF VARIOUS TYPE OF LASERS

CO_2 LASER- it emits infrared light that measures 10,640 nm in wavelength.

The effects of fractional CO_2 laser treatment on vaginal mucosa are increased thickness of the squamous stratified epithelium, increased levels of glycogen, and a huge number of glycogen-rich cells depositing at the epithelial surface. Increased Extra Cellular Matrix content which includes collagen and ground substance and activates fibroblasts were also observed in the connective tissue of the lamina propria. Additionally, undulated epithelium, newly formed connective tissue papillae, and blood capillaries penetrating inside the papillae were detected post-treatment.

ADVANTAGE

- It produces very high power with relative efficiency.
- CO2 laser offers low cost per watt in addition to good beam quality.
- Its efficiency is better than other laser types.
- It has a long life of about 20,000 Hours.
- Gives rapid healing with minimal discomfort and pain.

DISADVANTAGE

- One has to be well versed with this type of laser before operating it as high power can cause burns and contractures.

Er: YAG LASER – it emits an infrared light that measures from 1,064 to 2,940 nm in wavelength.

It leads to increased cellularity and thickness of surface epithelium and a compact lamina propria with dense connective tissue arrangement and increased elastin and collagen content. Mainly works on the surface epithelium.

ADVANTAGE

- Causes minimal residual thermal injury to the underlying tissue.
- Provides a milder less invasive treatment option.
- It is good for quick processing of thinner materials.
- Low cost of consumables.
- Short downtime.
- It offers higher energy output and a very high repetition rate.
- It is easy to operate and maintain.
- Purchasing cost is relatively lower.

DISADVANTAGE

- It has low absorption of radiation of lighter materials very close to the visible spectrum.
- Slow production is possible for thicker materials using this laser type. Hence it offers lower efficiency.

DIODE LASER – delivers wavelengths ranging from 810 to 1470 nm.

The mechanism of action is the same as the above two, heat causes collagen to denature and break into shorter collagen fibers. This partially denatured collagen stimulates the production of new collagen fibers which causes tissue tightening after the procedure.

ADVANTAGE

- The laser diode operates at lower power as compared to another laser.
- Gives higher power output as compared to other lasers.
- Easily portable due to its compact size.
- Operable for long hours.
- It offers excellent efficiency with a very high operation duration.
- It is comparatively easy to operate.

DISADVANTAGE

- They produce more divergent laser beams as compared to other lasers.
- Initial investment is expensive.

General Treatment Protocol

- Office procedure
- No Anaesthesia
- 2-3 passes of Entire Vaginal Canal
- 3 sessions
- 1-month interval
- 1 Memory Session after 1 year
- May require to repeat the full course after 2 years

Contraindications

- Active HPV/Herpes
- Abnormal PAP Smear
- Active Vaginal Infection
- Gynaecological Cancer
- Undiagnosed Vaginal Bleeding
- Uncontrolled Diabetes
- Pregnancy
- Recent Vaginal Injury
- Any Active Bleeding (Including Menses)

Adverse effects and complications

The effects of outpatient laser therapy appear well tolerated with most studies quoting low pain scores on visual analogue scale and high levels of patient satisfaction. Side effects appear to be mild and transient, ranging from mild vaginal and vulval edema, and vaginal irritation to urinary urgency and frequency. Symptoms usually subside after 2 weeks. Occasional vaginal bleeding can occur after treatment, which usually subsides after a few days.

Conclusion

The past decade has seen a substantial rise in technological advancements in terms of tissue functional restoration. The implementation of these modalities for vaginal rejuvenation has opened a new dimension. With this field rapidly evolving, procedures need to be standardized for safer practice. Studies suggest that laser treatment for the restoration of vaginal function might improve the quality of life of millions of women and many studies show that the procedure is effective and safe if appropriately applied. Yet long-term studies and outcomes are still awaited to validate the treatment protocols using these newer modalities in the emerging field of cosmetic gynecology.

REFERENCES

1. Kaplan I, Goldman J, Ger R: The treatment of erosions of the uterine cervix using the CO_2 laser. Obstet Gynecol 41: 795, 1973
2. Wilkie G, Bartz D. Vaginal rejuvenation: a review of female genital cosmetic surgery. Obstetrical & gynecological survey. 2018 May 1;73(5):287-92.
3. Barbara G, Facchin F, Buggio L, et al. Vaginal rejuvenation: current perspectives. International journal of women's health. 2017;9:513.
4. Garcia B, Scheib S, Hallner B, et al. Cosmetic gynecology—a systematic review and call for standardized outcome measures. International urogynecology journal. 2020 Oct;31:1979-95.
5. Bujnak A, Crowder CA, Krychman ML. Energy-Based Devices for Functional Vaginal Problems: Issues and Answers. Current Sexual Health Reports. 2021 Feb 26:1-3.
6. Tadir Y, Gaspar A, Lev-Sagie A, et al. Light and energy-based therapeutics for genitourinary syndrome of menopause: consensus and controversies. Lasers in surgery and medicine. 2017 Feb;49(2):137-59.
7. Ahluwalia J, Avram MM, Ortiz AE. Lasers and energy-based devices marketed for vaginal rejuvenation: A cross-sectional analysis of the MAUDE database. Lasers in surgery and medicine. 2019 Oct;51(8):671-7.
8. Zerbinati N, Serati M, Origoni M, et al. A. Microscopic and ultrastructural modifications of postmenopausal atrophic vaginal mucosa after fractional carbon dioxide laser treatment. Lasers Med Sci. 2015 Jan;30(1):429-36. doi: 10.1007/s10103-014-1677-2. Epub 2014 Nov 20. PMID: 25410301.
9. A.A. Bhide *et al*. The use of laser in urogynaecology Int Urogynecol J (2019)
10. G.A. Lapii *et al*. Structural reorganization of the vaginal mucosa in stress urinary incontinence under conditions of Er: YAG laser treatment Bull Exp Biol Med (2017)
11. Marta Barba, Alice Cola, et. Al. Efficacy of a Diode Vaginal Laser in the Treatment of the Genitourinary Syndrome of Menopause. doi: *10*(10), 1158; 2

RADIOFREQUENCY IN AESTHETIC GYNECOLOGY

Jignesh Vaghasia

Radiofrequency (RF) technology is often used in cosmetic gynecology for various procedures aimed at addressing a range of issues, including vaginal laxity, pelvic floor disorders, and urinary incontinence. The application of RF energy in this field has seen significant growth due to its non-invasive nature and its ability to stimulate collagen production, tighten tissues, and improve overall vaginal health. RF treatments in cosmetic gynecology are typically safe and can offer effective results with minimal downtime.

One of the primary uses of RF technology in cosmetic gynecology is vaginal resurfacing. This procedure, often referred to as RF vaginal tightening, aims to address issues such as vaginal laxity, decreased sensation, and mild urinary incontinence. RF energy is applied to the vaginal tissues, leading to the stimulation of collagen and elastin production, which can result in a tightening and strengthening of the vaginal walls.

Another common application of RF technology in cosmetic gynecology is for the treatment of pelvic floor disorders, including conditions such as stress urinary incontinence and pelvic organ prolapse. RF energy can be used to target the pelvic floor muscles, promoting tissue regeneration and improving muscle tone, which may help alleviate symptoms associated with these conditions.

Additionally, RF technology can be utilized for non-surgical labiaplasty procedures. By applying RF energy to the labial tissues, providers aim to improve the appearance of the external genitalia, addressing concerns related to asymmetry, sagging, or excess tissue. This non-invasive approach can be appealing to individuals seeking aesthetic improvements without undergoing traditional surgical interventions.

RF treatments in cosmetic gynecology are generally well-tolerated, and many patients appreciate the minimal discomfort and short recovery periods associated with these procedures. Additionally, RF technology is often suitable for individuals who are not good candidates for more invasive surgeries, providing them with alternative options to address their concerns.

HISTORY

- RF technology has been used in medicine for more than seventy years but it was used more as a cautery for cutting and coagulation. Later it was approved by the FDA, as a skin-tightening device. [1]
- It was the first breakthrough in nonsurgical facelift and off-face site technology [2]
- Nonablative RF was first explored to achieve tightening of the vaginal canal by Dillon and Dmochowski in 2009 [3]

RF HEATING MECHANISM

The heat generation is instantaneous and allows a rapid uniform and perfectly controlled process thus delivering outstanding results in terms of product quality, operational flexibility, and energy saving

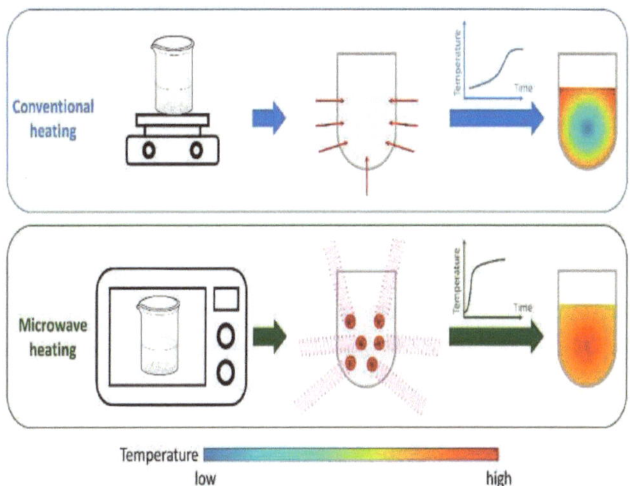

When an RF electromagnetic field is applied to materials it causes materials mass to generate heat directly inside the entire product mass that is why the related mechanism is called "endogenous".

Conventional Heating   **Dielectric (RF) Heating**

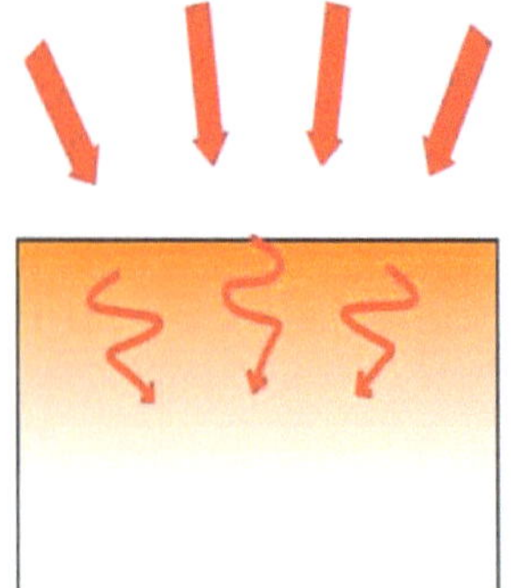
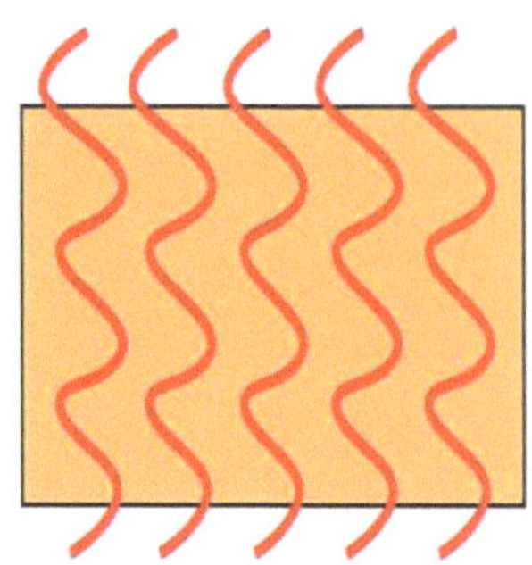

Heat slowly moves from the product surface to the center by conduction

Heat is generated instantly and consistently throughout the material

MODE OF ACTION

- The mode of action of radiofrequency technology involves heating the dermal layer of the vaginal mucosa to promote a cellular regenerative response. [4]
- Stimulate [Type 1] collagen remodeling and regeneration in the extracellular matrix.
- Contracture of elastin fibers
- Neovascularization
- Vaginal lubrication
- Recent studies also show an increase in the small nerve fiber density in the papillary dermis.[5]
- There is newly formed collagen, and increased elastin fibers in the submucosa in post-treatment biopsies [6]

HISTOPATHOLOGY CHANGES

Histologic studies have shown that heating this layer to between 42 -45* C activates heat so proteins and regenerative cellular pathways which ultimately increases collagen genesis neurogenesis elasticity and increased vascularity [7]

HIstologically, nonkeratinized squamous epithelium lines of the vaginal wall, but in the deep dermal layer the composition changes. This layer has increased deposition of dense connective tissue, smooth muscle, collagen, and elastin which imparts strength and elasticity to the tissue.[8] This is the layer that is predominantly targeted by radiofrequency devices.

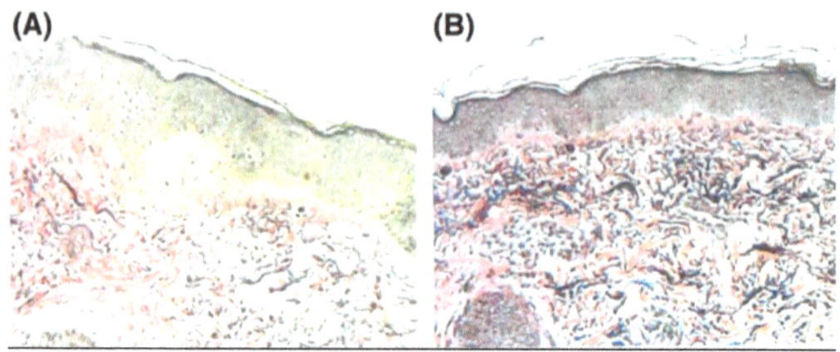

A: - Representative histology slid at baseline
B: - 3 months posttreatment showing increased network of collagen fiber and dermal elastic compared with baseline biopsy. [6]

COLLAGEN REMODELLING

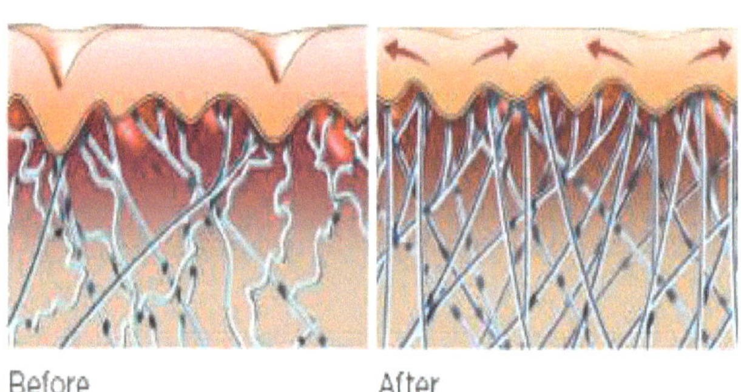

A: - Vagina pre –TTCRF (H&E) Thin epithelium
B Vagina post- TTCRF (H&E) thick epithelium

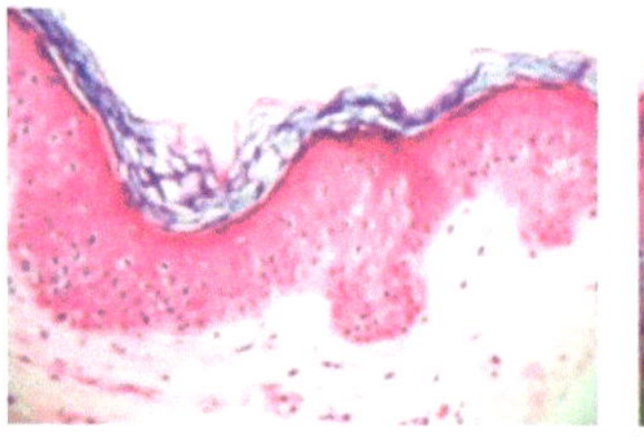
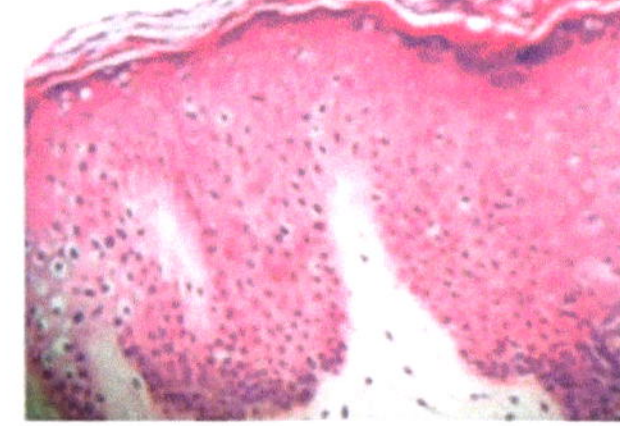

A: - Vagina pre –TTCRF (H&E) Thin epithelium
B Vagina post- TTCRF (H&E) thick epithelium

Types of RF

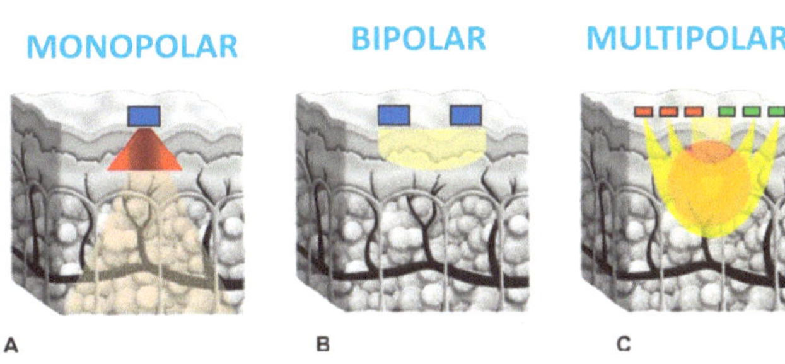

MONOPOLAR

- Monopolar RF wave is vertical penetration so it can go deeper.
- Deeper dermis level to rearrange collagen.
- Instant skin tightening which yet is just a small part of the results.
- Heat is generated at the surface where the monopolar RF head exactly touches the skin then the heat penetrates deep into the dermis and adipose tissue.

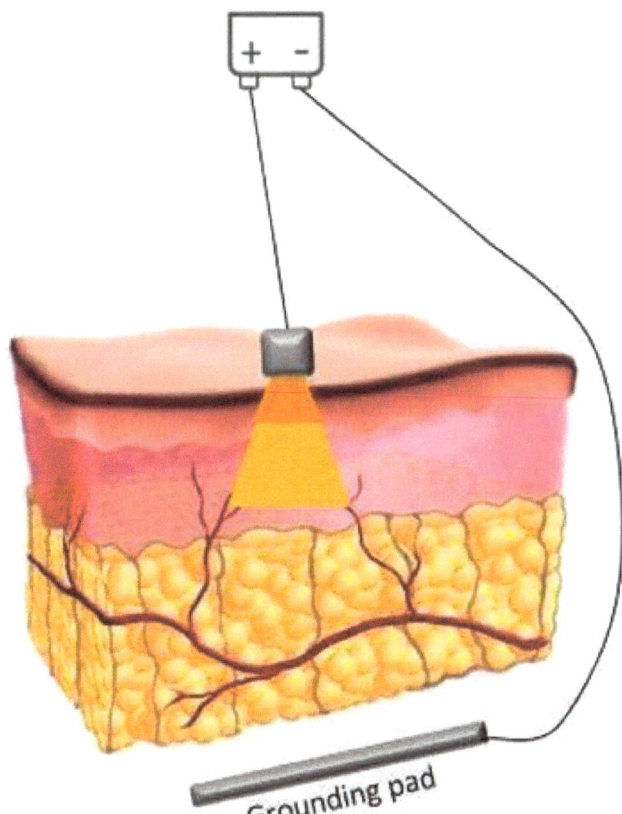

BIPOLAR

- Bipolar RF both delivery and return electrodes are incorporated in the handpiece.
- When the system is activated current flows between the handpieces in the kind of 'U' shape.
- Suitable for face.

More treatments and more minutes and sessions to obtain good results compared with monopolar therapy.

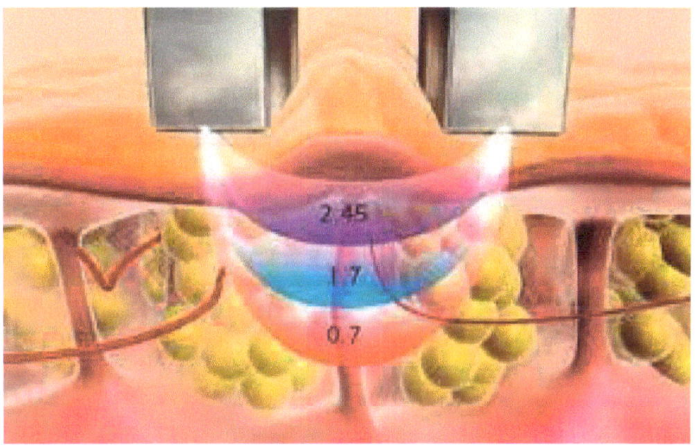

PROCEDURE

- OPD or lunchtime procedure
- Time taken 15-30 minutes
- Three sittings advocated each 2-4 weeks apart for most devices
- Touch-up sitting after 12-18 months

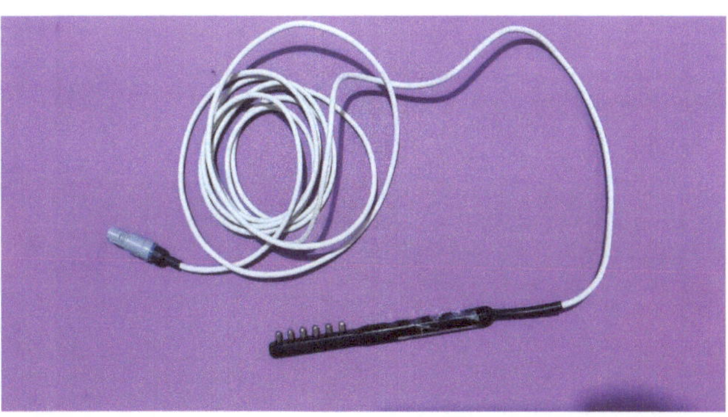

STERILIZATION

- Used probe immersed in 2% Betadine scrub + 2% Hydrogen peroxide/ 1 liter of water for a minimum of 5 minutes.
- Then brushed, washed, and kept on a clean cloth and then in CIDEX for another 20 minutes.
- Store in formalin chamber.

ADVANTAGES

- Painless-no anesthesia
- No downtime
- No medications
- Practically no side –effects

COMMONLY USED ENERGY DEVICES

Devices	Manufacturer	Number of Treatments
ThermiVa	ThermiAesthetics	3 at 4 -6 week intervals
ReVive	Viora	4-6 at 2 -3 week intervals
Pelleve	Cynosure	3-4 week at 4 week intervals
Viveve	Viveve Medical	1 at 1 time [9]
Protge intima	BTL Asthetics	2-4 week at 2-4 week intervals

Position Statement by Regulatory Agency

In July 2018, US FDA stated the indecisive use of radiofrequency devices for "vaginal rejuvenation" and other vaginal procedures and they have not approved any of these devices for specific gynecologic indications. [10]

ACOG published an opinion that insufficient high-quality data is supporting the effectiveness of these devices for vaginal treatments. So, patient should be counseled regarding potential complications such as pain, bleeding, scarring, adhesions, altered sensation, dyspareunia, and chronic pain. However, the overall risk appears to be low, and less than 1% of women will describe these problems when treatment is used correctly.

REFERENCES

1. Facial Plast Surg. Clin. North Am. 2011 May; 19(2):347-59

2. NS,Malerich AS,nassr AH, et al. Radiofrequency: an update on latest innovations. J Drug Dermtatol.2014;13(11):1331-5.

3. Dillon B., Dmochowski R. Radiofrequency for the treatment of stress urinary incontinence in women. Curr Urol Rep.2009;10(5):369-374

4. Pather k, Dilgir S, Rane A. The thermal in genital Hiatus Treatment(TIGHT) Study. Sex med.2021;9(6):100427.

5. Gold M, andriessen A. Bader A, et al. Review and clinical experience exploring evidence, clinical efficacy, and safety regarding nonsurgical treatment of feminine rejuvenation. J Cosmet Dermatol 2018;17(3);289-97

6. Dermatol Surg. 2023 jan 1;49(1):54-59.

7. Dayan E, Ramirez H, Theodorou S. Radiofrequency treatment of the labia minora and major; a minimally invasive approach to vulva restoration. Plast Reconstr Surg Glob Open. 2020;8(4):e2418

8. Photiou L, Lin MJ, Dubin DP, et al. Review of non-invasive vulvovaginal rejuvenation. J Eur Acad Dermatol Venereol,2020;34(4);716-26

9. Michal krychman et al. J Womens Health (Larchmt).2018;27(3):297-304

10. The US FDA Warns Against Use of EBDs to Perform Vaginal Rejuvenation or Vaginal Cosmetic Procedures: FDA Safety Communication; Available from: https://www.medsafe.govt.nz/safety/EWS/2018/EnergyBasedDevicesVaginal Rejuvenation. asp [Accessed February 28th, 2021]

HIFU & MFU IN COSMETIC GYNECOLOGY

Garima Srivastav

Unlike, laser or Radiofrequency, sound is not an electromagnetic wave but a form of acoustic energy travelling in waves.

- Audible sound range is 20Hz to 20,000Hz.
- Frequencies higher than the human ear are called ultrasound waves.
- Used for both diagnostic and therapeutic purposes.

MODE OF ACTION

Two main effects: Thermal and mechanical.

1-Thermal: energy is absorbed into the tissue and is converted into heat energy as temperature increases faster than dissipation.

2-Mechanical: effects are induced by HIFU that create cavitation, microstreaming, and radiation force.

Two types of focused ultrasound waves

HIFU: HIGH-INTENSITY FOCUSED ULTRASOUND

- Intense thermal effect of ultrasound, 47-59J/cm2 at 2 Mhz frequency.
- The ultrasound focal point can be as little as 1mm and reach deep in tissues up to 1.8 cm in depth.
- Causing thermal and mechanical effects.
- Used for ablating tumors, adipose tissue for body contouring.
- HIFU (High-Intensity Focused Ultrasound) is a non-invasive therapeutic technique that uses non-ionizing ultrasonic waves to heat tissue. HIFU can be used to increase the flow of blood or lymph or to destroy tissue, such as tumors, through several mechanisms.
- Treatment for symptomatic uterine fibroids became the first approved application of HIFU by the US Food and Drug Administration (FDA) in October 2004.

MFU: MICROFOCUSSED ULTRASOUND

- Utilizes lower ultrasound energy.
- More superficial
- Depth of 1.5-4.5 mm
- Thermal effect present with no cavitation.

- Producing coagulation points in the dermis and subdermal layer with sparing of overlying dermal and epidermal layers. (no cavitation).
- It has become one of the most popular treatments to tighten skin and elevate facial structure.
- It utilizes its capabilities to create controlled microthermal effects at the deeper dermis and subcutaneous tissue. Upto SMAS (SUPERFICIAL MUSCULOAPONEUROTIC SYYSTEM).
- Unlike Radiofrequency, it can be focused to target deeper tissues without affecting superficial tissues. For RF to achieve higher temperatures, surface cooling is needed to protect the skin.
- By using different transducers, energy can be delivered at various depths: 1.5,3.0,4.5 mm which covers the superficial dermis to the supra SMAS layer.
- FDA approved for eyebrow elevation.
- Can be used for skin laxity over eyes, face, submental area as well as neck, arms, thighs, and buttocks can be covered too.
- Treatment time 90 minutes.
- No downtime, minimal aftercare.
- C/I in open wounds, keloids, or lesions in the treatment area or implants in the treatment area.

MFU in Facial Rejuvenation

- The first reported use of MFU for aesthetic use was in 2008
- MFU was then approved by the Food and Drug Administration (FDA) in 2009 for brow lifts.
- The device was also cleared by the FDA in 2014 to improve lines and wrinkles of the upper chest and neckline (décolletage).
- The procedure is also used for overall facial rejuvenation, lifting, tightening, and body contouring

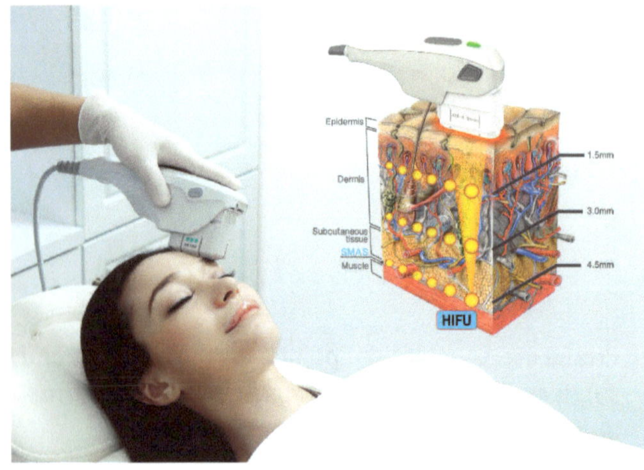

MFU in Vaginal Rejuvenation

- HIFU vaginal rejuvenation is the most powerful non-surgical treatment method, which treats the vaginal structure damaged by
- Aging
- Vaginal delivery
- Menopause, or
- By loss of basic elements such as collagen and elastin, and changes in the connective tissues

How does it work?

- MFU technology targets the dermal and SMAS layer of the skin, for both superficial and muscular tightening; generating new collagen, and causing the skin to tighten, tone, and lift continually for up to 90 days.
- MFU is a gold-class, non-surgical procedure, that targets internal skin structures at depths of 3mm & 4.5mm per treatment at a 360-degree rotation. This technique ensures consistent results with simultaneous toning and tightening.

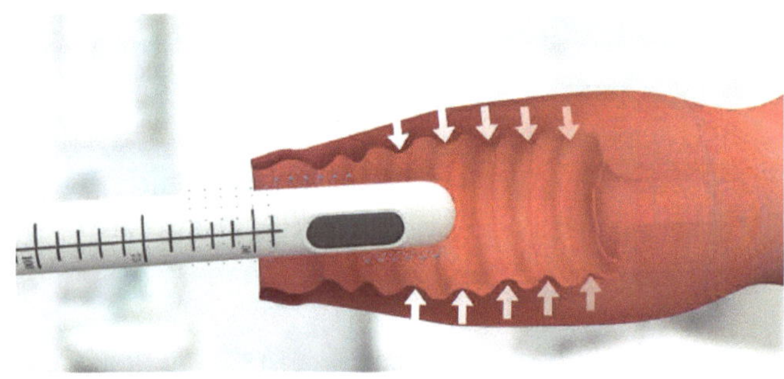

Benefits of MFU Vaginal Rejuvenation

- MFU vaginal rejuvenation has quickly become an advanced medical alternative to traditional Vaginoplasty for the following reasons:

- Immediate and long-term results
- Rsurfacing of vaginal tissue
- Tightening and toning of vaginal muscles
- Fast, virtually painless treatments
- No downtime

Treatment Methodology

- Ultrasound energy has a proven track record, in the field of medicine for over 50 years and achieves a staggering 20-25% instant result on average, with optimum results seen at approx. 3 months.
- 2-3 treatments are recommended for optimal results. Maintenance treatments are recommended.
- Results last on average between 2 and 4 years.
- Results vary from person to person and are based on factors such as age, lifestyle habits, and medical history.

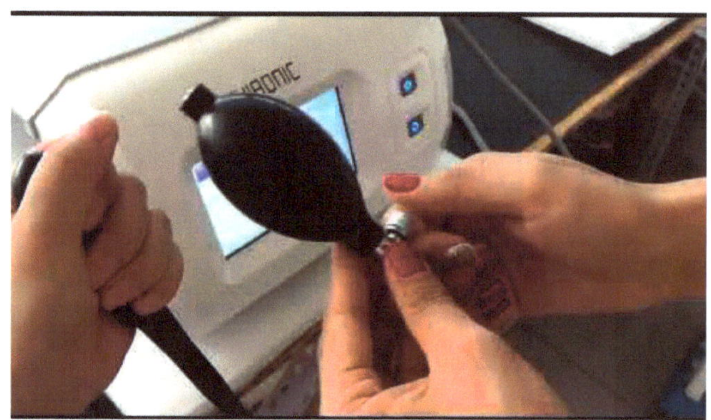

Treatment Methodology

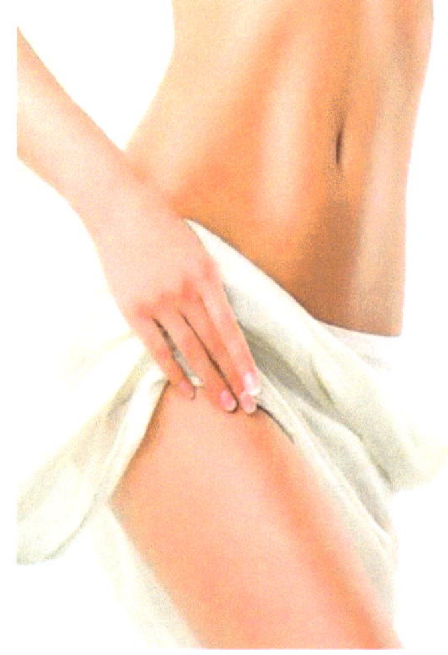

Applications

- Potent vaginal tightening and firming effect to improve sexual life.

- Increasing Vaginal lubrication and eliminating dryness.
- Improving vaginal sensitivity by cell regeneration.
- Comprehensive improvement of vaginal health and reducing infection.
- In GSM, UI, Vaginal atrophy.

MODE OF ACTION

- The Vagina Tightening HIFU System uses a non-invasive ultrasonic focusing technique to directly focus on the mucosal lamia and muscle layer.
- Using ultrasonic waves as the energy source and taking advantage of its penetration and locality, the system will send out ultrasonic energy focusing on the lamina propria and muscle fiber layer at a predetermined depth.
- A higher intensity of the ultrasonic region, called the focus region, is formed.
- In 0.1 seconds, the temperature of the region can reach above 65°C, so the collagen is reorganized and the normal tissue outside the focal region is undamaged.
- The heat causes the collagen to contract and denature resulting in shorter and thicker collagen. This results in the lifting and tightening of the skin.

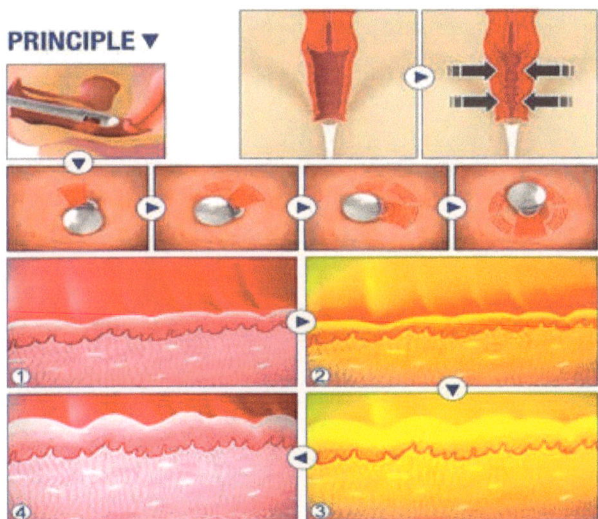

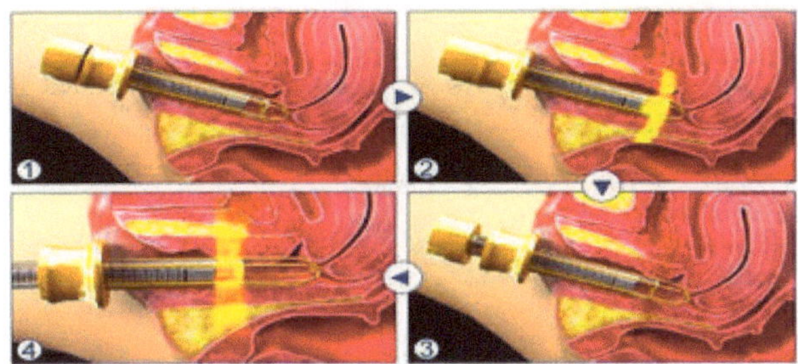

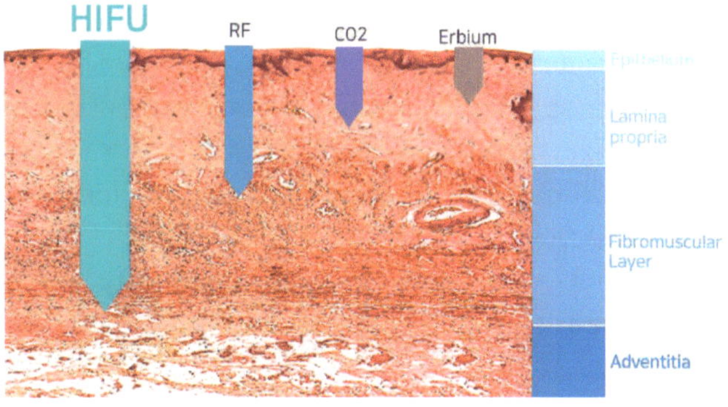

The schematic diagram represents the depth of various Energy-based Based Devices.

The diagram depicts MFU to penetrate the deepest of all vaginal layers depending on the probe used.

So, authors suggest, that due to unique technology, it may serve better than other EBDs to reach deeper layers than mucosa where SUI-related issues are rooted.

ADVANTAGES

- The treatment is painless, non-invasive, and lasts 20 minutes.
- No suggested recovery-time.
- Improved muscle strength, tone, and elasticity of vaginal muscles.
- Increased sensation during intercourse.
- Improved control over urinary incontinence.
- Vaginal tightening with HIFU requires no downtime, and clients can return to normal life immediately following the procedure. HIFU vaginal tightening is the perfect alternative to extensive, invasive surgery to restore the youthful look and function of the vagina.
- The most powerful benefit of this particular treatment is that there is no recovery time.
- Patients are free to return to their normal daily activities right away.
- HIFU gives you all the benefits of vaginal rejuvenation. without the high cost and high risk of surgery.

ULTRAVERA

- Gyeonggi, S. Korea is one of the very famous modified HIFU.
- Three handpieces for depths of 1.5, 3.0, and 4.5mm
- Energy levels are set between. 2-2 J/cm2.

EVIDENCE-BASED MEDICINE ON HIFU

- A prospective study of GSM and SUI in postmenopausal women by Elias et al demonstrated epithelial changes in mucosal histology such as stratification and increased glycogen in superficial keratinocytes.
- 6 patients also presented with hyperlaxity which improved at 6 months.

EVIDENCE-BASED MEDICINE

- Studies on the safety and efficacy of HIFU on vaginal laxity conducted by Sekiguchi in 2017 and 2018 concluded that all patients had improvement in vaginal laxity and treatment was safe without adverse effects.
- Since there is sparing of the epidermis and it is non-invasive, there is no post-procedure healing time.
- Patients can resume all activities immediately after the procedure.
- 3-4 treatments at intervals of 3-4 weeks are recommended with maintenance after 6-12 months.

CONCLUSION

- HIFU in treating GSM is comparable to lasers and RF.
- Due to unique technology it may serve better than other EBDs to reach deeper layers than mucosa where SUI-related issues are rooted.

REFERENCES

1. Phenix CP, Togtema M, Pichardo S, Zehbe I, Curiel L. High-Intensity Focused Ultrasound Technology, its scope and application in therapy and drug delivery. J Pharm Pharm Sci 2014;17(1): 136-53

2. Ter Haag G Intervention and Therapy. Ultrasound Med and Biol 2000;26(Suppl 1):S51-4

3. Zhou Y Principles and Application of therapeutic ultrasound in healthcare. 1st edition Boca Raton FL CRC Press;2015

4. Fatemi A, Kane MA.High-intensity Focused Ultrasound effectively reduces waist circumference by ablating adipose tissue from the abdomen and flanks: A retrospective case series. Aesthetic and Plastic Surg 2010;34(5): 577-82

5. Robinson DM, Kaminer MS, Baumann L, Burns AJ, Brauer JA,Jewell M, Lupin M, Narukar VA, Struck SK, HledikJ, Dover JS. High-intensity Focused ultrasound for reduction of subcutaneous adipose tissue using multiple treatment techniques. Dermatol Surg 2014;40(6):641-51

6. Yagel SHigh Intensity Focused Ultrasound: a revolution in noninvasive ultrasound treatment? Ultrasound Obstet Gynecol 2004;23(3):216-7

7. Elias MGJA, Corin G, Garcia PN, Sivo V, Nestor D, Nunez L. Management of vaginal atrophy, vaginal hyperlaxity, and stress urinary incontinence with intravaginal HIFU. Int J Obstet Gynecol Res 2019;18(11):1088

HIGH-INTENSITY FOCUSED ELECTROMAGNETIC TECHNOLOGY IN GYNECOLOGY

Garima Srivastav

The High-Intensity Focused Electromagnetic Technology (HIFEM) is a non-invasive technology for pelvic floor muscle strengthening. It has US FDA clearance for urinary incontinence in both men and women.

MODE OF ACTION

Electromagnetic fields are composed of both electric and magnetic fields. In which, electric fields are the result of electric charges, while magnetic fields are created given the movement of electric charges.

The electromagnetic phenomenon comprises basic principles that define its action.

Electric charges attract or repel each other with a force inversely proportional to the distance between them, magnetic poles act the same and exist in pairs.

In the case of HIFEM, a rapidly varying magnetic field induces an electric current to the target tissue.

HIFEM technology induces a simulative effect as the electromagnetic field passes non-invasively through the neuromuscular tissue to induce electric currents that stimulate muscle action.

It utilizes the principles of electromagnetic induction to depolarize motor neurons, thus stimulating intense involuntary contractions, bypassing the central nervous system.

Such intense muscle recruitment appears to trigger an exaggerated need for energy at the cellular level.

INDICATIONS IN GYNECOLOGY

The most common treatment for SUI to this date is rehabilitation of pelvic floor muscles (PFM) using physical exercise.

PFM is the anterior muscle in charge of bladder and urethral contraction, the middle muscle controlling the vagina and uterus, and the posterior muscles for rectal function.

Additional anatomic structures support these organs such as the pelvic diaphragm, urogenital diaphragm, and urethral /anal sphincters.

Both PFM and supporting muscle are subjected to electrical and electromagnetic stimulation.

Weakening of PFM Can promote urinary, and fecal incontinence, sexual disorders, or pelvic organ prolapse, generally termed pelvic floor dysfunction (PFD) as a result of aging or childbirth.

PFM enhancement was proven effective using physical exercise as training increases pelvic muscle tone, causes hypertrophy, and strengthens muscle fibers. To effectively achieve PFM re-education, hundreds of contractions are required and in a very specific manner to address proper muscles.

PFM can be stimulated by electric stimulation and more recently by using HIFEM technology.

Both technologies deliver electrical currents to PFM, which depolarize motoneurons to stimulate involuntary muscle contraction.

Electrical stimulation utilizes direct electric charge flow that does not spare skin surface while HIFEM uses electromagnetic induction to deliver current selectively to PFM.

As the magnetic field passes skin with no attenuation of energy, more energy is addressed to the target tissue, making it potentially superior it can induce more intense contractions that may result in favorable efficacy.

The high frequency of action potential leads not only to selective muscle contractions but also to a supramaximal muscle effect. In studies comparing HIFEM and electrical stimulation, HIFEM resulted as superior in the maximal voluntary contraction (MVC) and by patients' subjective evaluation of a decrease in symptoms.

In another study evaluating improvement in quality of life in a 3-month follow-up, patients reported significant improvement in their symptoms and reduced usage of pads. It is also shown to be promising for female and male sexual health function by improving PFM.

TECHNOLOGY

It works on the principle of patented High-Intensity Focused Electromagnetic Technology (HIFEM). This is an extremely powerful focused electromagnetic field. Its high intensity enables to reach supramaximal muscle contractions, while the patient comfortably sits on the chair.

US FDA cleared it, to provide entirely non-invasive electromagnetic stimulation of pelvic floor musculature for rehabilitation of weak pelvic muscles and restoration of neuromuscular control for the treatment of urinary incontinence in women.

CONTRAINDICATIONS

- Pregnancy
- Metal implants
- Cardiac pacemakers
- Implanted defibrillators, implanted neurotransmitters
- Electronic implants

THERAPY RECOMMENDATIONS

NUMBER OF THERAPIES

- 6 tx

FREQUENCY

- Scheduled twice a week

RESULTS DURABILITY

- Confirmed by 6-month follow-up

RIGHT CANDIDATE

- Stress, urge, and mixed urinary incontinence

Patients sit comfortably and clothed.

The electromagnetic energy causes 11200 kegel exercises of the pelvic muscles in 28 minutes.

Studies are using the chair to treat chronic pelvic pain as well in men and women.

Indications in men

- Sexual dysfunction
- Improving sexual function
- Better orgasms
- Chronic pelvic pain
- Chronic prostatitis, BPH, post radical prostatectomy (cancer)
- Fecal incontinence
- Constipation

Indications in women

- Urine incontinence
- Fecal incontinence
- Prolapse
- Chronic back pain
- Sexual dysfunction
- Constipation
- Post-childbirth (bladder control, muscle defects, perineal healing)
- Obesity
- Aging (Menopause)
- POP
- UI (nocturia, dribbling, hesitancy, urine retention)
- Chronic Pelvic Pain
- Surgery in the pelvic area (rehabilitation)

CONCLUSION

HIFEM is a newer technology, FDA-approved for incontinence (both stress and urge) and sexual dysfunction in both males and females.

It is still in early stage technology with scarce support in medical literature over short follow-up, lack of control groups, and objective, measurable tools.

HIFEM seems promising non-invasive technology for incontinence with no pain or discomfort.

The patient is fully clothed and sits comfortably in the chair.

Over the period, many companies have come up with similar technology.

CONSENT FORM

Diagnosis: ………………………………………

TREATMENT CONSIDERATIONS: You are scheduled for a series of non-invasive treatments with the …… device. ………………..

The therapy is intended to provide entirely non-invasive electromagnetic stimulation of pelvic floor musculature for rehabilitation of weak pelvic muscles and restoration of neuromuscular control for the treatment of urinary incontinence in women.

Your treatment provider will discuss your specific treatment needs.

The recommended number of treatments is 6.

The treatment is typically about 30 minutes per session, with sessions separated by at least 2 days, depending on your needs. Completing a full treatment series is necessary to maximize treatment efficacy. You may need additional treatments depending on the severity of your condition. The results will typically continue to improve over the next few weeks. There is typically no pain associated with your treatment and there is no anesthetic required. You will experience gradually increasing tingling feeling and muscle contractions. These sensations in the pelvic area are normal. You remain fully clothed during the treatment. On the day of the treatment, you are advised to wear comfortable clothes which allow flexibility for correct positioning and increased comfort during the treatment.

Initials……………………………………….

I am aware that pregnancy is contraindicated and pregnant women can't undergo the treatment. I

- I am aware that I can't undergo the treatment when menstruating.
- I understand there are certain risks associated with treatments and they include but are not limited to muscular pain, temporary muscle spasm, temporary joint or tendon pain, local erythema, or skin redness. I understand that the treatment may involve risks of complications or injury from both known and unknown causes, and I freely assume these risks.
- I am willing to fill in forms and/or anonymous questionnaires if requested, as this will help for medical evaluation of the results of the treatment. Information will be acquired for medical records or marketing purposes.
- I understand the results may vary from person to person and that an exact result cannot be predicted. It is very unlikely but it is possible that you will not feel any recognizable result after the procedure. I acknowledge the results may not meet my expectations.
- I certify that I have read this entire document and that I agree with all provisions. I certify that I have had the opportunity to ask questions and these questions have been answered in full to my satisfaction. I fully understand the treatment conditions, the procedure, and possible side effects.
- I have read the above information, and I request and give my consent to be treated with the procedure by the physician(s) in the below-stated practice and his/her designated staff.

My signature below indicates that the above information is accurate and current.

Patient signature: ……………………………………………… Date: ……………………………

Witness (in print): Signature: ……………………………… Date: ……………………………

Doctor Signature……………………………………………… Date: ……………………………

REFERENCES

1. Alexiades M. High-Intensity Focused Electromagnetic Fields (HIFEM) devices in dermatology J Drugs Dermatol.2019; 18(11):1088

2. Yamanishi T, Yasuda K, Suda S, Ishikawa N. Effect of functional continuous magnetic stimulation on urethral closure in healthy volunteers. Urology 1999;54(4):625-5

3. Voorham –van der Zalm PJ, pledger RC, Stiggerlbout AM, Elzevier HW, Lyklama a Nijeholt, G.A. effects magnetic stimulation in the treatment of pelvic floor dysfunction BJU Int 2006;97(5)1035-8

4. Strohbehn K Normal pelvic floor anatomy. Obstetrics Gynecology Clin N Am 1998;25(4)683-705

5. Faubion SS Shuster LT Bharucha AE.Recognition and Management of nonrelaxing pelvic floor dysfunction.Mayo Clin Proc 2012;87(2)187-93)

6. K pelvic floor muscle training is effective in the treatment of female stress urinary incontinence but how does it work? Int Urogynecol J Pelvic Floor Dysfunction 2004;15(2)76-84

7. Correia GN, Pereira VS, Hirakawa HS, Driusso P. Effects of surface and intravaginal electrical stimulation in the treatment of women with stress urinary incontinence: Randomized control trial. Eur J Obstet Gynecol Reprod Biol.2014;173:113-8.

8. Elena S, Dragana Z, Ramina S, Evegeniia A, Orazov M. Electromyographic procedure and electrical stimulation in women with pelvic floor dysfunction. Sex Med 2020;8(2):282-9

9. Samuels JB, Pezzela A, Berenholz J, Alinsod R. Safety and efficacy of noninvasive High intensity focussed electromagnetic (HIFEM) device for treatment of urinary incontinence and enhancement of quality of life. Lasers Surg Med 2019; 51(9)760-6

10. Hlavinka TC, Turcan P, Bader A,. The use of HIFEM technology in the treatment of pelvic floor muscles as a cause of female sexual dysfunction: a multicenter pilot study. J WomenHealth Care 2019;8:1

LOW-LEVEL LASER THERAPY (LLLT)

Fahad Usman

Low-level laser (light) therapy (LLLT) is a fast-growing technology used to treat a multitude of conditions that need
- stimulation of healing,
- relief of pain and inflammation
- restoration of function.

Wavelength (nm)	Colour Range	Penetration (mm)
150-380	UV	< 0.1
390-470	Violet to Deep Blue	~ 0.3
475-545	Blue – Green	~ 0.3 - 0.5
545-600	Yellow to Orange	~ 0.5 – 1.0
600-650	Red	~ 1.0 – 2.0
650-940	Deep Red- Near IR	2-3

Mechanism of Laser Therapy in Tissue Repair
- Skin responds well to red and near-infrared wavelengths.
- Photons are absorbed by mitochondrial chromophores in skin cells.
- Electron transport, adenosine triphosphate (ATP) nitric oxide release, blood flow, reactive oxygen species increase, and diverse signaling pathways get activated.
- Stem cells can be activated allowing increased tissue repair and healing

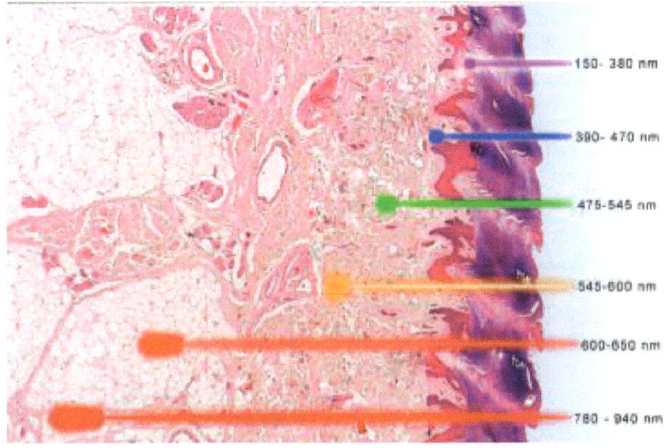

Figure 8: Tissue Penetration Depths of various wavelengths [1]

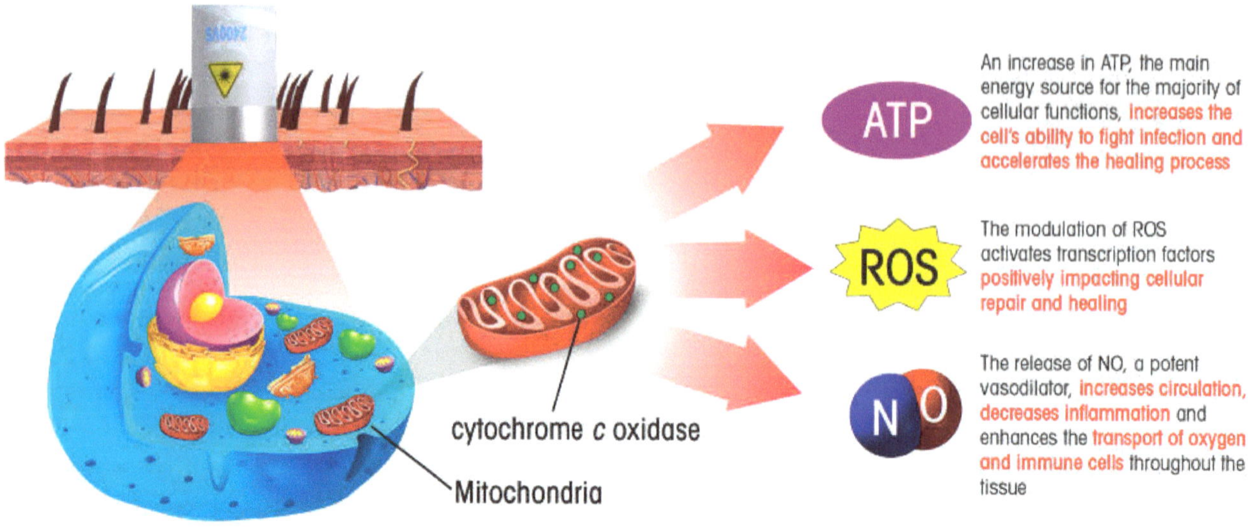

Figure 9: Mechanism of Laser Therapy in Tissue [2]

830 NM WITH 590 NM PHOTOSEQUENCING

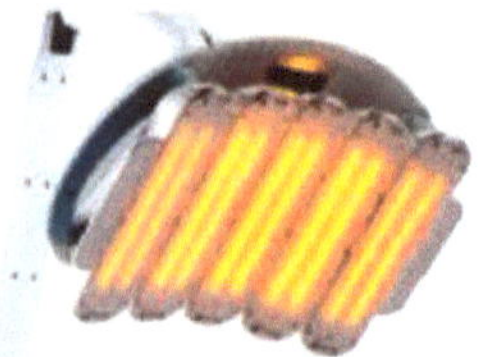

- Wound Healing*
- Pain Relief*
- Muscle and Joint Pain
- Arthritis
- Muscle Spasm
- Temporary Increase of Blood Circulation
- Hair Regrowth
- Acne Treatment*
- Skin Rejuvenation

633 NM

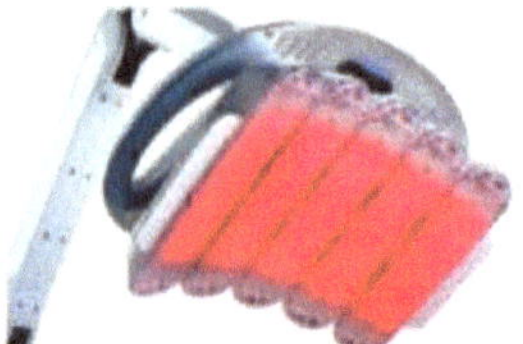

- Non-melanoma Skin Cancer (Exogenous PDT with 5-ALA)
- Skin Rejuvenation
- Hair Regrowth
- Additionally, Active Acne (Exogenous PDT with 5-ALA)

415 NM

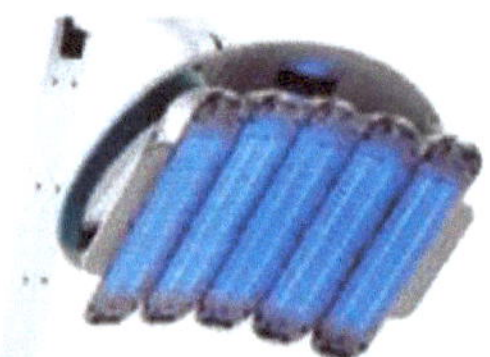

- Active Acne (Endogenous PDT)

*CE marked indications
Regional clearances may vary

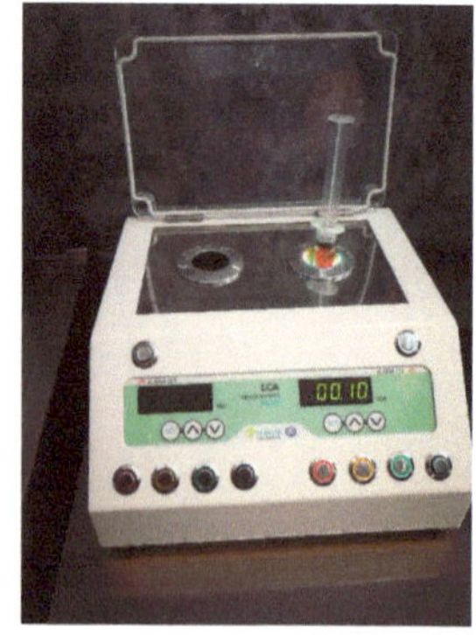

Figure 10: N-Biotek LED Cell Activator

EFFECTS OF LLLT

- Anti-inflammatory effect
- Tissue regeneration
- Pain relief
- Increase vascularity
- Anti-bacterial effect
- Treat neuropathies
- Analgesic effect
- Cell metabolism
- Accelerated wound healing

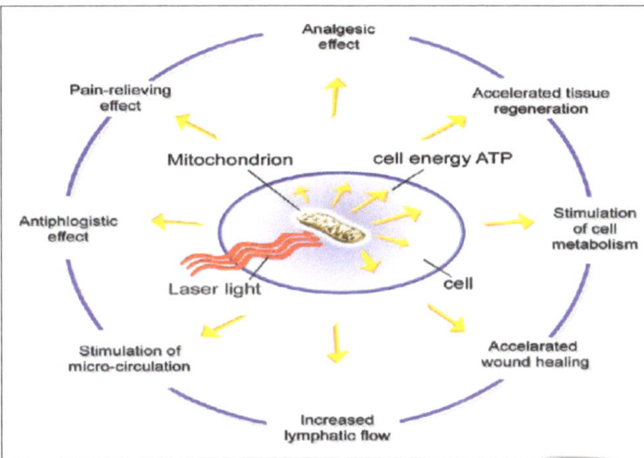

Figure 11: Mechanism of action of low-level laser therapy [3]

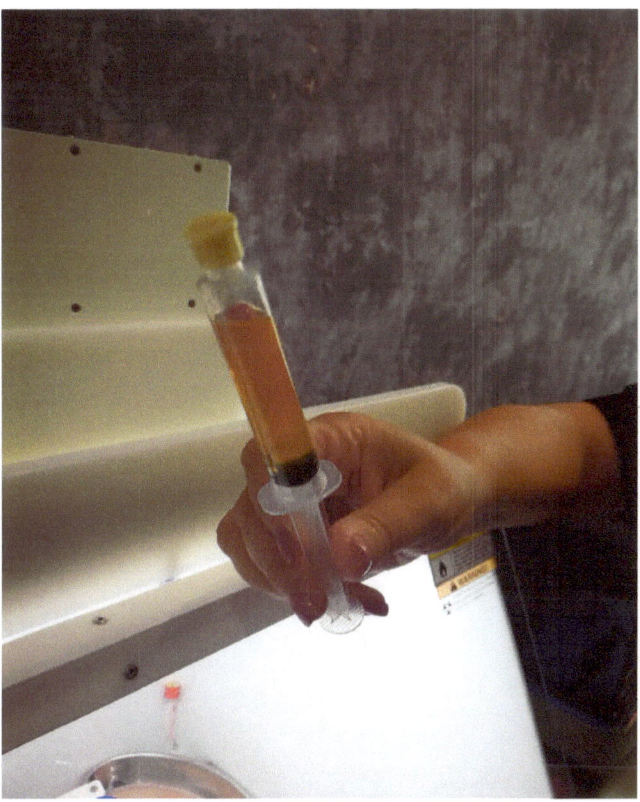

Figure 12: PRP After LED Cell Activator

BLUE AND RED LIGHT THERAPY (LLLT)

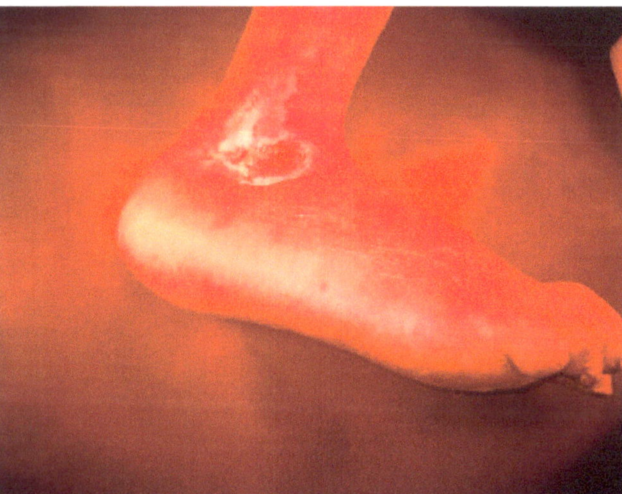

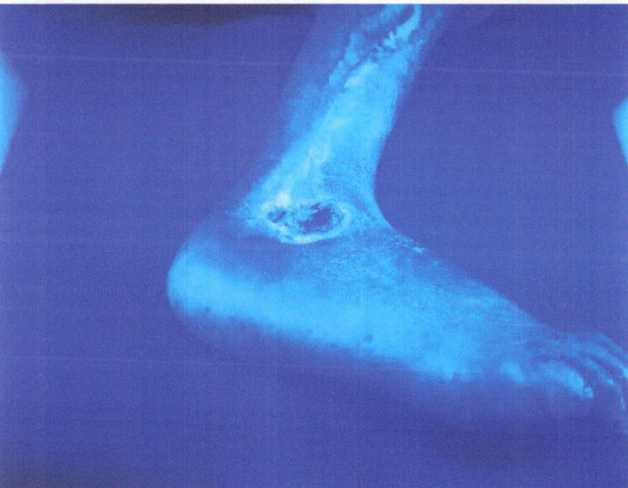

Figure 13: Carboxy Machine [1]

REFERENCES

1. https://www.researchgate.net/figure/Tissue-penetration-depths-of-various-wavelengths-Figure-courtesy-of-Wellman-Center-for_fig2_256835631
2. http://www.mdc-health.com/en/index.php?id=122
3. https://www.imbiodent.com/articulos/imagenes/articulos/pdfs/159/82-low-level_laser_therapy_on_postoperative_pain_after_mandibular_third_molar_surgery.pdf

CARBOXYTHERAPY

Fahad Usman & Garima Srivastav

Carboxytherapy involves the administration of medical-grade carbon dioxide gas beneath the skin through controlled injections. The process is relatively simple, with the gas triggering physiological responses within the treated tissues. Originally, used in the treatment of vascular conditions, carboxy therapy has found applications in various medical and cosmetic fields.

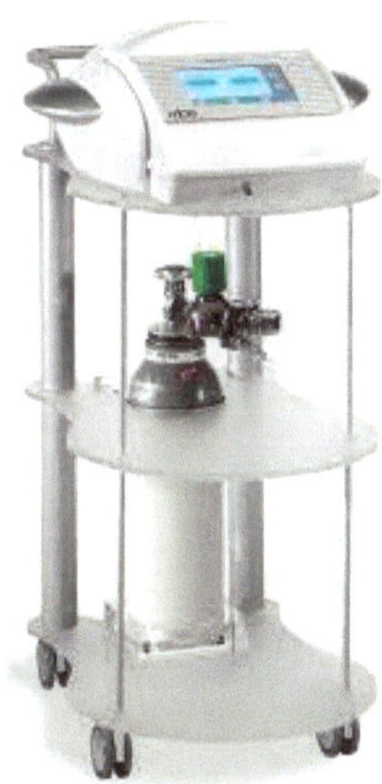

Characteristics of CO2 gas:
- The final product of organic metabolism, therefore does not present allergenic or toxic effects.
- It is a blood-soluble gas, i.e., not embolic.
- Colorless, odorless, soluble in water, heavier than air.
- High diffusion in tissues (close to 25X more than oxygen).

Physiological effects of CO2 gas:-
- Active arterial vasodilatation (direct action of CO2 on the vascular myocytes).
- Increases blood flow.
- Vascular endothelial growth factor (VEGF) induction.
- Increases microcirculation.
- Neo-angiogenesis.
- Bohr effect.

- Neo-collagenesis.
- Lipolysis.
- Regulation of the pH level.
- Stimulation of subcutaneous baroreceptors

MECHANISM OF ACTION

Bohr effect
- Hemoglobin's O2 binding affinity is inversely related both to acidity and to the concentration of CO2. That is, an increase in blood CO2 concentration, which leads to a decrease in blood pH will result in hemoglobin proteins releasing their load of oxygen. Conversely, a decrease in CO2 provokes an increase in pH, which results in hemoglobin picking up more O2.
- This effect facilitates O2 transport as hemoglobin binds to O2 in the lungs, but then releases it in the tissues, particularly those in most need of oxygen.

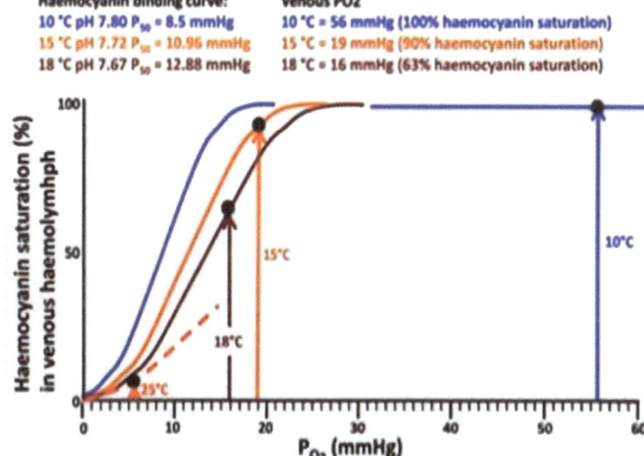

INDICATIONS OF CARBOXYTHERAPY
- Skin rejuvenation
- Periorbital area
- Cellulite
- Localized adipose tissue.
- Stretch marks
- Chronic wounds.
- Skin grafts

CARBOXYTHERAPY IN GYNECOLOGY

The role of carboxytherapy in genital restoration is overall trophic, functional, and sexual

- It enhances functionality, turgidity, hydration, and sensitivity, of the perineal area and vulvovaginal tissues and treats:
- Episiotomy scars
- Post caesarean scars
- Fissures
- Decreased lubrication
- Decreased sensitivity
- Skin laxity and sagging
- Muscular laxity
- Increased Ph level

Genitourinary syndrome symptoms.
- Genitourinary symptoms.
  - Dryness, burning, irritations, itching, discharge
  - unpleasant smell.
- Sexual symptoms.
  - Decreased/absent lubrication, dyspareunia, discomfort in intercourse, decreased libido, soreness, pos-coitus bleeding.
- Urinary symptoms.
  - Urgency, dysuria, nocturia, recurrent urinary tract infections, stress incontinence.
  - Vulvo Vaginal Atrophy (VVA) signs:
  - Loss of labial and vulvar fullness
  - Pallor of urethral and vaginal epithelium.
  - Pethechial atrophy.
  - Loss of urethral meatal turgor.
  - Less hydration.
  - Less elasticity.
  - Fissures.
  - Introitus retraction.

In cosmetic gynecology, carboxy therapy is employed to address several concerns, including vaginal laxity, stress urinary incontinence, and aesthetic improvements in the genital region. The introduction of carbon dioxide stimulates blood flow, leading to enhanced oxygenation and nutrient delivery. Additionally, it promotes collagen production, improving tissue elasticity and firmness.

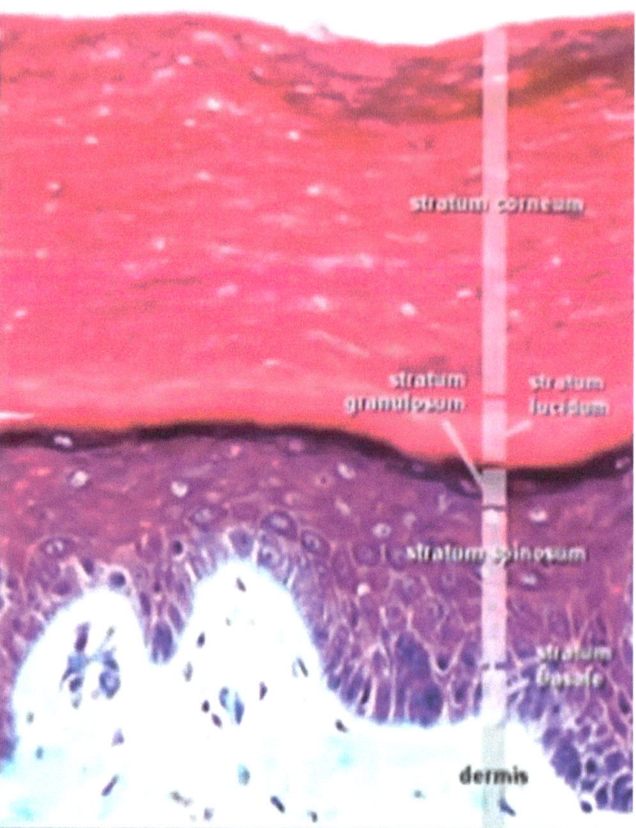

Importance of equipment:
- The treatments were conceived using a medical device designed to regulate and control the flow pressure and thermal of compressed sterile medical-grade CO2 gas.
- It allows to administration of reduced volumes of per cutaneously through hypodermic needles. gas
- It allows changes in the middle of the treatment changing the pressure of the flow.
- It allows tailored treatments.

SIDE EFFECTS
- There are no reports of adverse effects or complications, both local and systemic, in the medical literature on Carboxytherapy
- Moderate pain on the application site during treatment.
- Small bruises caused by puncturing with a 30G needle.
- Feeling of small subcutaneous emphysema at the application site, which disappears after a few hours

General contraindications

- Carriers of artificial pacemakers and/or any other implanted electronic device.
- Acute Myocardial Infarction - AMI less than 2 years ago
- Prior history of Cerebrovascular Accident
- Prior history of Transient Ischemic Attack
- Unstable angina
- Acute thromboembolism
- Congestive Cardiac Failure
- Coagulation disorders
- Under anticoagulant treatment

TREATMENT PROTOCOL VULVA

- Low flow: 20/30 cc/min,
- Needle 30G.
- Depth: only bevel.
- Total flow 70mL.
- 1 Session/week,
- N° of session: 8

Only heated gas devices.
- 2000cc is the maximum dose.
- More than that patient may feel dizzy, because of hypercapnia.

TREATMENT PROTOCOL: MONS PUBIS

- Use heated gas
- Low flow: 40cc/min.
- Needle 30G. 13 needle
- Depth: 3 mm.
- Total flow: 90 mL
- 1 Session/week.

- Number of sessions: 8

TREATMENT PROTOCOL: VAGINA

- Low flow: 20cc/min.
- Needle 32G.
- Depth: only bevel.
- Total flow depends on the mucosa's quality
- 1 Session/Week
- N° of sessions: 8
- Only heated gas devices

Contraindications for vulvovaginal treatment

- Pregnancy
- Lactation
- DST
- BDD
- Infection at the application site
- Current genitourinary diseases

DRAWBACKS

- Many sessions are required.
- Side effects like crackling, pain at the site of injection, and hematomas.
- Device may require maintenance.

CONCLUSION

- An innovative clinical treatment in vulva-vagina and perineal area to an outstanding performance.
- Lunchtime procedure, offers women a quick, painless office treatment, through a non-invasive method for improving vaginal health, sensation, sexual satisfaction, and resuming better QOL.
- Without need for recovery and no downtime!

PLASMA THERAPY IN COSMETIC GYNECOLOGY

Garima Srivastav

What is Plasma?

Plasma is the fourth state of matter next to solids, liquids, and gases. Despite making up 99% of the universe, it is not discussed much.

Plasma is formed when energy passes through the gas (such as air). During the heating that occurs, atoms in the hot gas are moving so fast that electrons can be knocked loose when they collide with each other. This process is called ionization.

- Plasma exeresis is used in non-surgical aesthetic procedures.
- Works by ionizing the gases in the space between the instrument and tissue.
- Uses voltage difference to create an electric arc.
- Causing sublimation of epidermis.
- Does not work when in contact with skin.

Plasma = ionized gas. As an aesthetic application, this refers to the use of plasma energy to create unique non-ablative thermal effects on the skin. According to the studies, this leaves a layer of dissected epidermis which acts as a natural bandage for idealized healing.

Tissue is not vaporized, treatment is not chromophore dependent and there is no easily discernable line of demarcation, making it dramatically different from the laser.

Histology has shown that even after a year, improvement in collagen production and reduced elastosis are still occurring. Outcomes are similar to low and medium fluence co2 lasers with minimum thermal necrosis and a favorable healing profile.

Pure plasma uses nitrogen gas plasma, emitted from the distal end of the handpiece, specifically chosen for its controlled and predictable delivery of thermal energy to the skin at depth.

This heats all tissue components even down to the reticular dermis creating a uniform physiological improvement. It targets water, so it penetrates deeply and heats consistently. Because it purges oxygen from the target area, there is no burning or charring.

INDICATIONS

Plasma does resurfacing, skin regeneration, and skin tightening very well. At higher settings, the epidermis and upper dermis are shed when new skin has formed, with recovery taking 7-10 days.

With fewer sittings and 1-3 days of recovery time, a more superficial effect is maintained.

Regardless the barrier remains intact, acting as an insulator and protection for the wound.

For skin tightening, the instantaneous skin heating by plasma occurs causing immediate tissue contraction, with the cascade of neocollagenesis, neovascularization, and fibroblast migration restoring skin function and health as well as appearance.

Acne, actinic keratosis, viral papilloma, atopic dermatitis, scars, rhytides, fine lines, and wrinkles can be treated by plasma therapy.

Pigmentation wrinkles around the eyes and mouth specifically around the eyes work well.

In Gynecology, it is used in vulval regeneration, treatment of warts, and labioplasty.

CLINICAL EFFECT

The clinical effect of plasma devices on the skin is dependent on several factors including the mechanical and electrical resistance of the tissue and the difference in potential between the tip and the skin. This is a feature of the device and the distance between the points and different energy outputs depends on the device being used.

The latest generation of plasma devices used in aesthetic medicine relies on high-frequency pulses as low frequencies would require a shorter tip gap and lead to unpleasant sensations including electro-muscular contractions and the sensation of electrocution. High frequencies are produced in a sine wave and often a step wave is introduced to produce a specific output where the energy produced is consistent and constant. The gap is defined as the distance between the tip and the target skin and relies on a potential difference between the two. The distance can be increased by increasing voltage or increasing frequency intensity to provide the ideal gap between the tip of the device and the patient, ensuring accurate targeting of the area or lesion to be treated.

Plasma medicine is a relatively new discipline that combines physics with medicine and already has quite a varied application, including sterilization of implants and surgical equipment, disinfection, wound healing, aesthetics, and treatment of skin cancers. The exact mechanism of action of plasma in clinical medicine is unknown, although the process of sublimation is likely to be important as part of the epidermis is converted from a solid state into a gaseous state thereby removing tissue without cutting or excision. The plasma also generates reactive oxygen species, reactive nitrogen species, free radicals, and UV photons which create injury to surrounding cells. It is thought that cells that are more susceptible to damage by these chemically reactive atoms and oxidative stress may be the reason plasma seems to be more selective in destroying bacteria and cancer cells. This process of selectively targeting bacteria may help to explain why plasma treatments offer an alternative approach to the treatment of acne.

In aesthetic medicine, plasma can successfully treat scarring, stretch marks, acne, dyskeratosis, xanthelasma, warts, verrucae, naevi, fibromas, seborrhoeic keratosis and a host of other skin lesions, however, the most exciting revolution for plasma technology for most patients is with non-surgical blepharoplasty.

There are a few contraindications with the use of plasma devices including pregnancy, breastfeeding, use of Roaccutane®, systemic illness, infection at the treatment site, open wounds, body dysmorphia, allergy to the anesthetic agent being used, immunosuppression, auto-immune disease and keloid / hypertrophic scarring (although plasma may be used to treat scarring, it is not recommended to treat other indications in patients who are prone to the development of keloid or hypertrophic scarring). Plasma does not tend to affect the melanocytes so is safe to use in all skin types, however, there may be increased healing time in darker skin types and some manufacturers recommend patch testing in Fitzpatrick skin types 4 and above. Following treatment with plasma, the skin does become more sensitive to the effects of UV radiation and patients must apply a high-factor, broad-spectrum SPF to the area treated to prevent prolonged redness or hyperpigmentation. Of course, skin that is sublimated may take a few weeks to develop the same level of pigmentation as the surrounding skin.

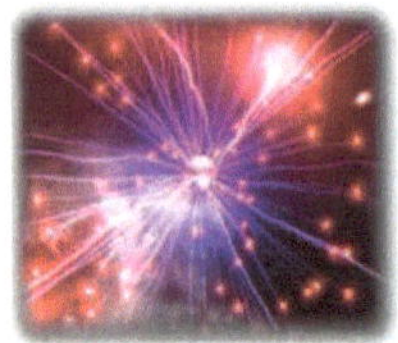

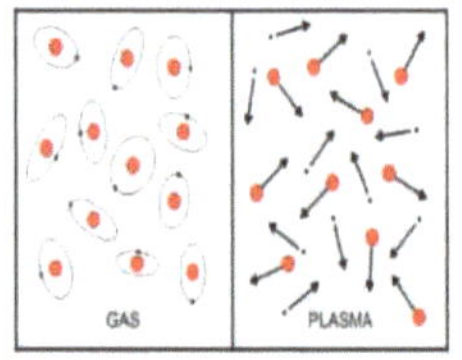

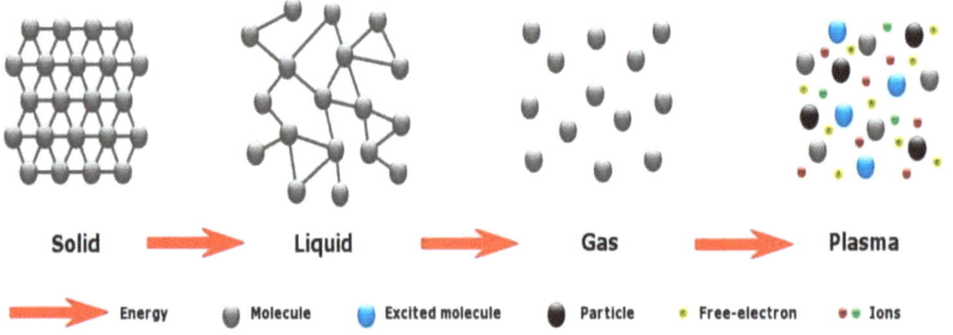

A pseudo sinusoidal signal in output
(High Voltage, Low Frequency and Low Current)

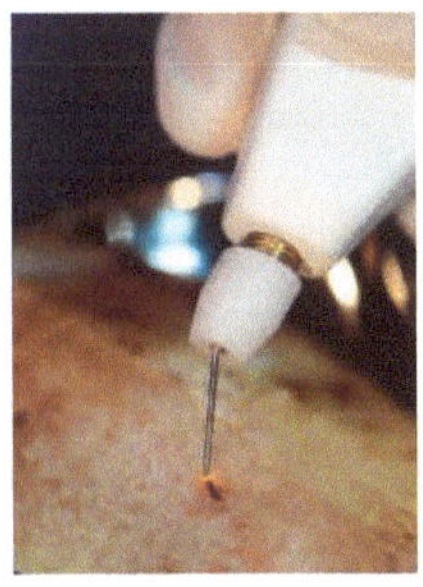

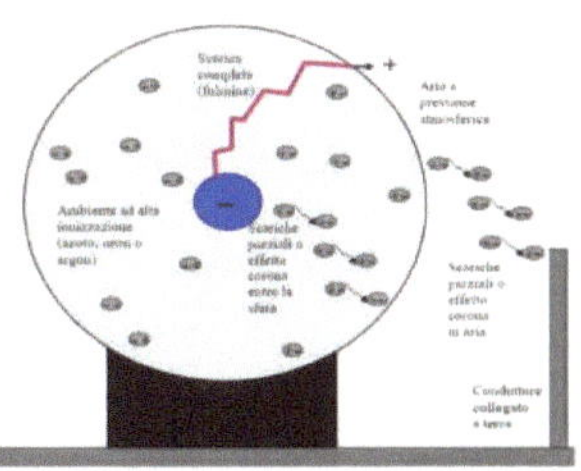

Difference in voltage
from the tip of the instrument and the skin

PLasma EXeResis

The ionization of the gases contained
in the air is obtained through an electric discharge,
as a result of this difference in voltage
between the tip of the instrument
and the patient's skin

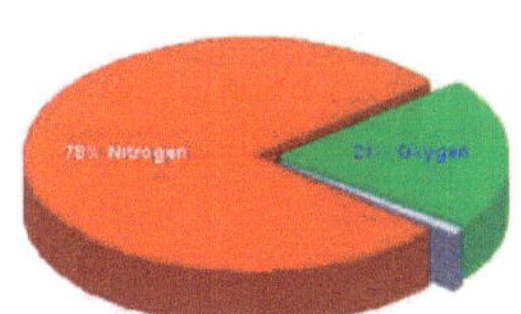

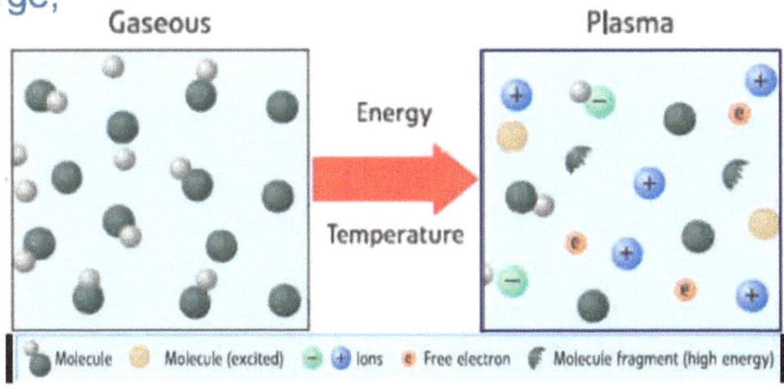

The ionization of the gases:
This energy as a difference in Voltage is delivered to Atoms (electrons + protons and neutrons)
contained in the air, producing an excitation of the electrons in the external shield.

Charged particles

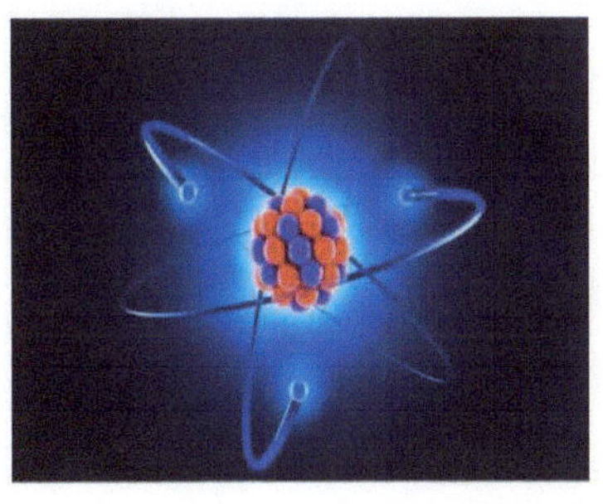

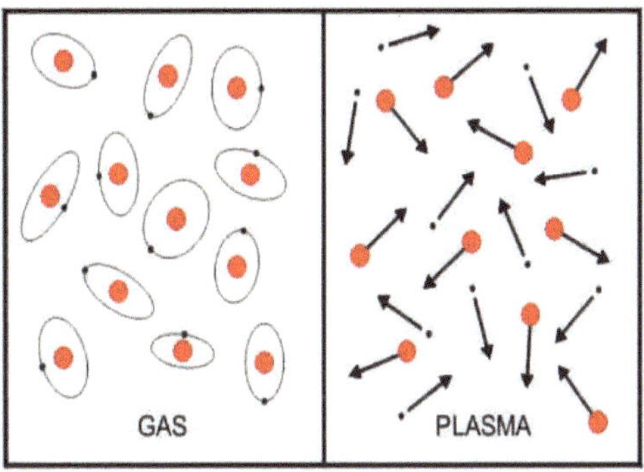

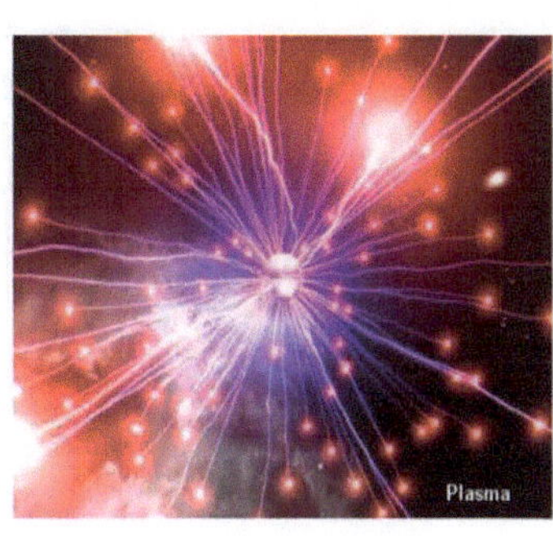

PLasma EXeResis

PLASMA GENERATOR

produces a controlled and focused micro-plasma beam due to the ionization of the gases contained in the air, a small electric arc similar to a minute lightning, useful to treat dermal and epidermal areas affected by aesthetic blemishes.

A micro-plasma beam to sublimate tissues

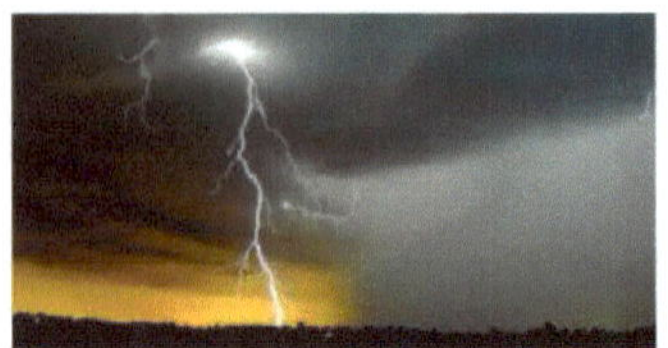

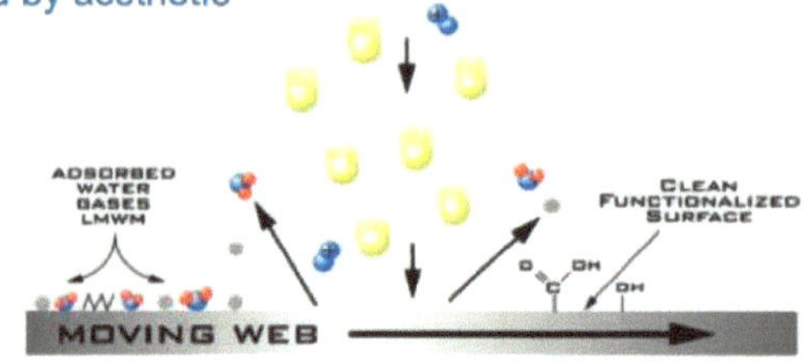

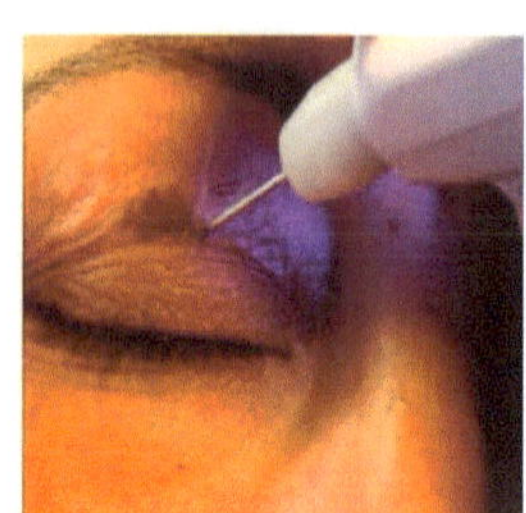

PLasma EXeResis

Sublimation:

passage from the solid state to the gaseous state of the tissues

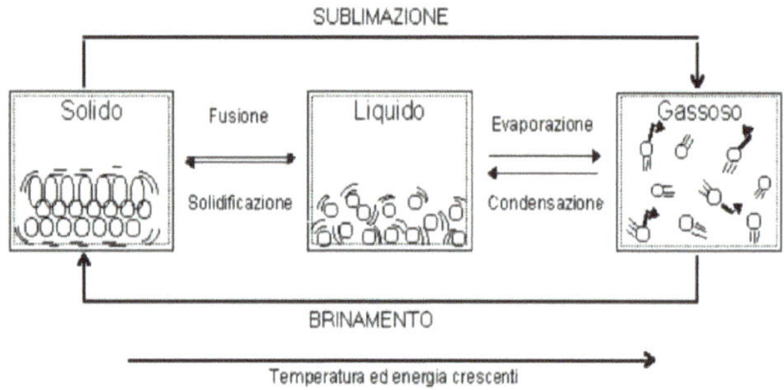

PLASMA GENERATOR = PLasma EXeResis

A medical device 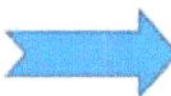 MICRO Plasma Generator

It isn't a Laser

- Different operating principle:

Laser uses photons to treat, vaporize and modify tissues

- Absorbed energy by the tissues in a different way
- Specific wavelengths to treat different kind of pathologies
  - Color Complementary
- Different interaction with the tissues

Differences Plexr & Laser CO$_2$

- ✓ Applications on risk areas (Tipe IV-V)
- ✓ **NO** Thermal damage
- ✓ No ground reference
- ✓ No safety glasses
- ✓ Different Recovery time, Inflammatory & reepithelialization reaction
- < Difference between treated areas and not

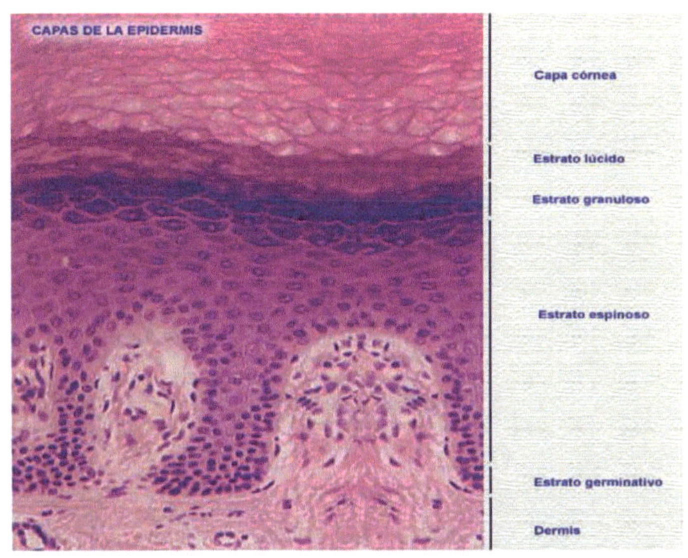

Plasma activity - Epidermic action
No thermal damages

Absence of necrotic layer and infiltrated inflammatory

SUBLIMATION EPIDERMIS

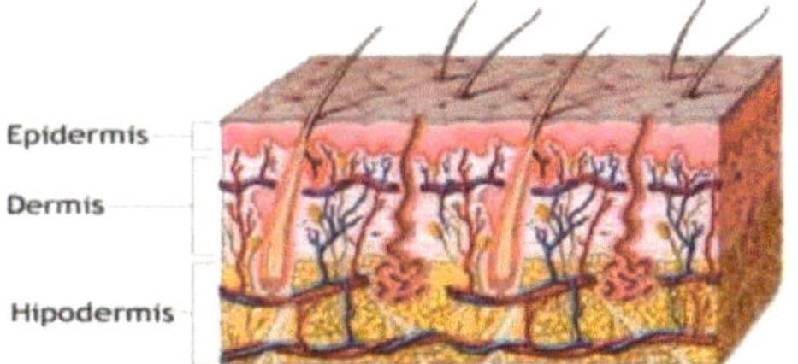

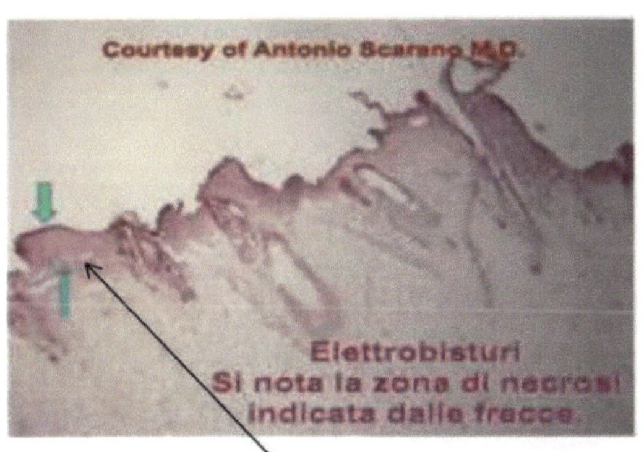

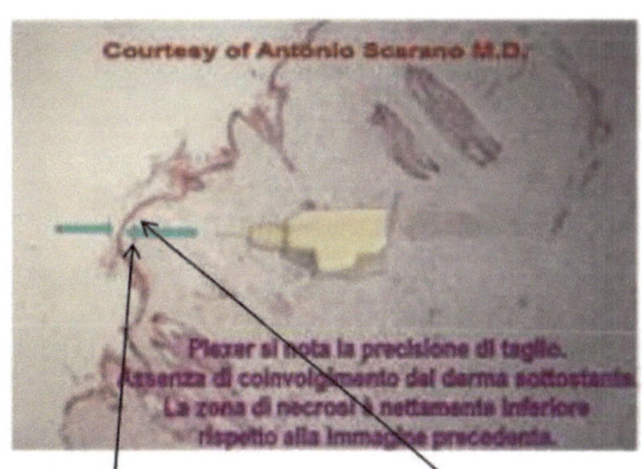

No thermical damage.

Absence of necrotic tissue

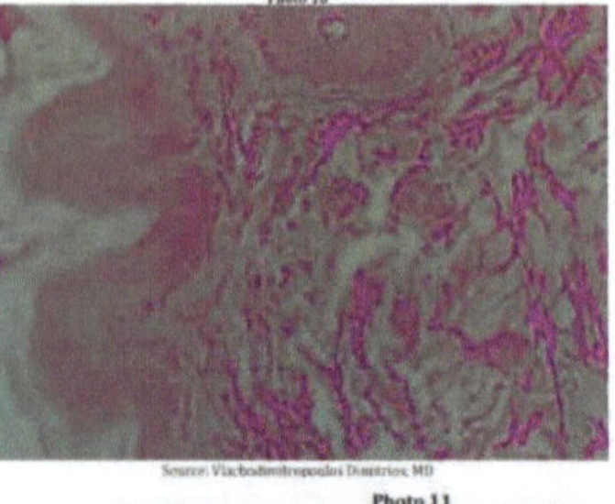

Normal skin

Treated skin Loss of epidermis, but not the basal membrane

The same area showing **fuzzyfication** and shrinkage of the elastic fibers x 200 (photo 12).

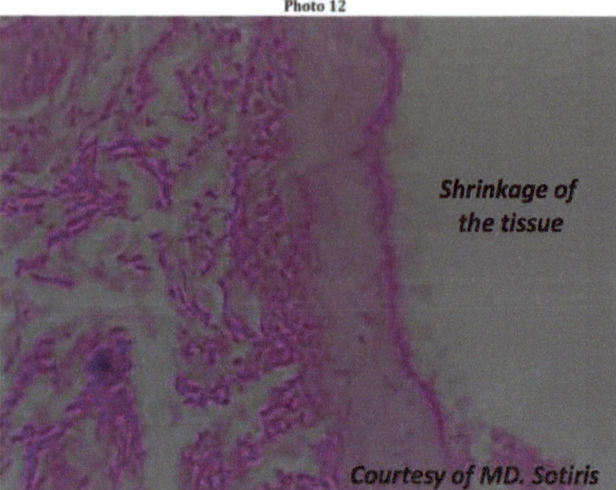

Source: Vlachodimitropoulos Dimitrios, MD

PLASMA GENERATOR = PLasma EXeResis

Sublimation and removal superficial corneocyte

> ➤ **Elastic Retraction**:
Non surgical Blepharoplasty , Face / body lifting, wrinkles, scars etc.
Tissue Shrinkage - Spot mode = each point is a hinge around which tissue curls

> ➤ **Removal of benign growths:**
fibroids, moles, warts, keloids, xanthelasmas, brown/white spots.
Spray mode = sublimation

- During treatments, visible smoke is produced (sublimation).
- A crust on the treated part is formed and will fall in a week leaving no bruising or scarring.
- No fibrosis or necrosis happens.

Neocollagenesis

After 30 days

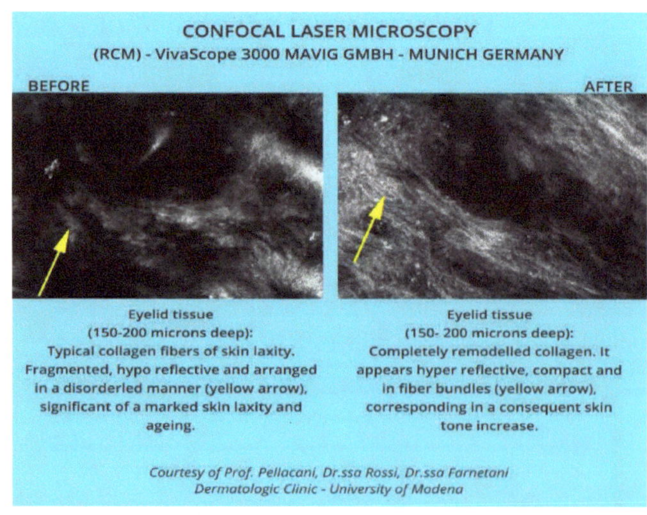

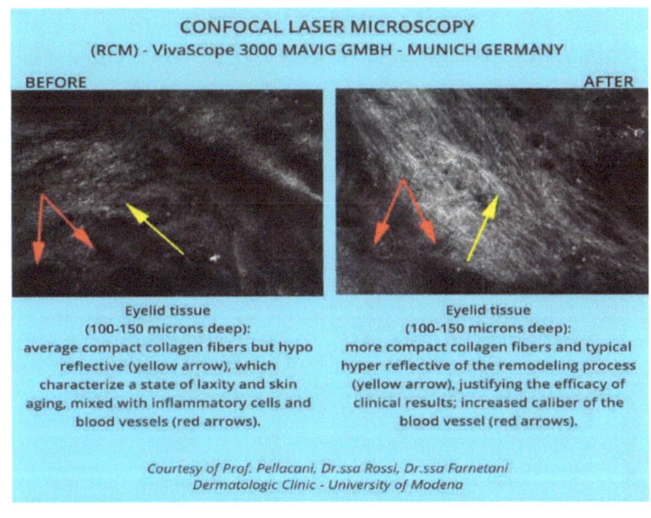

Indications

- Stretch marks
- Scars, keloids, warts, hyperpigmentation
- Coloured tattoos
- Moles
- Face, neckline, and body lifting
- Wrinkles
- Face, neckline, and body lifting
- Vaginal rejuvenation
- Vulvoplasty

PLASMA THERAPY IN GYNECOLOGY

- Labioplasty by sublimating the excess skin.
- Indicated in undesirable shape, length, or size of minor

Although plasma is a newer modality in gynecology, there have been various studies done.

Patients & methods

- 39 women (mean age 47,2 ± 6.3 years)
- Symptoms: dyspareunia, dryness, vaginal pain, burning, itching
- Exclusion criteria: previous use of systemic or topical estrogen-based preparations
- Visual Analog Scales
- Vaginal Health Index scoring

METHODS

- One plexer therapy was applied after topical local anesthetic.
- Outcomes were evaluated at baseline and 1 month following the therapy

- Participant satisfaction was measured on 5-point Likert scales (1 = very dissatisfied, 5 = very satisfied)

Visual Analogic Scale (VAS) mean scores of symptoms

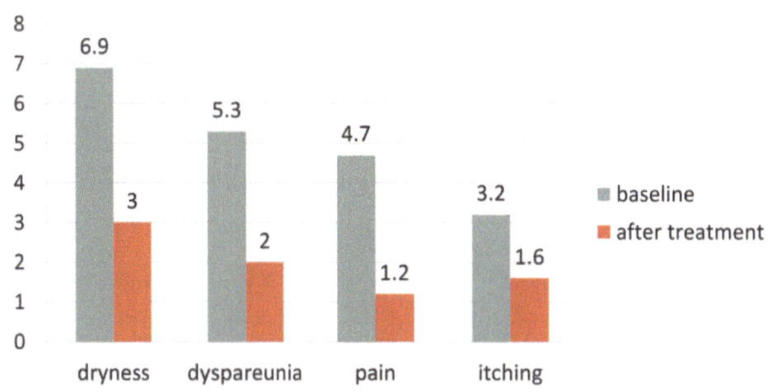

Wilcoxon signed-rank test: p < 0.0001

VAGINAL HEALTH INDEX (VHI) MEAN SCORES AT BASELINE AND AFTER TREATMENT

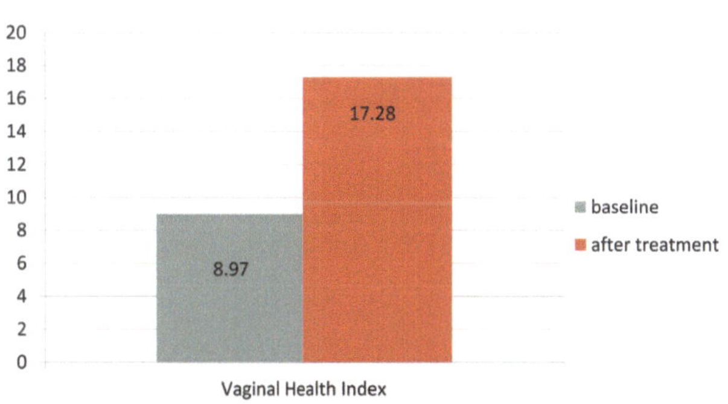

(Wilcoxon signed-rank test: p <0.0001)
5-point Likert scales

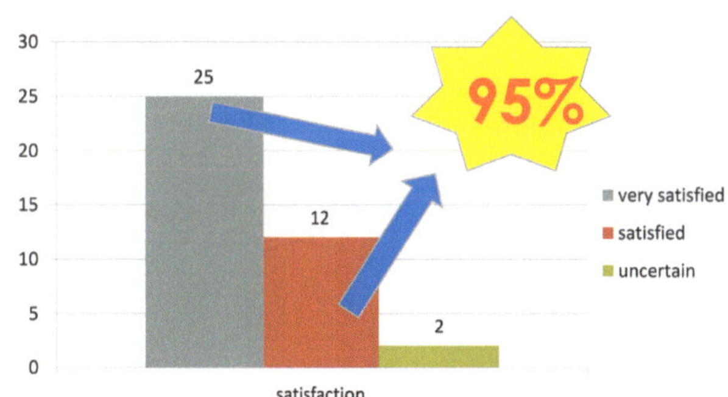

Conclusions

- Plasma is a good treatment option for VVA symptoms.
- Plasma therapy may improve genitourinary symptoms and clinical signs.

REFERENCES

1. Sotiris TG, Nikolaos G, Irini G. Plexr: the revolution in blepharoplasty. Pinnacle Medicine and Medical Sciences 2014;1(5):423-7.
2. Torvén S. Formation of double layers in laboratory plasmas. Astrophysics and Space Science Library 1976;74:109.
3. Gloustianou G, Sifaki M, Tsioumas SG, et al. Presentation of old and new histological results after plasma exercises (Plexr) application (regeneration of the skin tissue with collagen III). Pinnacle Medicine & Medical Sciences 2016;3(3):983-90.
4. Gay-Mimbrera J, García MC, Isla-Tejera B, et al. Clinical and biological principles of cold atmospheric plasma application in skin cancer. Advances in Therapy 2016;33(6):894–909.
5. Stamatina G, Sotiris TG, Aglaia V. Plexr in acne treatment. Pinnacle Medicine and Medical Sciences 2015;2(1):1-5.
6. Heinlin J, Morfill G, Landthaler M, et al. Plasma medicine: possible applications in dermatology. Journal of the German Society of Dermatology 2010;8(12):968-76.

MODULE 3

ADJUVANT THERAPIES

CHEMICAL PEELS AND VULVAL WHITENING

Fahad Usman

History

- **Ancient Egypt:** Cleopatra bathed in sour milk (lactic acid), and animal oils, and used Alabaster to exfoliate their skin.
- **Middle Ages: (Madame Pompadour France)** old wine with tartaric acid as its active ingredient was used
- **Turks: Fire** Fire to burn the skin
- **Indians:** Urine and pumice
- **1882, P.G. Unna** A dermatologist first described the properties of salicylic acid, resorcinol, phenol, and TCA
- **1903: McKee:** Chair of Dermatology NYU used phenol to treat acne scars
- **1961:** Baker and Gordon developed their deep peel to smooth, perioral wrinkles on one patient follow-up results in 3 month
- **1966:** Baker publishes results on 250 patients.
- **1980s:** to the present: many peels were introduced.
- **1990s:** Peels were the most popular aesthetic procedures. With the introduction of lasers and microdermabrasion ↓ in peels
- **2013:** Designer peels, new application methods to improve outcome

CHEMICAL PEELING

Chemical peeling is a cosmetic procedure that involves the application of a chemical solution to the skin to exfoliate and eventually peel off, revealing a smoother, regenerated skin layer. This process encourages the shedding of damaged or dead skin cells, promoting the growth of new, healthier skin. Chemical peels are commonly used on the face to address issues such as wrinkles, uneven skin tone, and acne scars, but they can also be adapted for use in intimate areas for intimate rejuvenation.

In the context of intimate rejuvenation, chemical peels may be used for various reasons:

Hyperpigmentation: Chemical peels can help address hyperpigmentation issues in intimate areas, such as dark spots or uneven skin tone, by promoting the growth of new, evenly pigmented skin.

Texture Improvement: Peels can improve the texture of the skin by reducing roughness or unevenness, providing a smoother and softer appearance.

Collagen Stimulation: Certain peels can stimulate collagen production, which is crucial for maintaining skin elasticity and firmness. This can be particularly beneficial in intimate areas where the skin may lose elasticity due to factors like aging or childbirth.

It's important to note that using chemical peels for intimate rejuvenation should be approached with caution. The skin in intimate areas is sensitive, and individual factors such as skin type, health status, and specific concerns should be taken into consideration.

CONSULTATIONS

- **Medical history:** cardiac, hepatic, or renal disease, recurrent herpetic outbreaks, keloid. Control medical problems (DM/collagen vascular disease)
- **Previous cosmetic procedures**
- **Allergy**
- **Smoking**
- **Medications:**
- ***Exogenous estrogens*** (OCP, supplements) ↑ photosensitizing → ↑ pigments
- ***Blood thinners*** (Plavix, coumadin, warfarin) ↑ bleeding from the peel site should be avoided in deep peels. Patients taking aspirin usually do not have complications, but, if the medication is not necessary, advise them to stop taking it 1 week before a deep peel.
- ***Oral isotretinoin*** ↑ photosensitizing and complications
- Set realistic expectations
- Before-and-after results should be shown
- Possible complications explained
- Plan the conditioning and peel choice a necessary chemoprophylaxis

Herpes:

- Acyclovir (400 mg) should be started 2 days before the peel and continued for 5 days after the peel to risk of recurrent herpes infection.
- Some dermatologists advise prophylaxis in all patients to avoid the risks of a herpetic outbreak.

Contraindications

- Pregnancy and lactation
- Allergy
- Active bacterial, viral, fungal, or herpetic infection
- Open wounds
- Photosensitizing drugs
- Inflammatory dermatoses: as psoriasis or atopic dermatitis
- Unrealistic expectations
- Uncooperative patient (patient is careless about sun exposure or application of medicine)
- For medium-depth and deep peels: history of abnormal scarring, keloids, atrophic skin, or isotretinoin use in the last 6 months

Depth of Peel Penetration

Superficial
- Penetrate epidermis only

Medium-depth
- Damage the entire epidermis and papillary dermis

Deep
- Mid-reticular dermis

Depth of Peel Penetration

- AHAs
- Retinoids
- Salicylic acid
- Jessner's solution
- Up to 30% TCA

Superficial

- 35-40% TCA
- Jessner's solution + 35%TCA

Medium

- Phenol peel
- Baker-Gordon
- TCA > 50%

Deep

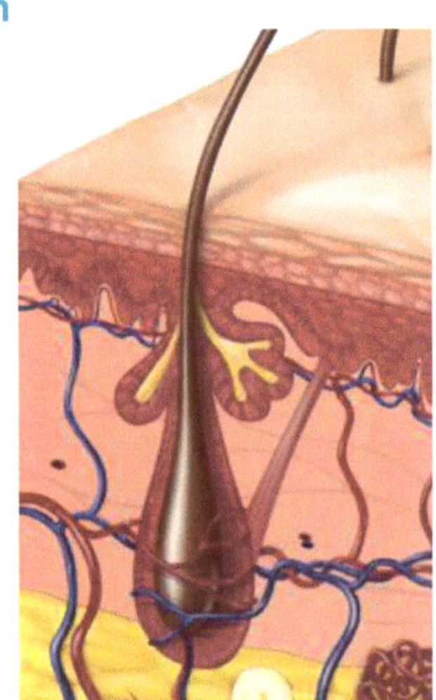

Skin Preparation

- Clean the skin
- **Degrease** with acetone, rubbing alcohol, Septisol, or a combination of these agents. (3 parts alcohol + 1 part acetone)
- Defatting allows even peel penetration as most agents are not lipid-soluble
- Peel the agent into a glass bowl.
- Applicators: Glove-Cotton-tipped applicators- 4 X 4-inch gauze
- Neutralizing agents in a spray bottle
- 1 bowl contains 10% sodium bicarbonate solution and the other contains cool water.

Technique of Chemical Peeling
Neutralization

An important step once the proper depth of the peel is achieved is determined by either the frost or how much time has elapsed.

This soothes the tingling discomfort caused by the peeling agent

Glycolic acid → Only peel to neutralize. Use bicarbonate spray.

Salicylic acid, Jessner solution, TCA, and phenol self-neutralize.

Follow Up

- For superficial peels, a follow-up appointment can be scheduled at the time of the next peel.

When to repeat?

- Most patients can tolerate a monthly superficial peel

Superficial peels

- Necrosis of the epidermis
- Healing time from 1-4 days
- Improve: Pigmentary irregularities / Minor surface changes
- For best results use a series of peels performed every 2-6 weeks

Agents:

- Jessner's solution
- Glycolic acid: 50%-70% → Keratinocyte dyscohesion Epidermolysis
- α-hydroxy acid peels: lactic acid, tartaric acid, and malic acid
- TCA: 10-20%

Alpha hydroxy acids

- Natural organic acids which function as exfoliating and hydrating agents

Source	Peel
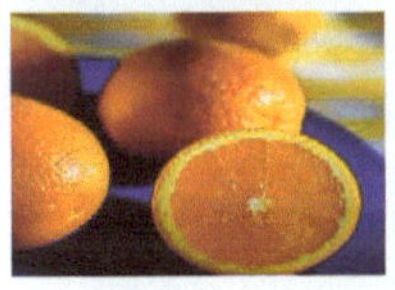	Glycolic Acid, derived from sugar cane
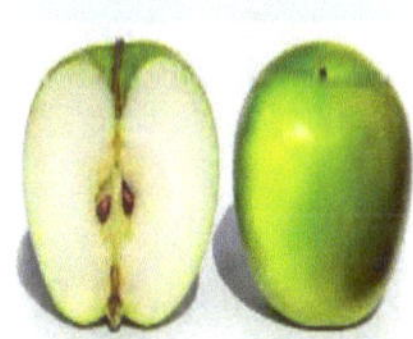	Lactic Acid, derived from sour milk
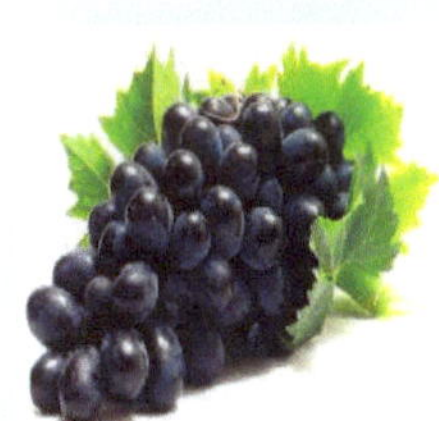	Citric Acid, from citrus fruits
	Malic Acid derived from apples
	Tartaric Acid, from grapes

Alpha hydroxy acids

- Weak fruity acids
- Mechanism: metabolic or caustic effect.
- **At low concentrations (< 30%):** they reduce sulfate and phosphate groups from the surface of corneocytes → ↓ corneocyte cohesion → exfoliation of the epidermis
- **At higher concentrations:** their effect is mainly destructive.
- Because of the low acidity, they do not induce enough coagulation of the skin proteins and therefore cannot neutralize themselves
- Must be neutralized using water or a weak buffer.

GLYCOLIC ACID

1. Safe. No systemic absorption.
2. Low cost. No big-ticket investment
3. Little or no downtime
4. Immediate visible results
5. Minimal discomfort
6. Performed by aestheticians

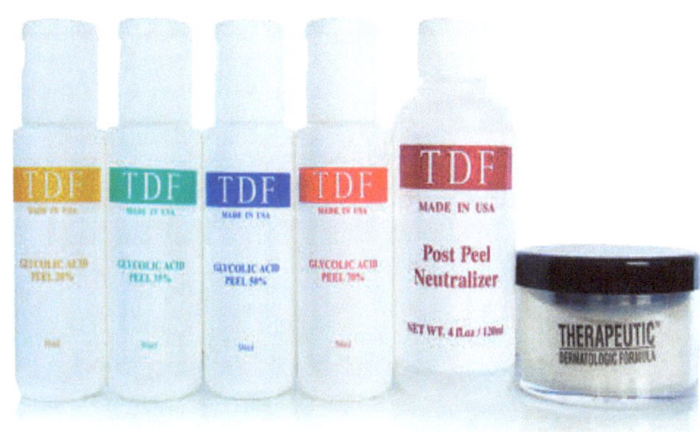

PHYSICAL PEELING
Microdermabrasion

- Developed in Italy in 1985; widespread in Europe before its introduction and popularity in the US.
- A mechanical medium used for exfoliation along with adjustable suction to produce a superficial epidermal ablation of stratum corneum
- Only effective for superficial scars

Advantages

- Performed in-office by a trained skin care professional
- No anesthesia required
- Painless
- Can be repeated at short intervals
- Simple
- Quick
- No downtime
- Good maintenance

Contraindications

- Keloids
- Undiagnosed skin lesions
- Recent herpes outbreaks
- Warts

REFERENCES

1. https://www.aboutplasticsurgery.com/skin/chemical-peels/
2. https://www.dermboston.com/dermatology-services-boston/cosmetic-treatments/chemical-peels/

VAGINISMUS AND BOTOX

Garima Srivastav

WHAT IS IT?

- Vaginismus is the involuntary tensing or contracting of muscles around the vagina.
- These unintentional muscle spasms occur when something — a penis, finger, tampon, or medical instrument — attempts to penetrate the vagina. The spasms may be mildly uncomfortable or very painful.
- Characterized by spastic, painful, and uncontrollable contractions of vaginal muscles which makes any attempt at penetration feel as if there is a wall or barrier to the vaginal canal

WHO MIGHT GET IT?

- Vaginismus symptoms may appear during the late teen years or early adulthood when a person has sex for the first time. The condition can also happen the first time a person tries to insert a tampon or has a <u>pelvic exam</u> at a healthcare provider's office.
- Some women develop vaginismus later in life. It can happen after years without any problems. Spasms or discomfort may occur anytime there's vaginal penetration. Or you may have them only at certain times, such as during sex or pelvic exams.

CAUSES

- Healthcare experts aren't sure why some people experience vaginismus. It can cause physical, psychological, and sexual issues. Bladder infections, <u>UTIs</u>, and <u>yeast infections</u> can worsen vaginismus pain.
- Factors that may contribute to vaginismus include:
- <u>Anxiety disorders</u>.
- Childbirth injuries, such as <u>vaginal tears</u>.
- Prior surgery.
- Fear of sex or negative feelings about sex, perhaps due to past sexual abuse, <u>rape</u>, or trauma.

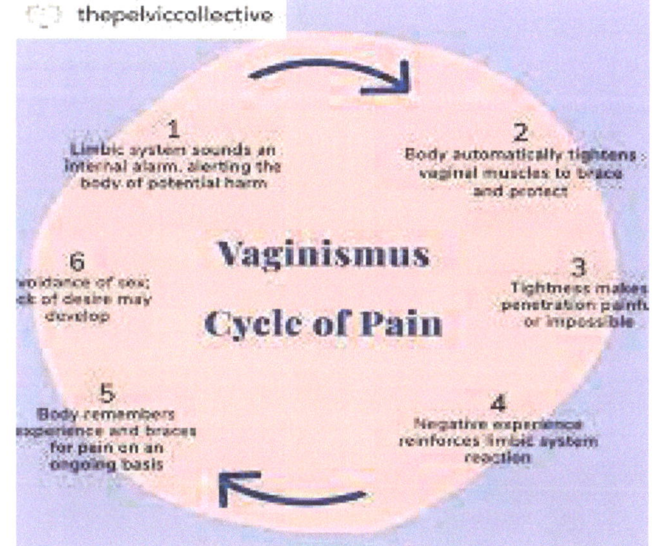

Vaginismus Pain Cycle is that experiencing or anticipating pain leads to fear, anxiety, and muscle tension that can be so intense and automatic that even the thought of vaginal penetration can cause you to feel reflexive pain and experience pelvic floor muscle tension.

Over time, this vicious cycle takes a toll on the physical, mental, romantic, and emotional well-being of individuals and couples.

When intercourse is impossible or painful, additional sexual attempts reinforce muscular response, further consolidating the negative mind and body reaction.

Additional sexual attempts result in discomfort, further reinforcing the limbic system response so that it is further intensified. The body experiences pain and reacts by bracing more on an ongoing basis, further entrenching this response and creating a vaginismus cycle of pain as illustrated in the diagram.

Prevalence

- Half of the world's population suffers from some kind of sexual dysfunction

- Vaginismus affects up to 7% of women, a figure that may be an underestimation
- Many of these patients tend to be quite reserved and do not share their health problem

Grading

- Minor 1: minor discomfort
- Grade 2: burning and tightness
- Grade 3: involuntary tightness
- Grade 4: significant pain

Effects of vaginismus

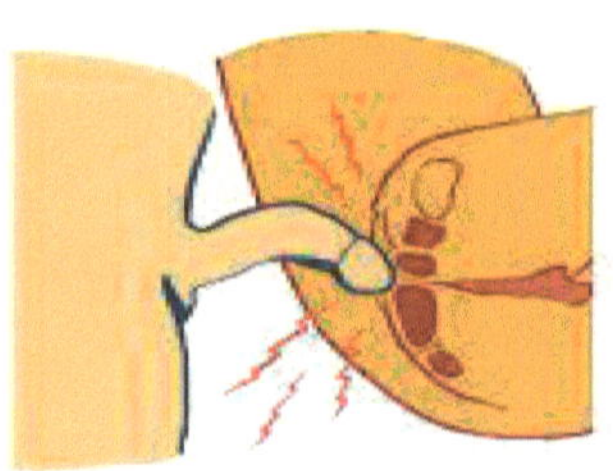
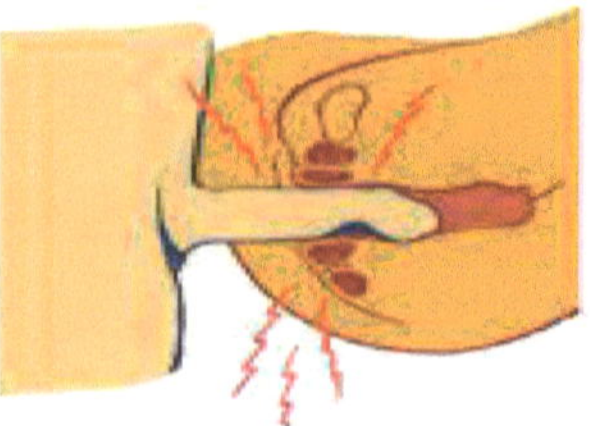

Muscles involved

- Bulbocavernosus, levator ani, pubococcygeus
- Muscles of lower 1/3 vagina, circumvaginal muscles

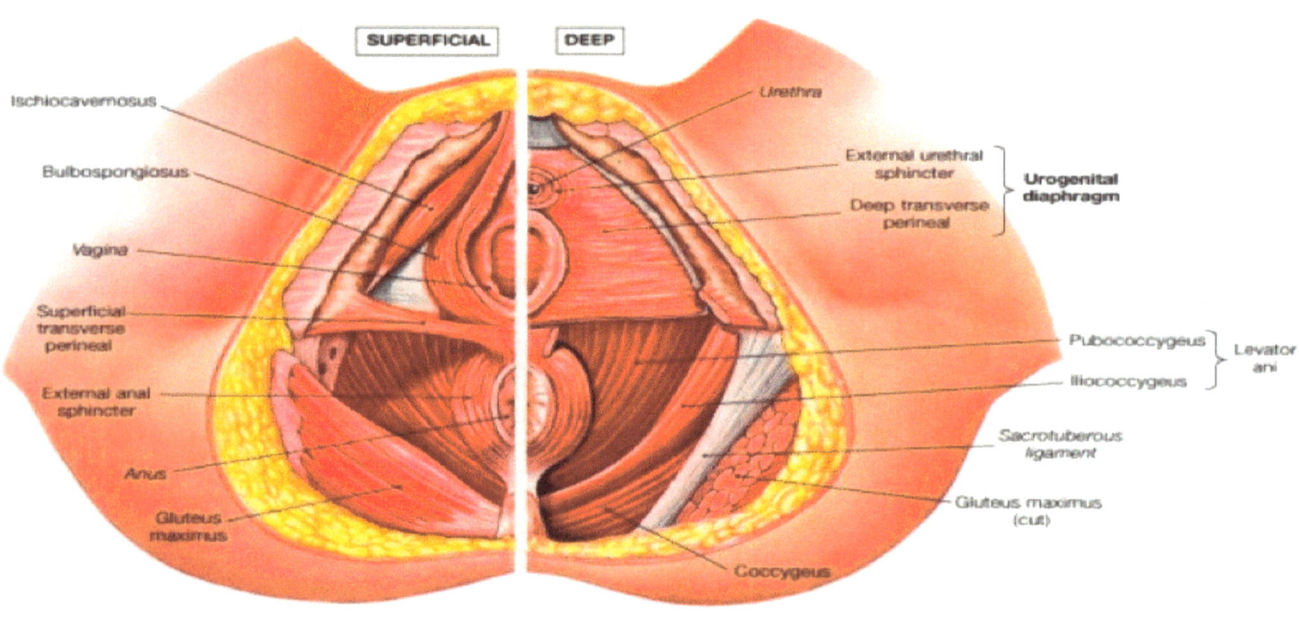

CONDITIONS MIMICKING VAGINISMUS

- These problems can cause symptoms similar to vaginismus:
- **Vaginal atrophy:** Lack of estrogen after menopause makes the lining of the vagina thinner and drier (vaginal atrophy).
- **Vulvar vestibulitis (provoked vestibulodynia):** This condition causes painful sex (dyspareunia). People may have pain from initial penetration throughout the entire experience.
- Vulvodynia

SYMPTOMS

- Signs of vaginismus include:
- Discomfort or pain during vaginal penetration.
- Inability to have sex or have a pelvic exam due to vaginal muscle spasms or pain.
- Painful intercourse.

CONVENTIONAL TREATMENT

- **Topical therapy:** Topical lidocaine or compounded creams may help with the pain associated with this condition.
- **Pelvic floor physical therapy:** A physical therapist will teach you how to relax your pelvic floor muscles.

- **Vaginal dilator therapy:** Vaginal dilators are tube-shaped devices that come in various sizes. Their primary purpose is to stretch the vagina. People with vaginismus use dilators to become more comfortable with, and less sensitive to, vaginal penetration. Your provider may recommend first applying a topical numbing cream to the outside of the vagina to make insertion easier.
- **Cognitive behavioral therapy (CBT):** CBT helps you understand how your thoughts affect your emotions and behaviors. It's an effective treatment for anxiety, depression, and post-traumatic stress disorder (PTSD).
- **Sex therapy:** Trained sex therapists work with individuals and couples to help them find pleasure again in their sexual relationships.

Success rate with the conventional treatment is 10-20%

Botox FDA-approved indications

- Strabismus
- Frontal headache
- Blepharospasms
- Cervical dystonia
- Glabellar complex
- Hyperhidrosis

Reconstitution and handling

Botox comes in an a vacum vial in a dose of 50 /100 U. It can be mixed with constituents of different cc, making different concentrations of the botox.

Why is Botox used for Vaginismus?

- Is a muscle relaxant that can weaken or stop any muscle's ability to contract including vaginal muscles.
- Procedure is done under nitrogen or GA to suppress fear and anxiety.
- It also facilitates progressive dilatation of the vagina for the insertion of larger dilators.
- Toxin dose is determined by the size of the target muscle, so larger muscles require larger doses.

Dose

- 100/150 units of Botox injected intravaginally into the bulbocavernosus, pubococcygeus, and puborectalis muscles along the lateral side walls, left and right as a one-time injection under anesthesia.
- Evenly injected at 3 points in the puborectalis muscle

Procedure

- One vial of frozen botox (100 IU) was diluted with 2 ml of saline without foaming or shaking the vial.
- Concentration of 50U/ ml or 2.5 U/.05 ml.
- Pediatric speculum and bending the needle at 30, botox 50 U (1 ml) was injected into the lateral submucosal surface of the bulbospongiosum marked by hymenal rings.
- Muscles contributing more to vaginismus are determined at the time of examination
- It can be injected into 1 or a combination of all 3 vaginal muscles responsible for vaginismus
- Only injected into vaginal side walls avoiding urethra and rectum
- Doesn't interfere with the efficacy of the procedure because these muscles envelop the entire vagina
- Weakening even a portion of muscles blocks their ability to fully contract and eventually go into a spasm
- The areas of maximum spasm of the vaginal muscles are identified under sedation to determine where the Botox should be injected.
- The injections done under anesthesia are followed by additional injections of a long-acting local anesthetic bupivacaine. (3 ml syringe. 25% bupivacaine total 18 ml, 9 ml each side from the cervix to introitus)
- After this the vagina is progressively dilated while the patient is still under anesthesia, and the dilators(4,5,6) are further coated with a topical anesthetic.
- All these measures allow the patient to wake up in the recovery room with the large dilator in place and no discomfort.
- Following this, supervised dilation continues so that the patient becomes comfortable moving the dilator in and out of the vagina. This supervised dilation continues for a total of two to three mornings.

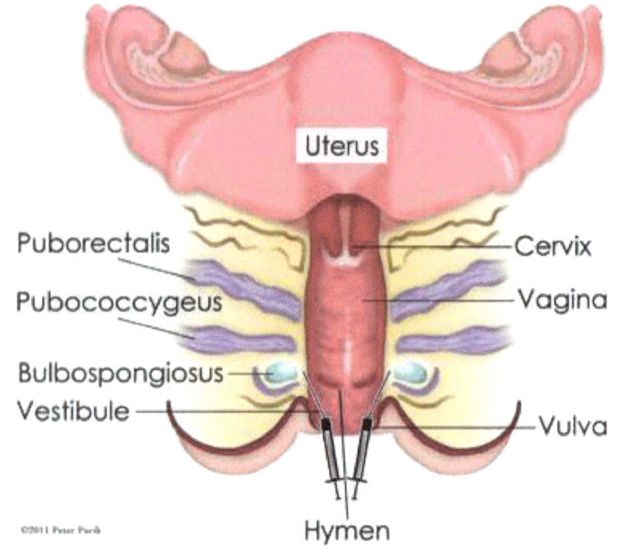

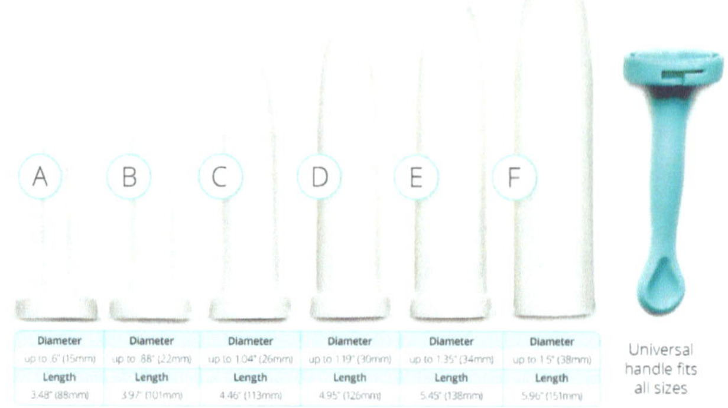

- With dilators in place intercourse becomes easier
- Although the patient may still have anxiety, it quickly subsides
- In most cases, a single treatment is sufficient
- Once it is relaxed and dilated for 12 months it is unlikely that it may spasm again
- Once injected it begins to take effect in 2-5 days

- Success rate with Botox is 90%

CONCLUSION

In conclusion, the botox for treatment of vaginismus is slowly finding its way as the last resort in severe cases of vaginismus.

In the personal opinion of the author, botox has been very successful in the treatment of vaginismus in her patients in the given methodology.

RECOMMENDATION OF BOTOX DOSE AND TECHNIQUE

VAGINISMUS GRADE	I	II	III	IV	V
DOSE (U)	25X2= 50	50X2= 100	75X2= 150	100X2= 200	
POINTS	2X2	3X2			

REFERENCES

1. Crowley T, Richardson D, Goldmeier D: Recommendations for the management of vaginismus: BASHH Special Interest Group for Sexual Dysfunction. Int J STD AIDS 2006;17:14–18.
2. Crowley T, Goldmeier D, Hiller J: Diagnosing and managing vaginismus. BMJ 2009;338:b2284.
3. Abdo CH, Oliveira WM Jr, Moreira ED Jr, Fittipaldi JA: Prevalence of sexual dysfunctions and correlated conditions in a sample of Brazilian women – results of the Brazilian study on sexual behavior (BSSB). Int J Impot Res 2004;16:160–166.
4. Lewis RW, Fugl-Meyer KS, Bosch R, Fugl-Meyer AR, Laumann EO, Lizza E, Martin-Morales A: Epidemiology/risk factors of sexual dysfunction. J Sex Med 2004;1:35–39.
5. Lewis RW, Fugl-Meyer KS, Corona G, Hayes RD, Laumann EO, Moreira ED Jr, Rellini AH, Segraves T: Definitions/epidemiology/risk factors for sexual dysfunction. J Sex Med 2010;7:1598–1607.
6. Spector IP, Carey MP: Incidence and prevalence of the sexual dysfunctions: a critical review of the empirical literature. Arch Sex Behav 1990;19:389–408.
7. Dogan S: Vaginismus and accompanying sexual dysfunctions in a Turkish clinical sample. J Sex Med 2009;6:184–192.
8. Kao A, Binik YM, Kapuscinski A, Khalife S: Dyspareunia in postmenopausal women: a critical review. Pain Res Manag 2008;13:243–254.
9. McGuire H, Hawton K: Interventions for vaginismus. Cochrane Database Syst Rev 2003:CD001760.
10. Brin MF, Vapnek JM: Treatment of vaginismus with botulinum toxin injections. Lancet 1997;349:252–253.
11. Pacik PT: Vaginismus: a review of current concepts and treatment using botox injections, bupivacaine injections, and progressive dilation with the patient under anesthesia. Aesthetic Plast Surg 2011;35:1160–1164.
12. Burgen AS, Dickens F, Zatman LJ: The action of botulinum toxin on the neuromuscular junction. J Physiol 1949;109:10–24.
13. Whittemore R, Knafl K: The integrative review: updated methodology. J Adv Nurs 2005;52:546–553.
14. Bax L, Yu LM, Ikeda N, Tsuruta H, Moons KG: Development and validation of MIX: comprehensive free software for meta-analysis of causal research data. BMC Med Res Methodol 2006;6:50.
15. DerSimonian R, Laird N: Meta-analysis in clinical trials. Control Clin Trials 1986;7:177–188.
16. Egger M, Davey Smith G, Schneider M, Minder C: Bias in meta-analysis detected by a simple, graphical test. BMJ 1997;315:629–634.
17. Sterne JA, Egger M: Funnel plots for detecting bias in meta-analysis: guidelines on choice of axis. J Clin Epidemiol 2001;54:1046–1055.
18. Shafik A, El-Sibai O: Vaginismus: results of treatment with botulin toxin. J Obstet Gynaecol 2000;20:300–302.
19. Fageeh WM: Different treatment modalities for refractory vaginismus in western Saudi Arabia. J Sex Med 2011;8:1735–1739.
20. Ghazizadeh S, Nikzad M: Botulinum toxin in the treatment of refractory vaginismus. Obstet Gynecol 2004;104:922–925.
21. Pacik PT: Botox treatment for vaginismus. Plast Reconstr Surg 2009;124:455e–456e.
22. Glass GV: Integrating findings: the meta-analysis of research. Rev Res Educ 1977;5:351–379.
23. Park AJ, Paraiso MF: Successful use of botulinum toxin type and in the treatment of refractory postoperative dyspareunia. Obstet Gynecol 2009;114:484–487.
24. Abbott JA, Jarvis SK, Lyons SD, Thomson A, Vancaille TG: Botulinum toxin type A for chronic pain and pelvic floor spasm in women: a randomized controlled trial. Obstet Gynecol 2006;108:915–923.
25. Yoon H, Chung WS, Shim BS: Botulinum toxin A for the management of vulvodynia. Int J Impot Res 2007;19:84–87.

PRP IN COSMETIC GYNECOLOGY

Fahad Usman

History of Platelet-Rich Plasma

- Platelet-rich plasma (PRP) is also known as platelet-rich growth factors (GFs).
- The concept and description of PRP started in the field of hematology. Hematologists created the term PRP in the 1970s to describe plasma with a platelet count above that of peripheral blood, which was initially used as a transfusion product to treat patients with thrombocytopenia.
- Ten years later, PRP started to be used in maxillofacial surgery as PRF. Fibrin had the potential for adherence and homeostatic properties, and PRP with its anti-inflammatory characteristics stimulated cell proliferation.

Use of PRP in Other Medical Fields

- Paediatric surgery,
- Gynaecology (Premature Ovarian Failure, Endometriosis and Cosmetic Gynaecology)
- Urology (Peyronie's disease, Erectile dysfunction)
- Plastic surgery
- Dermatology (Telogen Effluvium, Alopecia)
- Cardiac Surgery
- Orthopaedic (Arthritis)
- Sports Trauma (Musculoskeletal Problems — Accelerates healing of injured tendons, ligaments, muscles and joints)
- Burn
- Wound
- ophthalmology

PRP product-related terminologies and their abbreviations

A-PRF	Advanced Platelet-Rich Fibrin
ACP	Autologous Conditioned Plasma
AGF	Autologous Growth Factors
APG	Autologous Platelet Gel
C-PRP	Clinical Platelet-Rich Plasma
I-PRF	Injectable Platelet-Rich Fibrin
LP-PRP	Leukocyte-Poor Platelet-Rich Plasma
LR-PRP	Leukocyte-Rich Platelet-Rich Plasma
PFC	Platelet-derived Factor Concentrate
P-PRP	Pure Platelet Rich Plasma
PFS	Platelet Fibrin Sealant
PLG	Platelet-Leukocyte Gel
PRF	Platelet-Rich Fibrin
PRFM	Platelet-Rich Fibrin Matrix
PRGF	Preparation Rich in Growth Factors

PRP Method

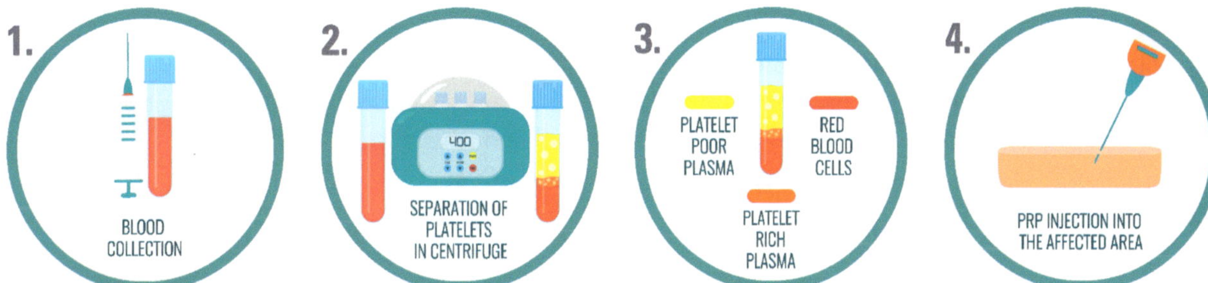

Figure 14: PRP Method [1]

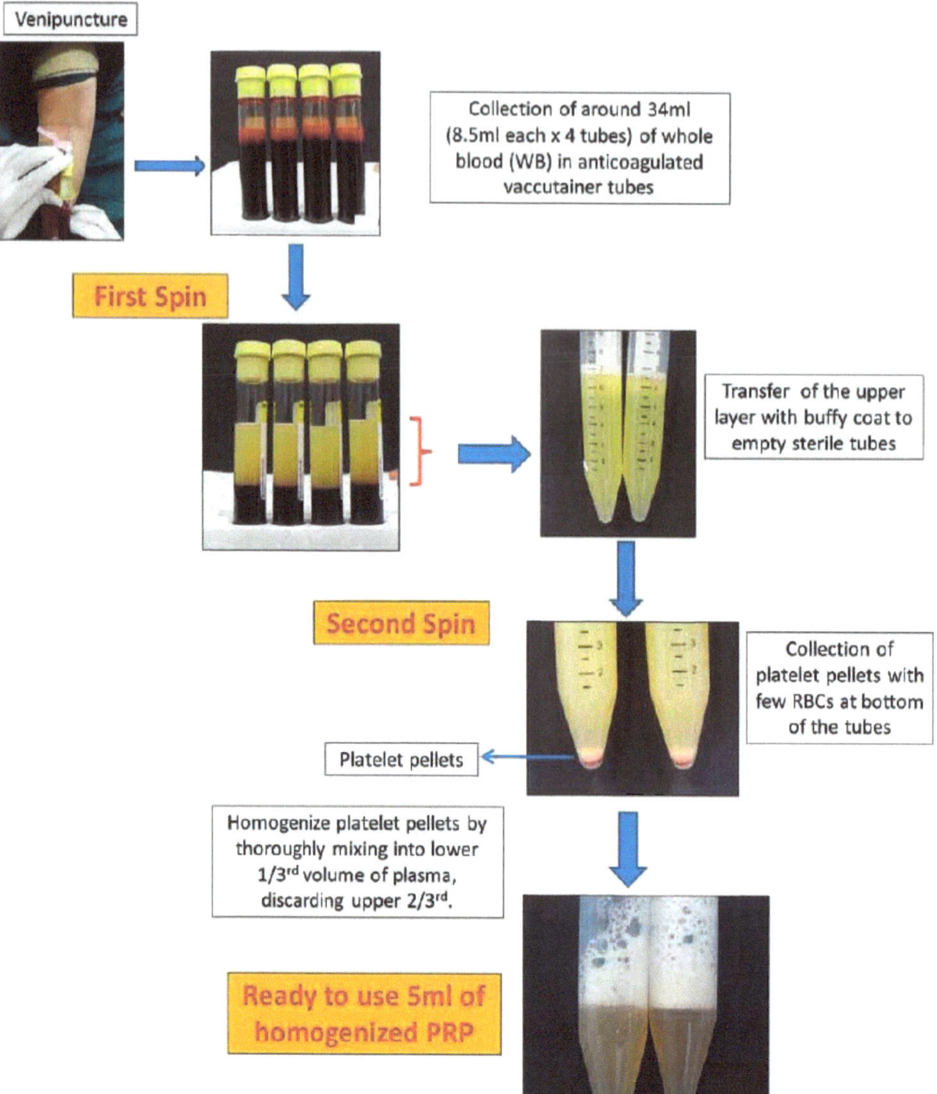

Figure 15: Flowchart describing the preparation of PRP [2]

- Obtain WB by venipuncture in acid citrate dextrose (ACD) tubes
- Centrifuge the blood using a 'soft' spin.
- Transfer the supernatant plasma containing platelets into another sterile tube (without anticoagulant).
- Centrifuge tube at a higher speed (a hard spin) to obtain a platelet concentrate.
- The lower 1/3rd is PRP and upper 2/3rd is platelet-poor plasma (PPP). At the bottom of the tube, platelet pellets are formed.
- Remove PPP and suspend the platelet pellets in a minimum quantity of plasma (2-4 mL) by gently shaking the tube.

PRP Composition

- Plasma - 55% of total blood volume
  - 91% water
  - 7% blood proteins (fibrinogen, albumin, globulin)
  - 2% Nutrients (Amino Acids, sugar, lipids)
  - Hormones (erythropoietin, insulin, etc.)
  - Electrolytes (sodium, potassium, calcium, etc.)
- Platelet Poor Plasma (PPP)
  - Very low number of **platelets** ($< 10 \times 10^3/\mu L$)
- Platelet Rich Plasma (PRP)
  - Platelets, Monocyte Macrophage, Fibroblast,
  - Endothelial cell, Keratinocyte
- Buffy Coat
  - White Blood Cells (7000-9000 per mm^3 of blood)
  - Platelets (250,000 per mm^3 of blood)

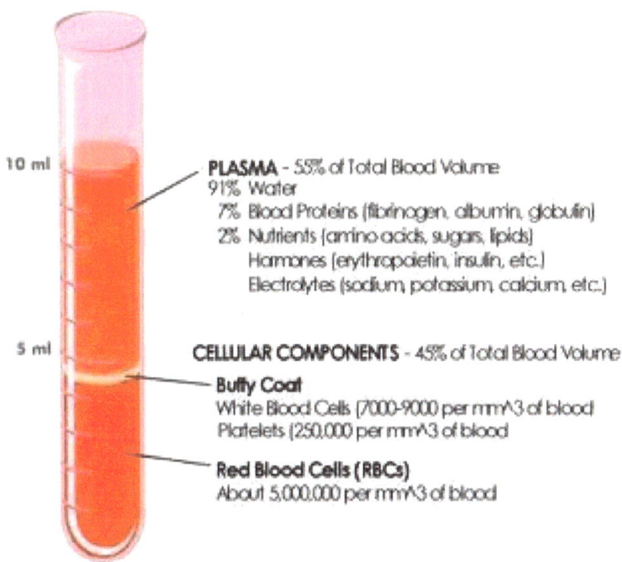

Figure 16: PRP Composition [3]

GROWTH FACTORS IN PRP

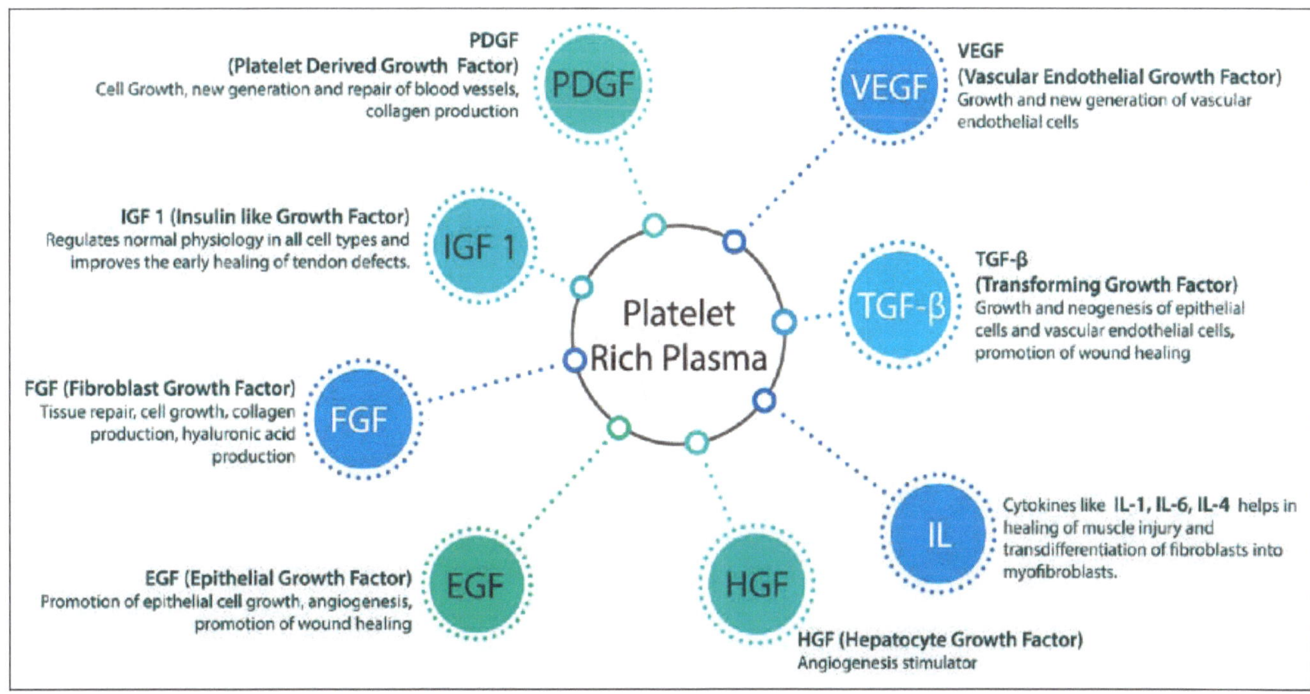

Figure 17: Growth factors and their functions [4]

PRP ACTIVATORS

- Calcium chloride, which are aggregation inducer, is used to activate platelets and stimulate degranulation, causing the release of the GFs
- Some doctors activate platelets, whereas others apply platelets without previously activating them, arguing that better results are obtained. Recent studies found that the use of such aggregators is not necessary because, at the time of administration, the platelets are automatically released and ready to exert their function.

USES OF PRP IN COSMETIC GYNECOLOGY / FUNCTIONAL GYNECOLOGY

- For the treatment of premature ovarian failure.
- Thin Endometrium
- Asherman Syndrome
- Peyronies disease
- Male Erectile Dysfunction
- O-Shot
- Intratesticular injection for non-obstructive Azoospermia
- Stretch marks treatment
- Intimate rejuvenation with PRP
- Wound management

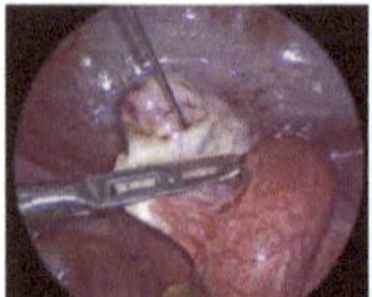
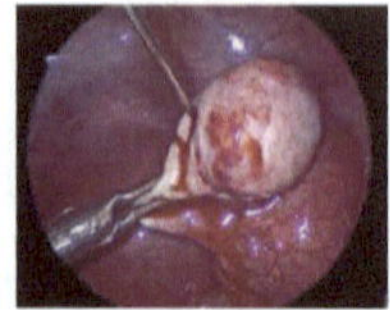

LAPAROSCOPIC PRP INJECTION FOR POF

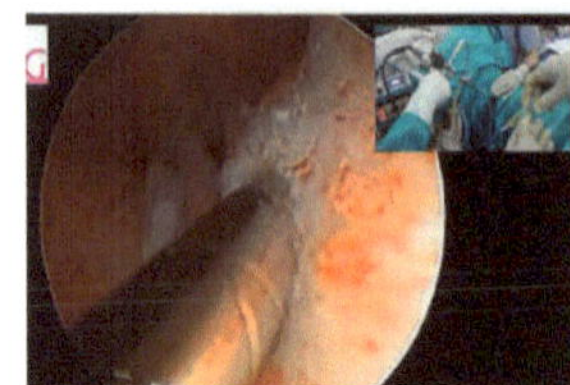
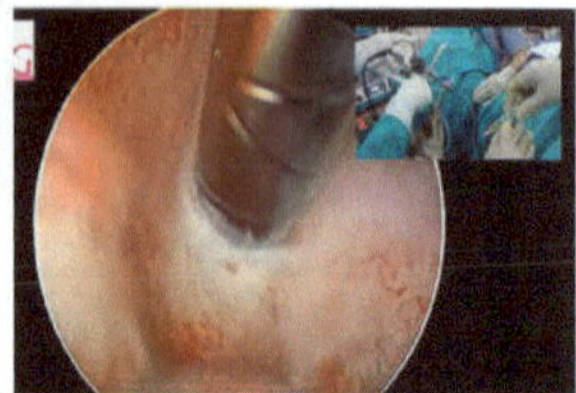

HYSTEROSCOPIC GUIDED PRP INJECTION FOR THIN ENDOMETRIUM

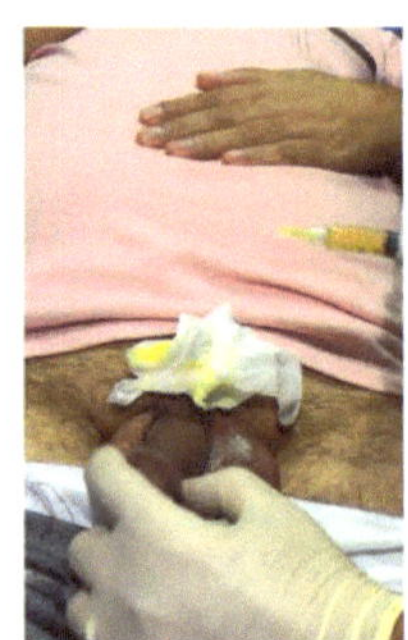
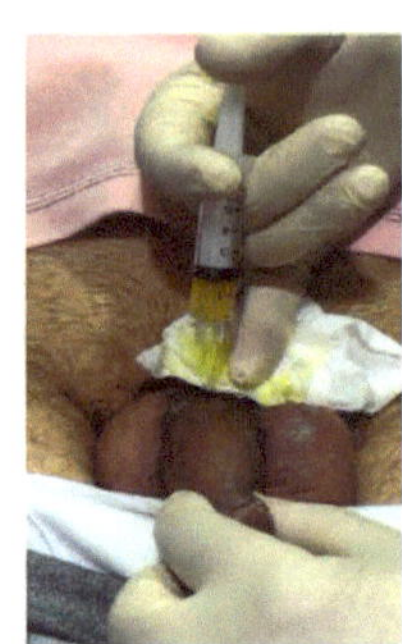

PRP INJECTION IN THE PENIS

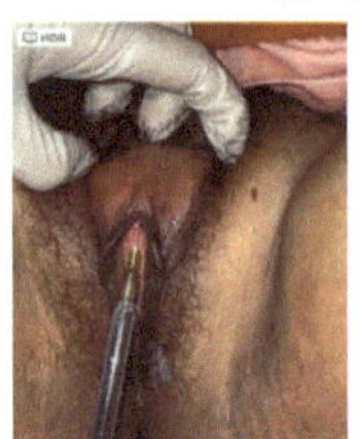
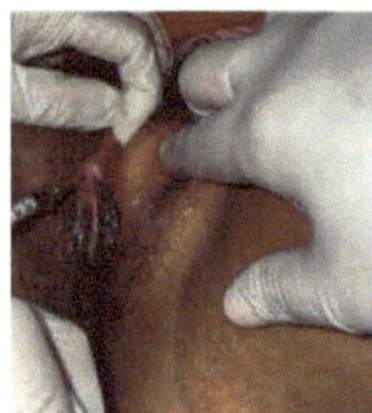
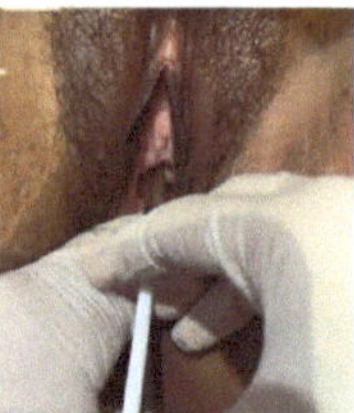

INJECTION OF PRP IN CLITORIS AND G-ZONE

REFERENCES

1. https://www.dermboston.com/dermatology-services-boston/cosmetic-treatments/prp/

2. Dhurat R, Sukesh M. Principles and Methods of Preparation of Platelet-Rich Plasma: A Review and Author's Perspective. Journal of Cutaneous and Aesthetic Surgery. 2014 Oct-Dec;7(4):189-197. DOI: 10.4103/0974-2077.150734. PMID: 25722595; PMCID: PMC4338460

3. https://r3stemcell.com/gilbert-az/orthopedic/treatments/prp-therapy/

4. Ramaswamy Reddy SH, Reddy R, Babu NC, Ashok GN. Stem-cell therapy and platelet-rich plasma in regenerative medicines: A review on pros and cons of the technologies. Journal of Oral and Maxillofacial Pathology: JOMFP. 2018 Sep-Dec;22(3):367-374. DOI: 10.4103/jomfp.jomfp_93_18. PMID: 30651682; PMCID: PMC6306612.

FEMALE SEXUAL DYSFUNCTION

Atiwut Kamudhamas & Nopwaree Chantawong

Female sexuality is multifactorial, including biological, psychological, sociocultural, and interpersonal relationship factors. Sexuality is also a multisystemic physiological response that depends on the integrity of the hormonal, vascular, nervous, muscular, connective, and immune systems. Female sexual health comprises three major dimensions: sexual identity, sexual function, and sexual relationships. Female sexuality varies throughout the life cycle and depends on both psychological and biological changes, which may be caused by age, parity, or illness. One-third to half of aged women find the problem distressing. Sexual disorders lead to poor quality of life, poor self-image and self-esteem, poor relationship quality, depression, and anxiety (1).

The Physiology of the Female Sexual Response Cycle

Nowadays, a variety of female sexual response models have developed including the DEOR model of Kaplan-Lif and Biopsychosocial female circular response cycle model of Rosemary Basson. In this chapter, the female sexual response cycle will be based on the EPOR model proposed by Master and Johnson due to the well explained in human physiology. The female sexual response consists of the excitement, plateau, orgasmic, and resolution phases (2-4).

Excitement Phase

The excitement phase, also known as the arousal phase, increases heart and respiratory rates and blood pressure. Vasocongestion occurs in the skin, breasts, torso, face, hands, soles of the feet, and possibly the entire body. Vasocongestion also occurs in the clitoris, labia minora, and vaginal walls. This is the so-called sex flush, which typically disappears soon after orgasm but may last up to two hours. During the excitement phase, Bartholin's and Skene's glands secrete mucin, which acts as a lubricant. In addition to vascular changes, the pubococcygeus muscle surrounding the vaginal opening tightens, and the uterus is elevated and size increases. At the same time, the breasts increase in size, and the nipples become erect. The excitement phase can last from several minutes to several hours.

Plateau Phase

The plateau phase is a continuation and progression of the changes that occur during the excitement phase. The clitoris becomes more sensitive and withdraws slightly under the clitoral hood, the glands produce more lubrication, the lower third of the vagina swells, and the pubococcygeus muscle tightens.

Orgasmic Phase

Orgasm is the culmination of the plateau phase. The heart rate increases further during this phase. Pelvic muscle contractions occur at approximately 0.8-second intervals and can last for 5–60 seconds. These contractions promote the feeling of orgasm, which creates a euphoric sensation. Orgasms are often associated with involuntary muscle spasms in other parts of the body. With effective stimulation, a woman can have multiple orgasms.

Resolution Phase

During this phase, the muscles relax, blood pressure decreases, and the body returns to a non-excitation state. The refractory period is part of the resolution phase. However, women experience a refractory period less commonly than men. With effective stimulation, a woman can have multiple orgasms.

Female sexual dysfunction (FSD) is defined as any problem that may cause the sexual response cycle to deviate from the normal range of functioning can affect sexual desire, arousal, and orgasm, and can cause dyspareunia (5). FSD can be a combination of psychological and biological disorders of varied severity and can afflict women of any age, impairing quality of life and relationship quality. The Diagnostic and Statistical Manual of Mental Disorders (DSM), first published in 1952, was developed by the American Psychiatric Association to provide standardized criteria for the classification of mental disorders. Its fifth edition, the APA itself called the DSM-5, was published in 2013 and contains extensive revisions (6) that are meaningful and clinically relevant. The DSM-5 specifies only three types of FSD. Female hypoactive desire dysfunction and female arousal dysfunction have been merged into a single syndrome called female sexual interest/arousal disorder (FSIAD). Similarly, dyspareunia and vaginismus, previously considered separate conditions, are now jointly called genito-pelvic pain/penetration disorder (GPPPD). Female orgasmic disorder (FOD) has been maintained. For establishing a sexual disorder diagnosis, the DSM-5 includes the requirement of experiencing the disorder 75%–100% of the time, with the notable exception of medication- or other substance-induced disorders, and a minimum duration of approximately six months. Moreover, the disorder must cause clinically significant distress. The three FSD diagnoses have specific symptomatologies, which are summarized in Criterion A (Table) and share three criteria (Table B, C, and D). The cohort studies report that 40%-43% of women experience sexual dysfunction (7-8). The prevalence of each isolated sexual problem is approximately 30% with the most common sexual problem being FSIAD and the less common being FOD and GPPPD respectively (7).

Table_ DSM-5 classification of female sexual dysfunction

Female orgasmic disorder (FOD)

Female sexual interest/arousal disorder (FSIAD)

Genito-pelvic pain/penetration disorder (GDP)

Substance/medication-induced sexual dysfunction (in women)

Other specified sexual dysfunction

Unspecified sexual dysfunction

DSM Diagnostic and statistical manual of mental disorders

Table_ DSM-5 Criterion A (symptomatology) of gender-specific female sexual dysfunctions

DSM-5 diagnosis	DSM-5 criterion A
Female sexual interest/arousal disorder	Lack of or significantly reduced sexual interest/arousal, as manifested by at least three of the following: 1. Absent/reduced interest in sexual activity 2. Absent/reduced sexual/erotic thoughts or fantasies 3. No/reduced initiation of sexual activity and typically unreceptive to a partner's attempts to initiate 4. Absent/reduced sexual excitement/pleasure during sexual activity in almost all or all (approximately 75–100%) sexual encounters (in identified situational contexts, or, if generalized, in all contexts) 5. Absent/reduced sexual interest/arousal in response to any internal or external sexual/erotic cues (e.g., written, verbal, visual) 6. Absent/reduced genital or nongenital sensations during sexual activity in almost all or all (approximately 75–100%) sexual encounters (in identified situational contexts or, if generalized, in all contexts)
Female orgasmic disorder	Presence of either of the following symptoms and experienced on almost all or all (approximately 75–100%) sexual encounters (in identified situational contexts or, if generalized, in all contexts) 1. Marked delay in, marked infrequency of, or absence of orgasm 2. Markedly reduced intensity of orgasmic sensations
Genito-pelvic pain/penetration disorder	Persistent or recurrent difficulties with one (or more) of the following: 1. Vaginal penetration during intercourse 2. Marked vulvovaginal or pelvic pain during vaginal intercourse or penetration attempts 3. Marked fear or anxiety about vulvovaginal or pelvic pain in anticipation of, during, or as a result of vaginal penetration 4. Marked tensing or tightening of the pelvic floor muscles during attempted vaginal penetration

*DSM Diagnostic and statistical manual of mental disorders

Table DSM-5 criterions B, C, and D

Criteria B	The symptoms in Criterion A have persisted for a minimum duration of approximately 6 months
Criteria C	Symptoms in criterion A cause clinically significant distress in the individual (based on the clinician's judgment)
Criteria D	The sexual dysfunction is not better explained by a nonsexual mental disorder or as a consequence of severe relationship distress (e.g., partner violence) or other significant stressors and is not attributable to the effects of a substance/medication or another medical condition

*DSM Diagnostic and statistical manual of mental disorders

Female Sexual Interest/Arousal Disorder (FSIAD)

In general, the assessment of sexual desire and arousal should comprise a complete sexual, medical, and psychosocial history, which can be obtained through interviews and validated self-administered questionnaires (9).

Validated measures include the Brief Index of Sexual Functioning for Women, the Changes in Sexual Functioning Questionnaire, the Derogatis Interview for Sexual Functioning, the Female Sexual Function Index, and the Sexual Satisfaction Scale. Questionnaires that specifically address relationship issues include the Dyadic Adjustment Scale, the Relationship Beliefs Scale, and the Locke-Wallace Marital Adjustment Test.

Since FSIAD is a new category, most available treatments are based on the treatment of hypoactive sexual desire disorder (HSDD) and female sexual arousal disorder (FSAD). FSIAD can be caused by biological, psychological, and social factors. Therefore, for optimal efficacy, it may be important to integrate psychological treatment with pharmacological treatment (10).

PHARMACOLOGICAL TREATMENTS
Androgen Therapy

Due to a lack of long-term safety studies on the potential risk of cardiovascular disease and breast cancer, no androgen therapy has been approved by the US FDA for treating FSD. Although systematic reviews of randomized trials involving perimenopausal and postmenopausal women have found that testosterone therapy improves sexual function, there is no consensus on the therapeutic levels of testosterone treatment for women. Contraindications include current cardiovascular disease, hepatic disease, endometrial hyperplasia/cancer, and breast cancer.

Estrogen/Tibolone

Estrogen treatment is particularly efficacious in treating reduced sexual desire caused by vulvovaginal atrophy. Tibolone has also been shown to increase sexual desire and lubrication (11). However, there are concerns that it may increase the risk of breast cancer recurrence (12) and stroke (13) in elderly women.

Flibanserin

Flibanserin (Addyi), a multifunctional serotonin agonist and antagonist approved by the FDA in 2015 for the treatment of diminished sexual desire in premenopausal women, acts on different neurotransmitters in the brain. In large trials involving women with a diagnosis of HSDD, flibanserin has been shown to result in a significantly greater increase in the number of sexually satisfying events per month compared to placebos (14–17). However, this drug must be used daily and has side effects, such as dizziness, somnolence, nausea, and fatigue. Moreover, it should not be used in combination with alcohol. The effects of long-term use are currently unknown.

Bremelanotide

Bremelanotide is a non-selective melanocortin receptor agonist but is thought to mainly act as an MC3R and MC4R receptor agonist. Bremelanotide is the most recent FDA-approved treatment for FSIAD. Bremelanotide has shown efficacy in improving sexual desire and increasing satisfaction with genital arousal (18). Bremelanotide can be given intranasally or subcutaneously with fewer side effects. The recommended dosage is 1.75 mg at the abdomen or thigh at least 45 min before sexual activity. It should be limited to only one dose every 24 hours and not more than 8 doses per month (19). The main adverse effects of bremelanotide Include pressure, nausea, headache, hyperpigmentation, and transient increases in systolic and diastolic blood (20). Bremelanotide is contraindicated in individuals with uncontrolled hypertension or cardiovascular disease (21).

Nonhormonal Centrally Acting Agents

Bupropion (Wellbutrin) is a norepinephrine–dopamine reuptake inhibitor that has been approved by the FDA as an antidepressant. When used to treat HSDD in nondepressed premenopausal women, bupropion has been shown to result in modest improvements in sexual interest and arousal (22). Buspirone (BuSpar), a partial serotonin 1A (5-HT1A) agonist prescribed to counteract the sexual side effects of SSRIs, has been found to significantly improve sexual function (23). Lybridos, a combination of sublingual testosterone and buspirone, was specifically developed for women who experience sexual inhibition during sexual stimulation or partnered sexual activity. A combination of testosterone and buspirone has been shown to result in a greater increase in sexual satisfaction among sexually dysfunctional women than a placebo (24). Bremelanotide injection, a melanocortin receptor agonist, has shown a clinically significant improvement in sexual function and sexual distress scores in a phase II trial (25).

Vasodilators/Phosphodiesterase Type 5 Inhibitors

Phosphodiesterase type 5 (PDE-5) inhibitors target increased vasocongestion and are likely to be most effective in women whose primary complaint is decreased genital responses (26). In women with reduced vaginal responses, an increase in sensation may also enhance general psychological arousal. Lybrido, a combination of sublingual testosterone and a PDE-5 inhibitor, has been associated with a significantly greater increase in sexual satisfaction than placebos (27- 28).

Topical Alprostadil

Alprostadil is a synthetic form of prostaglandin E1 (PGE1) used as a vasodilatory agent. In several trials, including phase III clinical trials, doses of 900 µg have shown statistically significant improvements in arousal, including lubrication and orgasm (29-31). However, some trials have failed to reproduce the results or have obtained inconsistent results (32).

Herbal Supplements

Studies have assessed the effects of several herbal supplements, including ginkgo biloba, ginseng, and maca, on female sexual desire and arousal. The obtained evidence suggests that none of them has sufficiently strong effects to be considered efficacious.

Non-Pharmacological Treatments

The sensitivity of the sexual response system depends on the meaning and intensity of real or imaginary stimuli. In a woman who has had predominantly negative sexual experiences—for example, sexual abuse—sexual stimuli may activate negative emotions, such as fear or disgust, instead of feelings of interest, arousal, and pleasure. Under such circumstances, medication cannot be expected to have a significant positive effect on improving sexual responsiveness. Cognitive behavioral therapy (CBT) techniques for reducing fear or disgust and sex therapy interventions for acquiring a positive perspective of sex can be helpful. Moreover, pharmacological facilitation of sexual interest and arousal may be more successful when treatment also focuses on psychological and relationship-related factors. Therefore, it is strongly recommended to treat a couple rather than only a woman with sexual interest and arousal problems and to combine psychopharmacological interventions with CBT and sex therapy (33). Psychological interventions include education about factors that affect sexual desire, relationship-building exercises (e.g., scheduling times for physical and emotional intimacy), communication training (e.g., sharing sexual needs and concerns), cognitive restructuring of problematic beliefs (e.g., accepting that a good sexual experience does not necessarily end with an orgasm), sexual fantasy training (e.g., exploring and developing mental imagery), and sensate focus. Sensate focus is a behavioral training technique that aims to achieve an increased focus on pleasurable sensations produced by touch and a decreased focus on goal-oriented sex (i.e., achieving orgasm). CBT may be useful when traditional sex therapy and education are ineffective. Mindfulness-based approaches, which aim to promote active awareness of the body and its sensations in the present moment in a nonjudgmental manner, have recently been suggested as potentially beneficial for women with FSIAD. Mindfulness training has also been found to increase vaginal lubrication and sexual desire, arousal, and satisfaction (34-37). The EROS clitoral therapy device (Urometrics, St. Paul, Minnesota, USA) is designed to improve arousal and has been approved by the FDA (38).

Female Orgasmic Disorder (FOD)

Difficulty in achieving orgasm is one of the most common sexual complaints among women (39-41). The DSM-5 (American Psychiatric Association, 2013) defines FOD according to three criteria: frequency, timing, and intensity. For a DSM-based diagnosis of FOD, orgasm must be delayed, attenuated, rare, or never experienced. Furthermore, difficulty experiencing orgasm must occur in most sexual situations over a significant period, of at least six months. A comprehensive assessment of women presenting with orgasm difficulties should include (1) partner-related factors, (2) relationship-related factors, (3) individual vulnerability, psychiatric comorbidity, or stressors, (4) cultural/religious factors, and (5) relevant medical factors. The Female Orgasm Scale (42) and the Female Sexual Function Index (FSFI) (43) are particularly useful as starting points for discussion in therapy, as well as for tracking treatment progress.

The treatment of orgasm difficulties should start with an assessment of the causes. Orgasm problems are often caused by insufficient stimulation. The current recommendation is that if a woman can orgasm through self-stimulation but not during partnered sex, the partner should be involved in therapy (40). The permission, limited information, specific suggestions, and intensive therapy (PLISSIT) model is a stepwise intervention for treating sexual concerns. Providing permission, limited information, and specific suggestions is the first-line approach, followed by intensive therapy if the problem is not resolved.

Effective treatment for women who experience orgasm difficulties centers on a combination of CBT and traditional sex therapy techniques, such as directed masturbation and sensate focus. CBT for anorgasmia focuses on promoting changes in attitudes and sexually relevant thoughts, decreasing anxiety, and increasing orgasmic ability and satisfaction (44). Education can be provided about how a woman becomes aroused, how long is needed for arousal, and what types of stimulation are commonly required to achieve orgasm.

While psychological treatments remain the most empirically validated methods, adjunctive options, including unsupported treatments, such as medications, mechanical devices, pelvic floor therapy, and Kegel exercises, have also been explored. The EROS Clitoral Therapy device is an FDA-approved clitoral vacuum that increases blood flow and engorgement and has been shown to improve orgasmic function (45).

There is currently no FDA-approved pharmacological intervention for women experiencing orgasm issues. However, studies have shown that hormonal therapy, such as tibolone, and PDE-5 inhibitors improve female orgasmic function (39-40,45). Moreover, a comprehensive history can determine whether medical conditions or other medications may inhibit orgasmic responses. A change in medication or the use of bupropion with an SSRI may help.

Genito-pelvic Pain/Penetration Disorder (GDP)

The three most frequently used terms to describe sexual pain in women are vulvodynia, dyspareunia, and vaginismus. Vulvodynia is defined as vulvar pain with no identifiable cause for at least three months. Vulvar pain may be caused by infectious, inflammatory, neoplastic, neurologic, traumatic, or iatrogenic (e.g., chemotherapy, radiation, or surgery) factors or hormonal deficiency. The 2015 Consensus Terminology and Classification of Persistent Vulvar Pain and Vulvodynia provide the following pain descriptors: localized (i.e., a portion

of the vulva) or generalized (i.e., the entire vulva), provoked or spontaneous, primary or secondary onset, and temporal patterns (e.g., intermittent).

The diagnosis of provoked vestibulodynia is based on allodynia findings (pain caused by normally unpainful stimuli) and varying degrees of erythema of the vestibule in the absence of a specific disorder. Vaginismus refers to involuntary contractions of the musculature of the vagina. The DSM-5 defines vaginismus as a vaginal penetration disorder of any form, making gynecological examinations, intercourse, and the use of tampons, fingers, and vaginal dilators painful or impossible. Vaginismus and vestibulodynia overlap, making a differential diagnosis based solely on an examination challenging. The severity of vaginismus is influenced by the intensity of vaginal spasms and the degree of related fear and anxiety. Dyspareunia and vaginismus have now been combined into GPPPD due to considerable overlap between the two conditions.

Table_Classification of severity (46-47)

Grade	Description
Lamont grade 1	The patient can relax for the pelvic exam
Lamont grade 2	The patient is unable to relax for the pelvic exam
Lamont grade 3	Buttocks lift off the table. Early retreat. Toes curl upward
Lamont grade 4	Generalized retreat: Buttocks lift, thighs close, patient retreats
Pacik grade 5	Generalized retreat as in Lamont level 4 plus visceral reaction which may result in any one or more of the following: Palpitations, hyperventilation, sweating, severe trembling, uncontrollable shaking, screaming, hysteria, wanting to jump off the table, a feeling of going unconscious, nausea, vomiting and even a desire to attack the doctor.

The assessment and diagnosis of genito-pelvic pain should include biological and psychosocial factors that may be involved in its onset and persistence. For this assessment, it is essential to create an open, validating, and nonjudgmental atmosphere. When a woman is in a committed relationship, her partner should be encouraged to participate in the assessment. The biological assessment should include inflammation, infection, estrogen fluctuations, endometriosis, mechanical trauma caused by intercourse in cases of vaginal dryness, intraorbital pain, and hyperactive pelvic floor muscle. The pain assessment should begin with a detailed evaluation of the pain, including (1) characteristics of the pain, such as onset, temporal patterns, pain duration, location (superficial or deep), quality of pain, and severity; (2) factors that may ameliorate or exacerbate the pain; (3) presence of comorbid issues (e.g., other sexual problems, other pain problems, and relationship-related and/or psychological distress); (4) personal explanations for the pain; and (5) previous treatment attempts and outcomes. The final component is an assessment of cognitive, affective, behavioral, and interpersonal factors.

Treatment of Vulvodynia

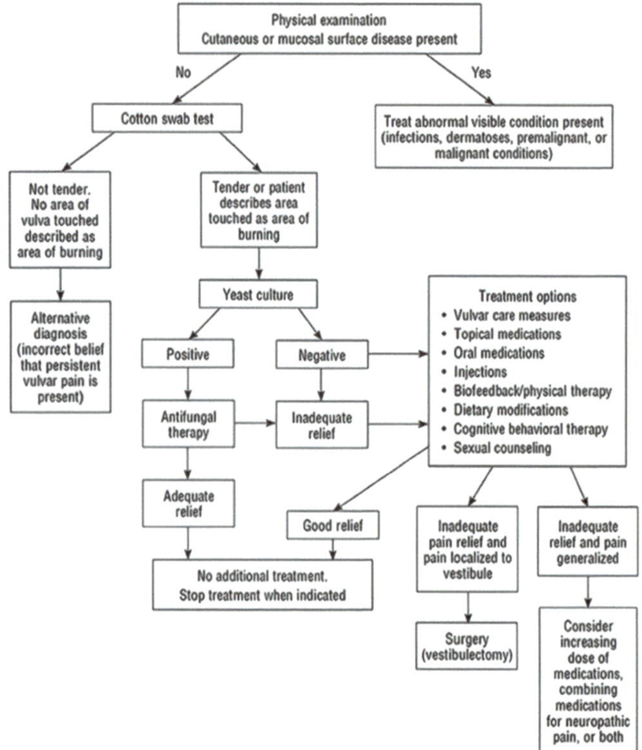

Figure_Persistent vulvar pain treatment algorithm (48)

A multidisciplinary approach is recommended for the treatment of vulvodynia (Figure_). The treatment should begin with vulvar care aimed at eliminating pads, fabric softeners, soap, and other allergens. Subsequent management depends on findings but usually includes physical therapy, relaxation therapy, and topical, oral, and/or injectable medications, which may be followed by surgery (vestibulectomy) if unsuccessful. Additional approaches include psychological treatments (CBT, psychotherapy, and mindfulness-based relaxation therapy), physical treatments (manipulative, myofascial physical therapy, EMG biofeedback, and dilators), and complementary/alternative treatments, such as acupuncture and hypnotherapy.

Medical options include topical application or injections of local anesthetics, injections of botulinum toxin A, and oral neuropathic pain medications, such as anticonvulsants or antidepressants (tricyclic antidepressants [TCAs] and serotonin and norepinephrine reuptake inhibitors [SNRIs]). Topical amitriptyline cream (TCA) avoids systemic side effects, such as drowsiness. Overall, there is insufficient evidence to support the efficacy of TCAs in treating vulvodynia (49), but in clinical practice, many women seem to benefit. Anticonvulsants (such as gabapentin) are useful for treating generalized vulvodynia and spontaneous localized vulvar pain. Lidocaine and methylprednisolone or betamethasone injections have been shown to significantly reduce local inflammatory reactions in 36% of patients (50), while injections of the long-acting anesthetics ropivacaine and bupivacaine have shown a 57% average improvement (51). Botulinum toxin A is recommended for pelvic floor hypertonus and vulvodynia if physical therapy and CBT are unsuccessful (52). Generalized vulvodynia often coexists with vestibulodynia and is managed similarly, apart from surgical excision.

Vestibulectomy, a minor day surgery involving the excision of about 2 mm of the lower part of the vulvar vestibule, is the most studied treatment for provoked vulvodynia. Recent studies have confirmed its positive outcomes, with success rates of 65%–70% or higher (53). However, vestibulectomy is recommended only if more conservative methods fail.

Treatment of Vaginismus

Non-pharmacological Treatment
Desensitization

The use of vaginal trainers (VTs), and the use of vaginal dilators of gradually larger sizes is one of the most recommended treatments for vaginismus. VTs may improve both the physical aspects of vaginismus and the fear of penetration. Psychological, sexual, and behavioral therapy in conjunction with VTs produces the best outcomes.

Psychological Interventions

CBT is systematic desensitization that can help reduce pelvic muscle contractions. It can be used in conjunction with physical therapy techniques, such as vaginal dilation, and sensate focus exercises. CBT is a complicated technique that is usually performed by a specialist. A practical systematic desensitization protocol developed by Thammasat Sexual Health Clinic has been shown to result in the disappearance of vaginismus in 50% of patients, partial improvement in 48% of patients, and no improvement in only 2% of patients. Moreover, the protocol is flexible and adjustable despite the hierarchy of anxiety stimuli. Techniques such as gradual exposure to the fearful object aimed at reducing the fear of penetration and avoidance behavior constitute another important avenue in the treatment of lifelong vaginismus (54).

Thammasat Sexual Health Clinic Protocol

Four different sizes of dilators (7/8mm, 9/10mm, 11/12mm, and 13/14mm sizes), and different depths from shallow to deep

Each dilator is given once a day for one to two weeks

Inform the patient that the whole process takes several months to a year

No arousal response is needed during the process

Water-based gel is recommended for any form of penetration to avoid friction.

Topical lidocaine is allowable in case

After all the dilators were successfully inserted, the index finger of the client was to be inserted.

Then change to dildo smaller to bigger and shallow to bigger

Then dildo that most mimics the partner's penis in color, shape, size, contour

Pharmacological Treatments

Anxiolytic medications, such as diazepam, or antidepressants, such as amitriptyline, in conjunction with psychotherapy, have been shown to resolve vaginismus symptoms. Botulinum toxin A is the most studied medication for vaginismus. Botulinum toxin A injection into the levator ani has been shown to improve vaginismus symptoms, such as an overactive muscle tone of the pelvic floor, pain, and vaginal spasms (55-57).

Aesthetic Interventions and Female Sexual Dysfunction

Lasers

Fractional CO_2 treatment can reduce bothersome Genitourinary Syndrome of Menopause (GSM) symptoms, such as dyspareunia, dryness, pruritus, dysuria, and urgency in patients with stress urinary incontinence and overactive bladders. At follow-up, there were improvements in somatic and social function and mental health, as well as in sexual arousal and satisfaction, urinary incontinence, enuresis, urgency, vaginal elasticity, vaginal fluids, and epithelial integrity, with results lasting up to one to two years (58-60).

A randomized trial involving sexually active premenopausal women showed that vaginal CO_2 laser therapy effectively improved sexual functioning, especially in terms of lubrication, orgasm, and satisfaction (61). It also found a statistically significant reduction in distress and reported that the sexually related emotions of women undergoing treatment improved after 12 months.

Radiofrequency

Radiofrequency can strengthen tissue and improve vaginal tightening, blood flow, vascularity, and moisture (62). The study found improvements in the ability to achieve orgasm, time to orgasm, vulvar and clitoral sensitivity, and vaginal lubrication and tightening (63).

Injections

Platelet-rich plasma (PRP) treatment is widely considered relatively safe, as it uses the patient's growth factors to stimulate tissue. PRP administration to the lower anterior vaginal wall has shown significant improvements in the FSFI's total score and all subdomain scores, including the orgasm score (64). Intramucosal injections of PRP combined with Hyaluronic acid have been shown to increase vaginal secretions, elasticity, and epithelial thickness and to decrease vaginal pH, improving patients' sex lives (65). PRP injected into the clitoris and upper vaginal wall has become known as the orgasm shot or O-shot. This procedure is believed to increase sexual gratification and ameliorate urinary incontinence by stimulating and promoting the growth of healthy vaginal tissue (64,66).

REFERENCES

1. Porst H, Buvat J (eds) (2010) Standard Practice in Sexual Medicine. Wiley-Blackwell

2. Lipshultz LI, Pastuszak AW, Goldstein AT, Giraldi A, Perelman MA (eds) (2016) Management of sexual dysfunction in men and women: An interdisciplinary approach, 1st ed. Springer, New York, NY

3. Levin RJ (2008) Critically revisiting aspects of the human sexual response cycle of Masters and Johnson: correcting errors and suggesting modifications. Sex Relation Ther 23:393–399

4. Costantini E, Villari D, Filocamo MT (eds) (2018) Female sexual function and dysfunction. Springer International Publishing, Cham, Switzerland

5. Sobczak JA (2009) Female sexual dysfunction: knowledge development and practice implications. Perspect Psychiatr Care 45:161–172

6. (2013) Diagnostic and statistical manual of mental disorders. American Psychiatric Association, Arlington, VA

7. Shifren JL, Monz BU, Russo PA, Segreti A, Johannes CB (2008) Sexual problems and distress in United States women: Prevalence and correlates. Obstet Gynecol 112:970–978

8. Nazareth I (2003) Problems with sexual function in people attending London general practitioners: cross-sectional study. BMJ 327:423–420

9. Ishak WW (ed) (2017) The textbook of clinical sexual medicine, 1st ed. Springer International Publishing, Basel, Switzerland

10. Both S (2017) Recent developments in psychopharmaceutical approaches to treating female sexual interest and arousal disorder. Curr Sex Health Rep 9:192–199

11. Nijland EA, Weijmar Schultz WCM, Nathorst-Boös J, Helmond FA, Van Lunsen RHW, Palacios S, Norman RJ, Mulder RJ, Davis SR, LISA study investigators (2008) Tibolone and transdermal E2/NETA for the treatment of female sexual dysfunction in naturally menopausal women: results of a randomized active-controlled trial. J Sex Med 5:646–656

12. Kenemans P, Bundred NJ, Foidart J-M, et al (2009) Safety and efficacy of tibolone in breast-cancer patients with vasomotor symptoms: a double-blind, randomized, non-inferiority trial. Lancet Oncol 10:135–146

13. Cummings SR, Ettinger B, Delmas PD, et al (2008) The effects of tibolone in older postmenopausal women. N Engl J Med 359:697–708

14. Katz M, DeRogatis LR, Ackerman R, Hedges P, Lesko L, Garcia M Jr, Sand M, BEGONIA trial investigators (2013) Efficacy of flibanserin in women with hypoactive sexual desire disorder: results from the BEGONIA trial. J Sex Med 10:1807–1815

15. Derogatis LR, Komer L, Katz M, Moreau M, Kimura T, Garcia M Jr, Wunderlich G, Pyke R, VIOLET Trial Investigators (2012) Treatment of hypoactive sexual desire disorder in premenopausal women: efficacy of flibanserin in the VIOLET Study. J Sex Med 9:1074–1085

16. Thorp J, Simon J, Dattani D, Taylor L, Kimura T, Garcia M Jr, Lesko L, Pyke R, DAISY trial investigators (2012) Treatment of hypoactive sexual desire disorder in premenopausal women: efficacy of flibanserin in the DAISY study. J Sex Med 9:793–804

17. Jaspers L, Feys F, Bramer WM, Franco OH, Leusink P, Laan ETM (2016) Efficacy and safety of flibanserin for the treatment of hypoactive sexual desire disorder in women: A systematic review and meta-analysis. JAMA Intern Med 176:453–462

18. Diamond LE, Earle DC, Heiman JR, Rosen RC, Perelman MA, Harding R (2006) An effect on the subjective sexual response in premenopausal women with sexual arousal disorder by bremelanotide (PT-141), a melanocortin receptor agonist. J Sex Med 3:628–638

19. Edinoff AN, Sanders NM, Lewis KB, Apgar TL, Cornett EM, Kaye AM, Kaye AD (2022) Bremelanotide for treatment of female hypoactive sexual desire. Neurol Int 14:75–88

20. Mayer D, Lynch SE (2020) Bremelanotide: New drug approved for treating hypoactive sexual desire disorder. Ann Pharmacother 54:684–690

21. White WB, Myers MG, Jordan R, Lucas J (2017) Usefulness of ambulatory blood pressure monitoring to assess the melanocortin receptor agonist bremelanotide. J Hypertens 35:761–768

22. Segraves RT, Croft H, Kavoussi R, Ascher JA, Batey SR, Foster VJ, Bolden-Watson C, Metz A (2001) Bupropion sustained release (SR) for the treatment of hypoactive sexual desire disorder (HSDD) in nondepressed women. J Sex Marital Ther 27:303–316

23. Landén M, Eriksson E, Agren H, Fahlén T (1999) Effect of buspirone on sexual dysfunction in depressed

patients treated with selective serotonin reuptake inhibitors. J Clin Psychopharmacol 19:268–271

24. van Rooij K, Poels S, Bloemers J, et al (2013) Toward personalized sexual medicine (part 3): testosterone combined with a Serotonin1A receptor agonist increases sexual satisfaction in women with HSDD and FSAD, and dysfunctional activation of sexual inhibitory mechanisms. J Sex Med 10:824–837

25. Clayton AH, Althof SE, Kingsberg S, et al (2016) Bremelanotide for female sexual dysfunctions in premenopausal women: a randomized, placebo-controlled dose-finding trial. Womens Health (Lond Engl) 12:325–337

26. Basson R, Brotto LA (2003) Sexual psychophysiology and effects of sildenafil citrate in oestrogenic women with acquired genital arousal disorder and impaired orgasm: a randomized controlled trial. BJOG 110:1014–1024

27. Poels S, Bloemers J, van Rooij K, et al (2013) Toward personalized sexual medicine (part 2): testosterone combined with a PDE5 inhibitor increases sexual satisfaction in women with HSDD and FSAD, and a low sensitive system for sexual cues. J Sex Med 10:810–823

28. van der Made F, Bloemers J, Yassem WE, Kleiverda G, Everard W, van Ham D, Olivier B, Koppeschaar H, Tuiten A (2009) The influence of testosterone combined with a PDE5-inhibitor on cognitive, affective, and physiological sexual functioning in women suffering from sexual dysfunction. J Sex Med 6:777–790

29. Heiman JR, Gittelman M, Costabile R, Guay A, Friedman A, Heard-Davison A, Peterson C, Dietrich J, Stephens D (2006) Topical alprostadil (PGE1) for the treatment of female sexual arousal disorder: in-clinic evaluation of safety and efficacy. J Psychosom Obstet Gynaecol 27:31–41

30. Kielbasa LA, Daniel KL (2006) Topical alprostadil treatment of female sexual arousal disorder. Ann Pharmacother 40:1369–1376

31. Kielbasa LA, Daniel KL (2006) Topical alprostadil treatment of female sexual arousal disorder. Ann Pharmacother 40:1369–1376

32. Islam A, Mitchel J, Rosen R, Phillips N, Ayers C, Ferguson D, Yeager J (2001) Topical alprostadil in the treatment of Female Sexual Arousal Disorder: a pilot study. J Sex Marital Ther 27:531–540

33. Peterson ZD (ed) (2017) The Wiley handbook of sex therapy. John Wiley & Sons, Ltd, Chichester, UK

34. Brotto L, Barker M (2014) Mindfulness in sexual and relationship therapy. Taylor & Francis, Abingdon, UK

35. Brotto LA, Basson R (2014) Group mindfulness-based therapy significantly improves sexual desire in women. Behav Res Ther 57:43–54

36. Brotto LA, Erskine Y, Carey M, et al (2012) A brief mindfulness-based cognitive behavioral intervention improves sexual functioning versus wait-list control in women treated for gynecologic cancer. Gynecol Oncol 125:320–325

37. Brotto LA, Heiman JR (2007) Mindfulness in sex therapy: Applications for women with sexual difficulties following gynecologic cancer. Sex Relation Ther 22:3–11

38. Billups KL, Berman L, Berman J, Metz ME, Glennon ME, Goldstein I (2001) A new non-pharmacological vacuum therapy for female sexual dysfunction. J Sex Marital Ther 27:435–441

39. Ishak WW, Bokarius A, Jeffrey JK, Davis MC, Bakhta Y (2010) Disorders of orgasm in women: a literature review of etiology and current treatments. J Sex Med 7:3254–3268

40. Laan E, Rellini AH, Barnes T, International Society for Sexual Medicine (2013) Standard operating procedures for female orgasmic disorder: consensus of the International Society for Sexual Medicine. J Sex Med 10:74–82

41. Binik YM, Hall KSK (eds) (2020) Principles and practice of sex therapy: Sixth edition, 6th ed. Guilford Press, London, England

42. Fisher TD, Davis CM, Yarber WL (2013) Handbook of sexuality-related measures. https://doi.org/10.4324/9781315881089

43. Rosen R, Brown C, Heiman J, Leiblum S, Meston C, Shabsigh R, Ferguson D, D'Agostino R Jr (2000) The Female Sexual Function Index (FSFI): a multidimensional self-report instrument for the assessment of female sexual function. J Sex Marital Ther 26:191–208

44. Meston CM, Hull E, Levin RJ, Sipski M (2004) Disorders of orgasm in women. J Sex Med 1:66–68

45. Carpenter KM, Williams K, Worly B (2017) Treating women's orgasmic difficulties. The Wiley Handbook of Sex Therapy 57–71

46. Lamont JA (1978) Vaginismus. Am J Obstet Gynecol 131:633–636

47. Pacik PT (2011) Vaginismus: a review of current concepts and treatment using botox injections, bupivacaine injections, and progressive dilation

with the patient under anesthesia. Aesthetic Plast Surg 35:1160–1164

48. Haefner HK, Collins ME, Davis GD, et al (2005) The vulvodynia guideline. J Low Genit Tract Dis 9:40–51

49. Leo RJ, Dewani S (2013) A systematic review of the utility of antidepressant pharmacotherapy in the treatment of vulvodynia pain. J Sex Med 10:2497–2505

50. Segal D, Tifheret H, Lazer S (2003) Submucous infiltration of betamethasone and lidocaine in the treatment of vulvar vestibulitis. Eur J Obstet Gynecol Reprod Biol 107:105–106

51. McDonald JS, Rapkin AJ (2012) Multilevel local anesthetic nerve blockade for the treatment of generalized vulvodynia: a pilot study. J Sex Med 9:2919–2926

52. Abbott JA, Jarvis SK, Lyons SD, Thomson A, Vancaille TG (2006) Botulinum toxin type A for chronic pain and pelvic floor spasm in women: a randomized controlled trial: A randomized controlled trial. Obstet Gynecol 108:915–923

53. Landry T, Bergeron S, Dupuis M-J, Desrochers G (2008) The treatment of provoked vestibulodynia: a critical review. Clin J Pain 24:155–171

54. ter Kuile MM, van Lankveld JJDM, de Groot E, Melles R, Neffs J, Zandbergen M (2007) Cognitive-behavioral therapy for women with lifelong vaginismus: process and prognostic factors. Behav Res Ther 45:359–373

55. Ferreira JR, Souza RP (2012) Botulinum toxin for vaginismus treatment. Pharmacology 89:256–259

56. Ghazizadeh S, Nikzad M (2004) Botulinum toxin in the treatment of refractory vaginismus. Obstet Gynecol 104:922–925

57. Bertolasi L, Frasson E, Cappelletti JY, Vicentini S, Bordignon M, Graziottin A (2009) Botulinum neurotoxin type A injections for vaginismus secondary to vulvar vestibulitis syndrome. Obstet Gynecol 114:1008–1016

58. Salvatore S, Nappi RE, Parma M, Chionna R, Lagona F, Zerbinati N, Ferrero S, Origoni M, Candiani M, Leone Roberti Maggiore U (2015) Sexual function after fractional microablative CO_2 laser in women with vulvovaginal atrophy. Climacteric 18:219–225

59. Franić D, Fistonić I (2019) Laser therapy in the treatment of female urinary incontinence and genitourinary syndrome of menopause: An update. Biomed Res Int 2019:1–9

60. Adabi K, Golshahi F, Niroomansh S, Razzaghi Z, Ghaemi M (2020) Effect of the fractional CO2 laser on the quality of life, general health, and genitourinary symptoms in postmenopausal women with vaginal atrophy: A prospective cohort. J Lasers Med Sci 11:65–69

61. Lou W, Chen F, Xu T, Fan Q, Shi H, Kang J, Shi X, Zhu L (2022) A randomized controlled study of vaginal fractional CO2 laser therapy for female sexual dysfunction. Lasers Med Sci 37:359–367

62. Le C, Murgia RD, Noell C, Weiss M, Weiss R (2022) Female genitourinary treatments in aesthetics. Clin Dermatol 40:259–264

63. Alinsod RM (2016) Transcutaneous temperature controlled radiofrequency for orgasmic dysfunction. Lasers Surg Med 48:641–645

64. Sukgen G, Ellibeş Kaya A, Karagün E, Çalışkan E (2019) Platelet-rich plasma administration to the lower anterior vaginal wall to improve female sexuality satisfaction. J Turk Soc Obstet Gynecol 16:228–234

65. Hersant B, SidAhmed-Mezi M, Belkacemi Y, et al (2018) Efficacy of injecting platelet concentrate combined with hyaluronic acid for the treatment of vulvovaginal atrophy in postmenopausal women with a history of breast cancer: a phase 2 pilot study. Menopause 25:1124–1130

66. Vanaman M, Bolton J, Placik O, Fabi SG (2016) Emerging trends in nonsurgical female genital rejuvenation. Dermatol Surg 42:1019–1029

FILLERS IN COSMETIC GYNECOLOGY

Fahad Usman

CHAPTER 17

History

- **19th century to 1950:** Paraffin
- **1970:** Silicone
- **1981:** Bovine collagen (bull)
- **1985:** Cross-linked bovine collagen
- **1989:** Hyaluronic acid from cock's comb
- **1990:** Human collagen
- **1995:** Hyaluronic acid from bacteria
- **2000:** Polymers
- **2005:** Biphasic fillers
- **2006:** Ca Hydroxlapetite

Hyaluronic acid introduction

- Found in most tissues: skin, cartilage, and synovial fluid
- Naturally occurring polysaccharide carbohydrate polymer.
- Hygroscopic > 1,000 times it's weight → Volume expander
- Attract water within extracellular space, hydrating the skin
- Involved with the transport of essential nutrients to the skin
- Involved in wound healing
- Joint protection in synovial fluid

- HA degrades progressively with age

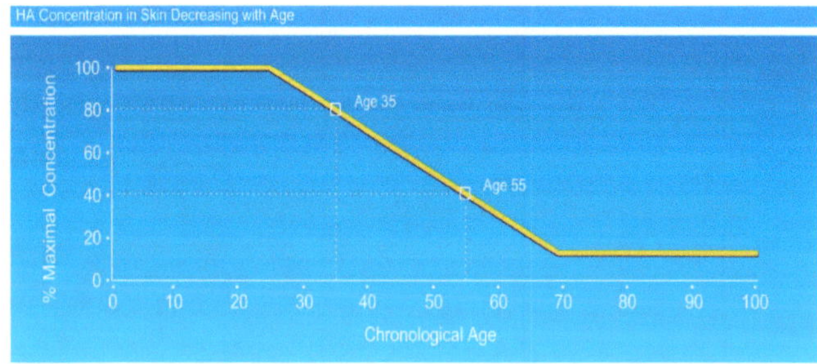

Figure 1: HA Concentration in Skin Decreasing with Age

Hyaluronic acid functions

- Important extracellular space component
- Attract water within extracellular space, hydrating the skin
- Maintain structure and functions of tissues:
  - Create volume by high water binding capacity
  - Lubrication of joints and tendons
  - Regulation of protein distribution
  - Nutrient distribution to and from cells
- Affect cellular integrity, mobility, and function
- Involved with the transport of essential nutrients to the skin
- Involved in wound healing

Dermal fillers Injection techniques

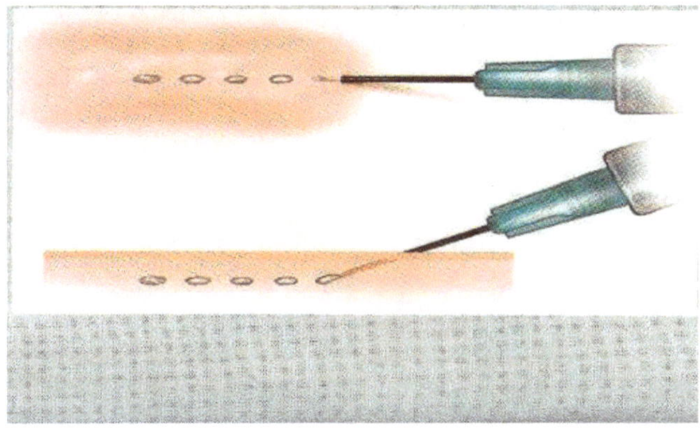

Serial Puncture Technique

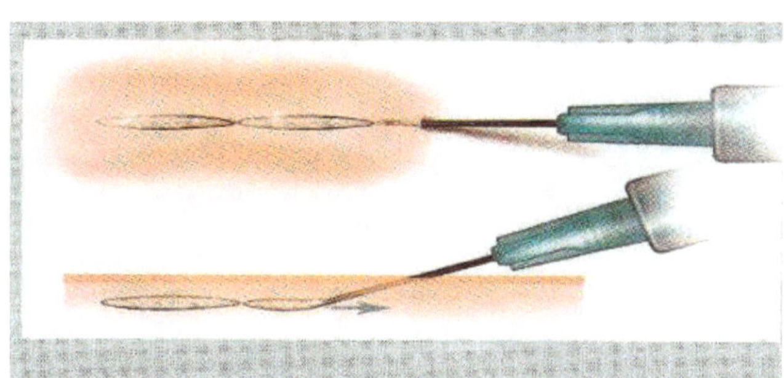

Serial Threading Technique

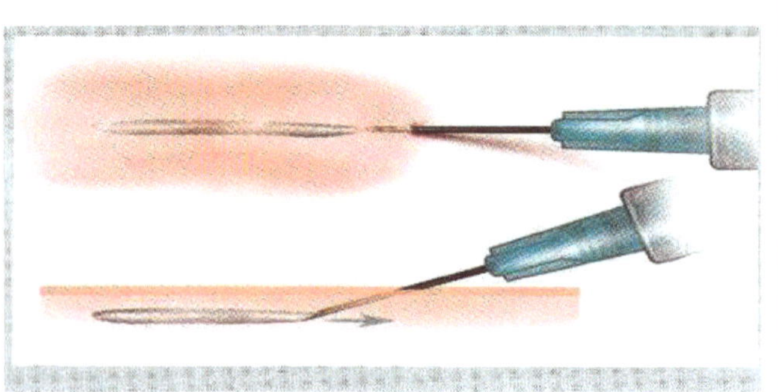

Linear Threading Technique

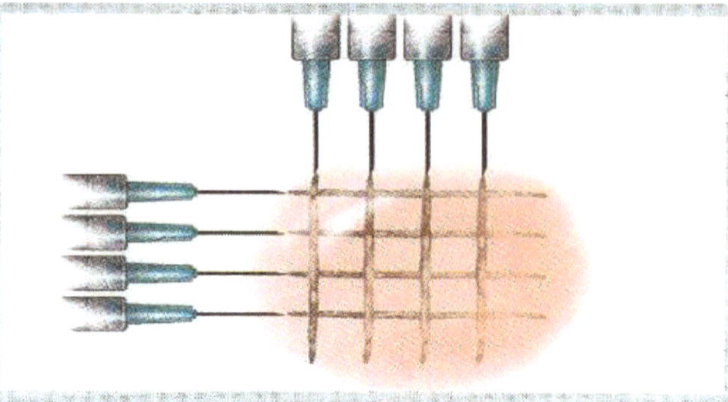

Cross-Hatching Technique

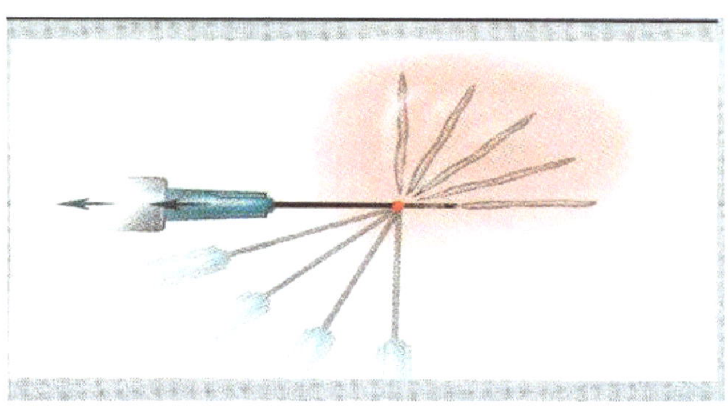

Fanning Technique

Figure 2: Injection Techniques [1]

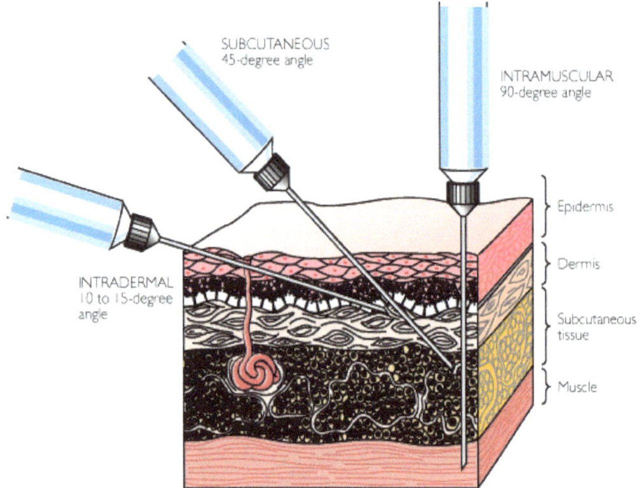

Figure 3: Filler Injection Technique [2]

Dermal fillers cannula Injection techniques

- Plan your access point
- Make entry with 20 G Needle with swift puncture to ↓ pain
- Utilizes 2-inch 25 G Blunt cannula
- Insert Cannula at 45°
- Before injection perform gentle tunneling
- Aspirate
- Deposit filler in a retrograde linear fashion
- Pull back → rotate (Fanning)
- Reassess with patient's feedback
- Touch up
- Massage

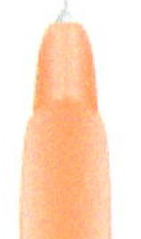

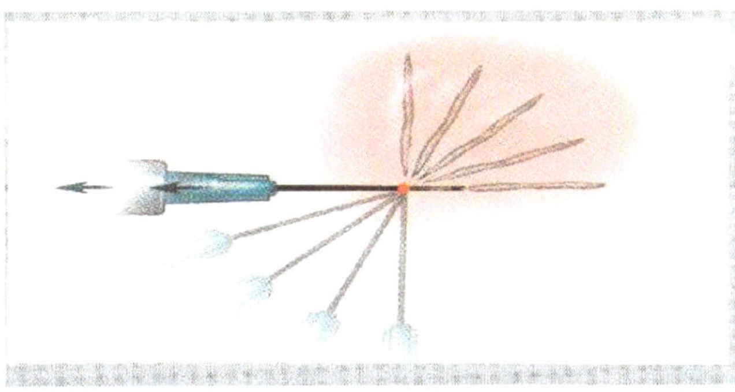

Figure 4: Cannula

Intimate Rejuvenation Procedures

- 14mg/ ml. non-cross-linked Hyaluronic Acid (HA)
- Injectable moisturizer
- Quickly absorbed into introitus skin
- Replenishes HA lost due to vaginal aging
- Hydrates skin and mucosa
- Restores elasticity
- Improves texture and tone
- Apply numbing cream for 20 min
- Use a 30 G needle
- Inject 1 ml per labia majora / 1ml into vaginal mucosa
- May use 0.25 mm Needling device and local application
- Protocol: once per month for 4 months
    LABIA MAJORA AUGMENTATION
- Filler Injection can provide:
- Aesthetically enhanced and youthful labia majora
- Additional cushion at the pubic bone to correct fat loss
- Mask minor hypertrophy of labia minora
- Improve skin sagging
- Apply numbing cream for 20 min
- Use 1% lidocaine with epinephrine for entry point
- Using an 18 G needle create a portal for cannula entry
- Use a 22G 50 mm blunt cannula
- Injected at the upper pole of both labia majora
- Use 2-3 ml of HA on each side
- Retrograde deposition of the filler
- Gentle bimanual massage

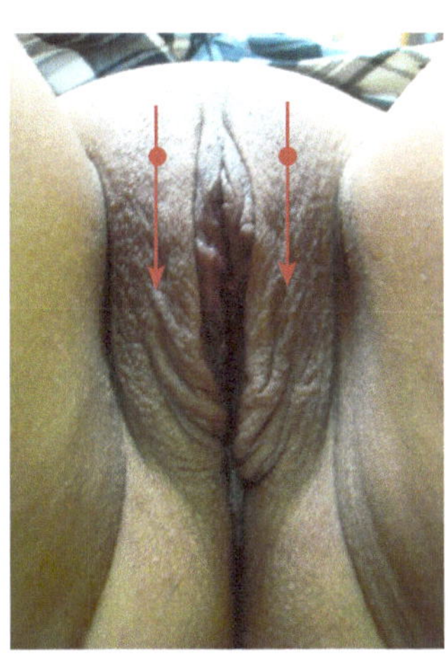

Figure 5: Point of injection

BEFORE & AFTER

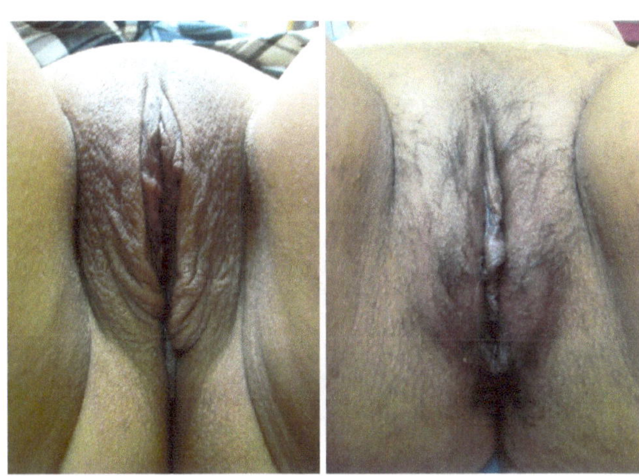

Figure 6: Before & After pictures of Fillers in intimate area.

REFERENCES

1. https://plasticsurgerykey.com/hyaluronic-acid-injectable-filler/
2. https://www.rroij.com/open-access/methods-and-guidelines-in-the-medication-and-drug-administration-a-review-.php?aid=78041

MOMMY MAKEOVER

Salman Khan

Pregnancy and breastfeeding can lead to significant hormonal changes, leading to alteration in the body's fat distribution. These in turn cause changes in breast volume, shape, abdominal skin, and fat accumulation on hips, thighs, and love handles. A mommy makeover is a combination of plastic surgery procedures, such as breast augmentation, breast lift, breast reduction, tummy tuck, and liposuction, to restore pre-pregnancy appearances. Additional treatments may be performed based on the patient's specific concerns.

The candidate as Mommy Makeover

Mommy makeover surgery is a highly individualized combination of procedures and is specifically tailored for any patient after a thorough consultation with a plastic surgeon.

- Mommy makeovers are generally recommended for individuals who have completed their family and do not plan to have more children.
- Candidates should have specific fat pockets that do not decrease despite weight loss, exercise, and lifestyle modifications.
- Candidates should be in overall good health with no uncontrolled medical conditions.
- It's advisable for candidates to be at or near their ideal weight.
- Candidates are generally advised to quit smoking (or ex-smoker for more than 12 months)
- Candidates should have realistic expectations about the outcomes of the procedures.
- A mommy makeover can provide significant improvements, but it's important to understand the limitations and potential risks.

Abdominoplasty

A tummy tuck, or abdominoplasty, is a surgical procedure that removes excess fat and skin from the abdomen area. It will also tighten weakened and loose abdominal muscles to give the abdomen a flatter, firmer appearance. (5)

Traditional or Full Abdominoplasty: This is the standard abdominoplasty procedure. It involves a horizontal incision just above the pubic hairline, extending between the hip bones. Excess skin and fat are removed, and the abdominal muscles are tightened by rectus plication. Recommended for those with significant skin laxity and muscle diastasis, often after significant weight loss or pregnancy

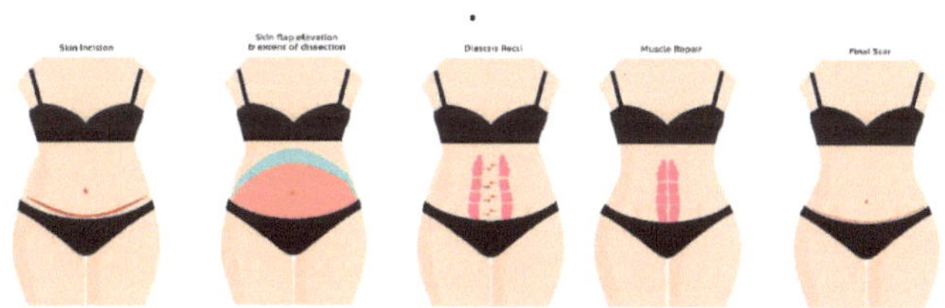

Fig 1: Full abdominoplasty Procedure Step by Step

Mini Abdominoplasty: This is a less extensive version of the traditional abdominoplasty. It typically involves a smaller incision and is focused on the lower abdomen.

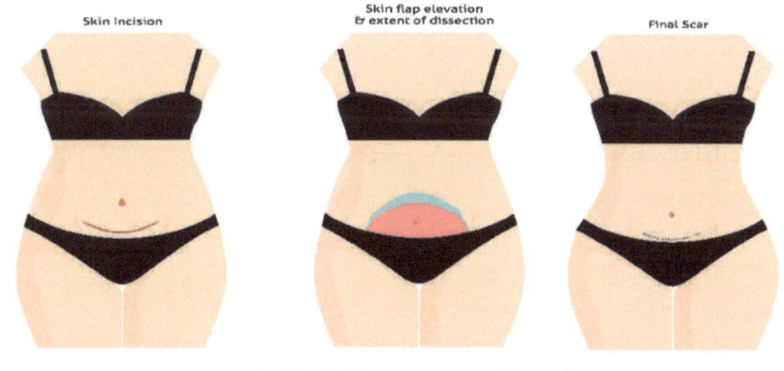

Fig 2: Mini abdominoplasty procedure

The Procedure

A tummy tuck, or abdominoplasty, is a surgical procedure to remove excess skin and fat from the abdomen and, in some cases, tighten the abdominal muscles. While the specific steps may vary depending on the surgeon's approach and the extent of the procedure. Following the pre-marked guidelines:

- **Anesthesia:** The patient is administered either general anesthesia or intravenous sedation to ensure they are comfortable and pain-free during the procedure.
- **Incisions:** The surgeon will make an incision just above the pubic area. Typically, this incision is placed low enough so that the resulting scar can be hidden easily by undergarments or a bathing suit. (5) A second incision is made around the navel to free it from the surrounding tissue.
- **Skin and Fat Removal:** Excess skin and fat are removed, and the remaining skin is pulled taut to create a smoother, flatter abdominal profile.
- **Closing Incisions:** After addressing the abdominal muscles (rectus plication) closure process begins. The placement and appearance of the new umbilicus are carefully considered. Skin is closed in layers, starting with the deeper layers (muscles and tissues) and progressing to the surface. (5)

Complications:

- Surgical site infection
- In some cases, the incisions may heal poorly, leading to issues such as delayed wound healing, widened scars, or skin loss.
- Bleeding/ hematoma
- Seroma formation
- Scars may fade over time but will remain visible.

Recovery: After the surgery, the patient is monitored in a recovery area. It's essential to follow post-operative care instructions, which may include wearing compression garments and avoiding strenuous activities.

Clinical Case: A 35-year-old female patient, let's call her Sarah, has recently lost a significant amount of weight through diet and exercise. While she is thrilled with her weight loss, she is left with excess skin and weakened abdominal muscles. She schedules a consultation with a plastic surgeon to discuss her concerns and explore the possibility of abdominoplasty, commonly known as a tummy tuck.

The procedure begins with the administration of anesthesia. An incision is made along the lower abdomen, carefully concealing it within the bikini line. The excess skin is then removed, and the abdominal muscles are tightened to create a firmer and flatter contour. Liposuction may also be performed to address any remaining pockets of fat. Once the desired changes are made, close the incisions with sutures. Pain medication is administered to manage any discomfort and is provided with post-operative care instructions. The surgeon may recommend wearing a compression garment to minimize swelling and support the healing process. Over the next several months, the client experiences a transformation in her abdominal appearance. The scars gradually faded, and the contour of her abdomen was improved.

Breast Augmentation

Post-pregnancy, women often experience dissatisfaction with their breast appearance due to the physical demands of childbirth and nursing. Some experience sags and loss of volume, requiring breast augmentation, lift, or implants. Others experience excessively large breasts, necessitating a reduction for more balanced and shapely results.

Breast augmentation with Implants

- **Saline breast implants:** Saline breast implants are filled with sterile salt water. If the implant shell leaks, a saline implant will collapse and the saline will be absorbed and naturally expelled by the body. Saline breast implants provide a uniform shape, firmness, and feel, and are FDA-approved for augmentation in women age 18 or older.
- **Structured saline breast implants:** These implants are filled with sterile salt water, and contain an inner structure that aims to make the implant feel more natural.
- **Silicone breast implants:** Silicone breast implants are filled with silicone gel. The gel feels a bit more like natural breast tissue. If the implant leaks, the gel may remain within the implant shell or may escape into the breast implant pocket. A leaking implant filled with silicone gel will not collapse. Silicone breast implants are FDA-approved for augmentation in women aged 22 or older.
- **Gummy bear breast implants:** Form-stable implants maintain their shape even when the implant shell is broken. Shaped gummy bear breast implants have more projection at the bottom and are tapered toward the top.

Breast augmentation with fat (Autologous fat transfer):

Liposuction is used to extract fat from the abdomen, love handles, back, or other parts of your body and is then injected into breasts for augmentation. This is a good option for ladies who want a slight increase in breast size and desire natural results as shown in Figure 2.

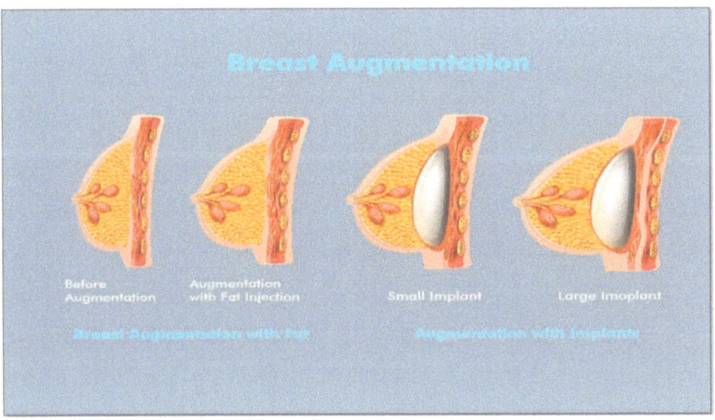

Fig 3: Breast Augmentation with Implants and with Autologous Fat

Breast Augmentation Procedure

An important decision involved in breast augmentation is whether to use silicone or saline implants both silicone and saline implants are available in similar shapes, sizes, and textures but they differ in the composition filling the implant. (9) Breast implants can be inserted either behind the glandular tissue, known as sub-glandular placement, or behind the muscle, known as sub-muscular placement. Additionally, there is a hybrid option called the dual-plane placement shown in Figure 3.

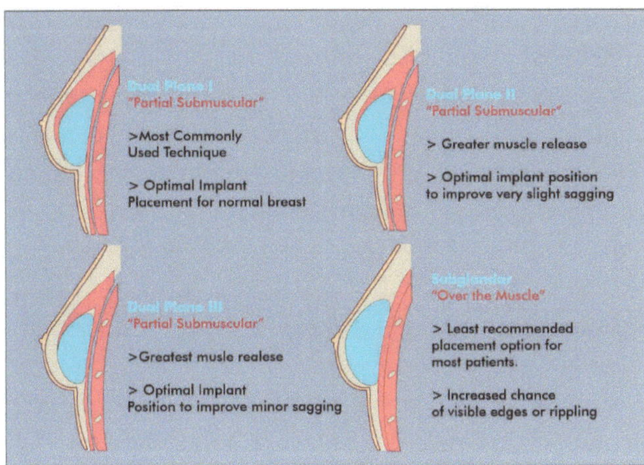

Fig 4: Breast Implants for Breast Augmentation

Submuscular Placement: In this placement, the breast implants are positioned beneath the chest muscle (Pectoralis major). It provides more natural-looking results, especially in thin individuals, as the muscle provides additional coverage over the implants.

Sub glandular Placement: In this placement, the breast implants are positioned above the chest muscle and below the breast gland. It is generally, a shorter and less painful recovery period and results in a more direct and prominent projection of the breasts.

Dual-Plane Placement: This is a hybrid placement that combines elements of both sub-muscular and sub-glandular placement. It allows for the natural coverage of the upper part of the implant by the muscle while placing the lower part under the breast gland. (10)

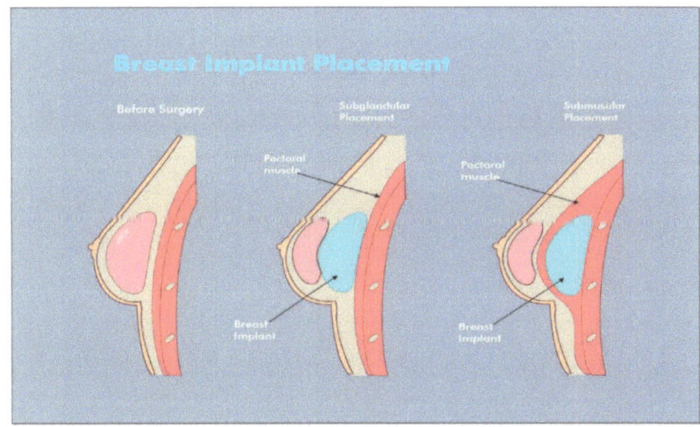

Fig 5: Breast Implants before surgery and with implants

Incisions for Breast Augmentation:

- **Inframammary Incision:** This incision is made along the inframammary fold, which is the natural crease under the breast. It allows direct access to the breast pocket, providing better visibility for precise implant placement.
- **Trans axillary Incision:** Incision is made in the natural folds of the armpit. It provides access to create a pocket for implant placement and is suitable for saline and some types of silicone implants. (12)
- **Trans umbilical Incision (TUBA):** This incision is made through the navel (belly button). Through this single incision in the belly button, a tunnel is created to the breast area for the placement of breast implants. (12)

Mommy makeover surgery:

The length of the surgery will depend on the number of procedures combined but can take between 4-6 hours to complete. An abdominal compression garment and supportive bra will be worn after the procedure to help reduce swelling and assist in shaping and contouring. (12)

The tummy tuck, liposuction, and breast augmentation procedure are performed under general anesthesia. In most breast implant surgeries, the nipples and areolas remain attached. It is essential to preserve the shape of the original breast when performing breast implant surgery. The breast implants will most likely be inserted using an inframammary incision. This is the most commonly used incision and is made below the breast fold. (13) This incision is generally less concealed and may cause fewer breastfeeding difficulties than the periareolar incision option. If a breast "lift" mastopexy is required the "lollipop" incision will most likely be used to lift the breast. This includes two incisions. One is a circular incision made around the border of the areola to reposition the nipple to a higher anatomical placement. The second incision is a straight vertical cut from the bottom of the areola to the breast fold.

Incisions for the tummy tuck will generally be made below the bikini line if possible. However, this is not always the case as it usually depends on the extent of the surgery. Most commonly, incisions are made from hip to hip along the public bone. (14) The incision length and exact locations will depend on the specific areas that require treatment as well as the amount of excess skin that needs removing. From the incision to the lower ribs, the skin and underlying fat are lifted free of the underlying vertical abdominal muscles. The rectus muscles are then surgically tightened by stitching the anterior rectus sheath into position. This will strengthen the abdomen and result in a smaller, shapelier waistline. During this procedure, if necessary, a small amount of targeted liposuction in the love handles or back will get rid of stubborn fat deposits to achieve a more contoured shape. (15) Once the skin is removed and the remaining skin is pulled tighter, the naval is stitched into its new position. The long incision is closed with stitches, and the dressing is applied. Plastic drain tubes will be inserted to drain fluid from the area. (15, 16) These will likely remain for up to 7 days after the procedure.

Complications after mommy makeover:

- Bleeding/ hematoma
- Surgical site infection.
- Seroma formation
- loss of nipple sensation
- Capsular contracture
- Anaplastic large cell lymphoma
- Recurrent looseness of skin
- Fat necrosis
- Cardiac and pulmonary complications
- Persistent pain,
- Contour deformity

Why breast augmentation with autologous fat is considered the best technique?

Fat transfer provides a more natural look and feel compared to breast implants. The augmented breasts feel like natural breast tissue because they are composed of the patient's fat. It is a minimally invasive procedure compared to breast implant surgery. It involves liposuction to harvest fat from areas with excess, and then the fat is injected into the breasts. The liposuction component of the procedure allows patients to contour other areas of their body while enhancing their breasts. Common donor areas include the abdomen, thighs, or flanks. (17) Since the augmentation is achieved with the patient's fat, there are no foreign objects (implants) in the body, reducing the risk of complications associated with implants. The results of fat transfer tend to be subtle and natural-looking. The augmentation is achieved by strategically placing fat to enhance the breasts, creating a more gradual and realistic change. Fat transfer eliminates the risk of implant rupture or leakage, which can occur with breast implants. The augmented breasts consist of the patient's tissue. (18)

Clinical Case: A 32-year-old mother of two who has recently completed her family. Despite maintaining a healthy lifestyle, she is frustrated with the changes in her body that occurred during and after pregnancy. Her major concerns were sagging breasts, loss of breast volume, excess abdominal skin, and weakened abdominal muscles. She decides to consult with a plastic surgeon to discuss the possibility of a mommy makeover.

The surgeon recommends a breast augmentation to restore lost volume and a breast lift to address sagging. Silicone implants were used to achieve the desired fullness. Periareolar incisions for implant placement and additional incisions for the breast lift. To address the excess abdominal skin and weakened muscles, abdominoplasty was proposed. For this a horizontal incision is made above the pubic area, extending between the hip bones. The patient was recommended to wear compression garments to support healing and reduce swelling post-operatively. Several months post-surgery, her breasts are fuller and lifted, and her abdomen is firmer and more toned.

Advantages and Disadvantages of Fat Augmentation

PROS:

- One of the most facilitated advantages of fat augmentation surgery is the removal of fat from the body parts with unwanted fat such as thighs, waist, hips, abdomen, etc. which contours the body and can minimize unwanted fat areas.
- Breast augmentation with fat transfer is a far less invasive procedure with smaller incisions (~ 4 mm) and is an ideal choice for sagging breasts.
- The fat transfer surgery involves injecting fat into the breasts that leaves almost no scarring and results in quick and comfortable recovery.
- Breast augmentation with a fat transfer has a better safety record and relatively fewer postoperative complications than breast implants.

- As compared to breast implants, breasts feel and look more natural as their own body's fat is injected and that's why it's also called "natural breast augmentation surgery with fat transfer."

CONS:

- There may be limitations of an increase in breast size restricted to about one cup size. To achieve a significant change in breast volume and curvy cleavage, fat transfer surgery is not a great option.
- Changes may develop such as non-cancerous benign breast cysts (breast calcification) which are small deposits of calcium in the breast tissue.
- Liposuction is not good for lean patients because there isn't enough adipose tissue to use in the fat transfer technique.
- Fat survival is typically 50-70%, but body reactions may result in some fat absorption, requiring more fat injections for desired enhancement.
- Unlike breast implants, sagging happens with age, considerable weight loss, pregnancy, etc., which can't be prevented after a fat transfer procedure.

REFERENCES

1. Iribarren-Moreno R, Cuenca-Pardo J, Ramos-Gallardo G (2019) Is plastic surgery combined with obstetrical procedures safe? Aesthet Plast Surg 43(5):1396–1399. https://doi.org/10.1007/s00266-019-01448-9

2. Sinno S, Shah S, Kenton K et al (2011) Assessing the safety and efficacy of combined abdominoplasty and gynecologic surgery. Ann Plast Surg 67(3):272–274. https://doi.org/10.1097/SAP.0b013e3181f9b245

3. Matarasso A, Smith DM (2015) Combined breast surgery and abdominoplasty: strategies for success. Plast Reconstr Surg 135(5):849e–860e. https://doi.org/10.1097/PRS.0000000000001238

4. Hodgkinson EL, Smith DM, Wittkowski A (2014) Women's experiences of their pregnancy and postpartum body image: a systematic review and meta-synthesis. BMC Pregnancy Childbirth. https://doi.org/10.1186/1471-2393-14-330

5. Bjelica A, Cetkovic N, Trninic-Pjevic A, Mladenovic-Segedi L (2018) The phenomenon of pregnancy—a psychological view. Ginekol Pol 89(2):102–106. https://doi.org/10.5603/GP.a2018.0017

6. Tan EK, Tan EL (2013) Alterations in physiology and anatomy during pregnancy. Best Pract Res Clin Obstet Gynaecol 27(6):791–802. https://doi.org/10.1016/j.bpobgyn.2013.08.001

7. Edmondson SJ, Ross DA (2021) The postpartum abdomen: psychology, surgery and quality of life. Hernia 25(4):939–950. https://doi.org/10.1007/s10029-021-02470-0

8. Stevens WG, Cohen R, Vath SD, Stoker DA, Hirsch EM (2006) Is it safe to combine abdominoplasty with elective breast surgery? A review of 151 consecutive cases. Plast Reconstr Surg 118(1):207–212. https://doi.org/10.1097/01.prs.0000220529.03298.42

9. Simon S, Thaller SR, Nathan N (2006) Abdominoplasty combined with additional surgery: a safety issue. Aesthet Surg J 26(4):413–416. https://doi.org/10.1016/j.asj.2006.06.004

10. Saad AN, Parina R, Chang D, Gosman AA (2014) Risk of adverse outcomes when plastic surgery procedures are combined. Plast Reconstr Surg 134(6):1415–1422. https://doi.org/10.1097/PRS.0000000000000738

11. Goldwyn RM (1986) Abdominoplasty as a combined procedure: added benefit or double trouble? Plast Reconstr Surg 78(3):383–384. https://doi.org/10.1097/00006534-198609000-00018

12. Agrawal NA, Hillier K, Kumar R, Izaddoost SA, Rohrich RJ (2022) A review of venous thromboembolism risk assessment and prophylaxis in plastic surgery. Plast Reconstr Surg 149(1):121E-129E. https://doi.org/10.1097/PRS.0000000000008663

13. Davis MJ, Lopez JP, Turner A, Abu-Ghname A, Davies LW, Buchanan EP (2022) Sharing the operating room: a descriptive study of combined and collaborative plastic surgery cases. Plast Reconstr Surg 149(5):1009E-1013E. https://doi.org/10.1097/PRS.0000000000009028

14. Cardoso de Castro C, Cupello AM (1990) Analysis of 60 cases of simultaneous mammaplasty and abdominoplasty. Aesthetic Plast Surg 14(1):35–41. https://doi.org/10.1007/BF01578323

15. Grieco M, Grignaffini E, Simonacci F, Raposio E (2015) Analysis of complications in postbariatric abdominoplasty: our experience. Plast Surg Int 2015:1–5. https://doi.org/10.1155/2015/209173

16. Iglesia CB. From Vaginal Mesh to Mommy Makeovers: Lessons on Safely Introducing New Technologies in Gynecologic Surgery. Urogynecology. 2023 Oct 1;29(10):785-6.

17. Toto V, Scarabosio A, Alessandri-Bonetti M, Albanese R, Persichetti P. Combined Surgery (Mommy-Makeover) Compared to Single Procedure (Abdominoplasty) in After-Pregnancy Women: A Prospective Study on Risks and Benefits. Aesthetic Plastic Surgery. 2023 Aug 23:1-0.

18. Ørholt M, Larsen A, Hemmingsen MN, Mirian C, Zocchi ML, Vester-Glowinski PV, Herly M. Complications after breast augmentation with fat grafting: a systematic review. Plastic and Reconstructive Surgery. 2020 Mar 1;145(3):530e-7e.

G-SPOT AUGMENTATION

Sandhya Deora

The G-spot remains elusive to many, men more than women, but those who have found it cannot refute its existence. Great pioneers in the field of human sexuality like Sigmund Freud, Alfred Kinsey, and his coworkers had different theories about female orgasm. While Freud told us that the mature woman is vaginally responsive and should give up her childish interest in her clitoris(1), Kinsey and his coworkers concluded that the clitoris is sensitive and the vagina is not(2). This concept was reinforced by the work of Masters and Johnson, whose research claimed that all female orgasms involve the clitoris and are physiologically indistinguishable(3).

In 1950, Grafenberg(4) published a seminal paper: "The Role of the urethra in female orgasm". His main statement was that "an erotic zone always could be demonstrated on the anterior wall of the vagina along the course of the urethra" and that this area swells with sexual stimulation, reaching its maximum at the end of the orgasm. He also wrote that "we can almost say that there is no part of the female body which does not give a sexual response, the partner has only to find the erotogenic zones." Dr. John Perry and Beverly Whipple(5) named this area of the urethra the Grafenburg spot or the G-spot. This area on the anterior wall of the vagina is 10-20mm in diameter and is said to be approximately 5 cm above the ostium of the urethra(6). Although anatomical and biochemical studies have failed to provide evidence regarding the G-spot and only case studies and anecdotal observations support its presence(7), the demand for surgical G-spot augmentation is increasing.

TYPES OF ORGASM

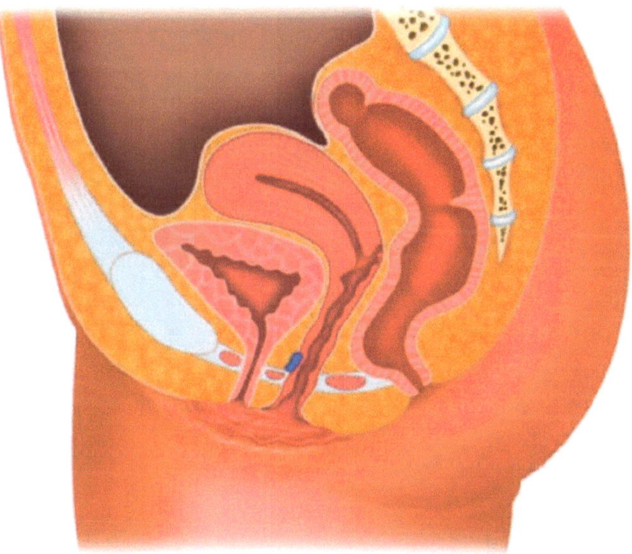

Before we dive into the details of augmentation, we should first understand the types of orgasms. Women have two kinds of orgasms, "clitorally activated" versus "vagnally activated"(via G-spot). Jannini et al(8) showed that orgasms resulting from direct clitoral stimulation have been reported to be sharp, bursting, short-lasting, superficial, and more localized, confined only to the pubic area. (9,10) By contrast, vaginally activated orgasms have been described as more diffuse, whole body, radiating, psychologically more satisfying, and longer lasting(8-10). It has been further shown that women who have both types of orgasms have even deeper, more powerful, blended orgasms resulting from contractions in both areas at once.

ANATOMY OF THE G-SPOT

The search for this mysterious, highly erogenous vaginal region, the G-spot has produced important data, substantially improving understanding of the complex anatomy and physiology of sexual responses in women. The anatomical relationships and dynamic interactions between the clitoris, urethra, and anterior vaginal wall have led to the concept of a clitourethrovaginal complex, which when properly stimulated could induce intense orgasms.

Gravina et al(11) examined the urethrovaginal space along a line drawn between the border of the smooth muscle, the mucosal-submucosal layer of the urethral wall, and the border of the vaginal wall and its lumen. The three-dimensional reconstruction of the urethrovainal space had a glandlike aspect with small feeding vessels.

Komisaruk et al(12) confirmed the presence of several different organs in this highly complex body region. They stated that this area may include the anterior vaginal wall, the urethra itself, the Skene glands (including the periurethral glands, also known as the female prostate gland), perhaps the other glands in this region (vestibular glands and Bartholin glands), the surrounding muscle and connective tissue, and possibly the crura of the clitoris.

In addition to the potentially important role of engorgement of the vascular erectile components of the clitorourethrovaginal complex during sexual arousal(13), these tissues were located superficially below the mucosal layer of the vagina in a cadaveric autopsy study. (14) These findings suggest that the filler should be placed closer to the urethra than to the vaginal wall.

In a recent study by anatomic dissection of fresh frozen cadavers, Ostrzenski(15) identified the G-spot as an elongated structure lying on the superonasal perineal membrane at an oblique angle of 35 degrees dorsal (that is, vaginalward) to the urethra, with the perineal-ward pole lying 3mm from the urethra, the cervicalward pole 15mm from the urethra, and the whole structure parallel to the urethra(Fig?? 14-2

WHY AUGMENTATION

As described above, the nonspecific, deep location of the G-spot and lack of sexual satisfaction in women lead to the search for ways to help them achieve the bliss of vaginal orgasms. Hence, came the concept of G-spot augmentation or amplification as one of the options.

The idea behind this is to increase the size of the fabled area to the size of the marble, protruding inside the vagina so that it is stimulated during intercourse.

TYPES OF AUGMENTATION

Fillers used for this purpose are hyaluronic acid, human collagen, autologous fat, and even silicone by some experts.

Filler injections for G-spot enhancement treatment have become known as the G-spot shot. The G-Shot®, as demonstrated by its inventor, David Matlock, is given either just into the subvaginal mucosa (that is, between the G-spot and the vaginal mucosa) or into the G-spot in the urethrovaginal septum (that is, directly into the G-spot itself).

Autologous fat transplantation has also been used to amplify the G-spot area. In a book article, Gress (16) describes an amelioration of sexual stimulation after autologous fat transplantation in 52% of his patients. In these patients, a 5–12-cc fat graft had been injected. Lipofilling to amplify the G-spot area is appealing because the long-term persistence of the fat is expected to be very good. Exact volumetric measurements are missing; however, because of the very good vascularity of the vaginal mucosa, volume survival rates should be superior to the breast tissue, where survival rates of >70% have been demonstrated using magnetic resonance imaging volumetry (17).

Christian Herold et al report a case of autologous fat transplantation where 8cc of fat from the trochanteric area was injected and the patient was satisfied with the procedure with no side effects. (18)

As we know, the vaginal wall or mucosa is made of connective tissues which have collagen. It is supposed that restoring the collagen in the G-spot will stimulate the enhancement of the size and sensitivity of the area which will result in improved sexual reactivity. The synthetic human collagen or hyaluronic acid is injected directly into the location of the G-spot in the front vaginal wall. The collagen or hyaluronic acid will accumulate more water or hydration in the tissues which will increase their volume and so it will enhance the size of the G-spot as well as sensitivity. The procedure's drawback is that the body absorbs collagen within six to eight months and hence, to maintain the effect, the injections must be repeated.

Christine A. Hamori(19) reports the usage of yet another permanent filler called Macroplastique. "I achieve this by injecting 1.5 to 2.5 ml of Macroplastique®

(Cogentix Medical) transurethrally using a Storz Viscous Fluid Injection Set. Macroplastique is placed just under the muscularis of the urethra, above the previously determined G-spot to cause the G-spot to bulge vaginalward. Alternatively, the Macroplastique Implantation Device can be used, which involves a blind procedure and requires that the G-spot be palpated transvaginally to make sure that the tip of the device is in the urethra at the correct position. The needle is inserted and the injection is completed. Macroplastique is medical-grade silicone that is thermogravimetric analysis (TGA)– approved for periurethral and periureteric injection for various urologic indications. It is permanent and does not migrate or lose any appreciable volume. Macroplastique lasts forever, and if it is inadvertently placed incorrectly, it is fairly easy to remove. By contrast, hyaluronic acid is temporary, lasting only 12 to 18 months; if it is combined with Botox, it may last 2 to 2 1/2 years. It can be diminished by injecting hyaluronidase to dispel it, but 100% removal takes time. Allergy to hyaluronic acid occurs occasionally, whereas silicone allergy has never been reported, to my knowledge." The only reported complication was urinary obstruction which was managed with an indwelling catheter for 12 hours.

PROCEDURE

G-spot augmentation is intended for sexually active women with normal sexual function and is performed at the doctor's office under local anesthesia. A physical examination, apart from a standard general examination, requires a vaginal examination that includes locating the patient's G-spot. With the fingers gently inserted into the vagina about 5 to 6 cm past the introitus and beneath the pubic bone, pressure on the anterior vaginal wall roughly midway between the pubic bone and the cervix will initially cause a desire to micturate. After releasing and reapplying pressure, the patient will eventually report that this produces erotic and pleasing feelings. The examiner should stop at this point, record the depth of the G-spot about a fixed anatomic landmark such as the urethral orifice, and continue to inform the patient verbally. The recorded depth of the G-spot will be useful later during G-spot augmentation

The whole procedure will take less than 30 minutes, where most of the time taken is for examining and locating the G-spot. As it is, an outpatient non-surgical process, no recovery time is required. It will be painless and scar-free. However, abstinence is suggested for 2-3 days after the procedure, so that the fillers can settle down.

So, in conclusion there is ample evidence of the existence of the G-spot and the benefits of its augmentation. Though many refute it, the procedure performed in expert hands and with the patients in whom the G-spot is located produces excellent results. The lack of enough data is probably due to the stigma associated with female sexual gratification. Doctors as well as patients continue to grow and explore more, hence, so will the G-spot.

REFERENCES

1. Freud, Sigmund. (1931b). Female sexuality. SE, 21: 221-243

2. Kinsey, Alfred C; Pomeroy, Wardell B; Martin, Clyde E; and Gebhard, Paul H. Sexual Behaviour in the Human Female. Philadelphia: W. B. Saunders Co, 1953

3. Masters WH, Johnson EV, eds. Human Sexual Response. Boston: Little Brown, 1996.

4. Grafenberg E. The role of urethra in female orgasm. Int J Sexology 3:145, 1950

5. Perry JD, Whipple B. Pelvic muscle strength of female ejaculators: evidence in support of a new theory of orgasm. J Sex Res 17:22, 1987

6. Gravina GL, Brandetti F, Martini P, Carosa E, Di Stasi SM, Morano S, et al. Measurement of the thickness of the urethrovaginal space in women with or without vaginal orgasm. *J Sex Med.* 2008;5:610–8. http://dx.doi.org/10.1111/j.1743-6109.2007.00739.x. [PubMed] [Google Scholar]

7. Hines TM. The G-spot: a modern gynecologic myth. *Am J Obstet Gynecol.* 2001;185:359–62. http://dx.doi.org/10.1067/mob.2001.115995. [PubMed] [Google Scholar]

8. Janini EA, d'Amati G, Lenzi A. Histology and Immunohistochemical studies of female genital tissue. In Goldstein I, Maston C, Davis S, et al, eds. Women's Sexual Function and Dysfunction Study, Diagnosis and Treatment. London: Taylor and Francis, 2006.

9. Komisaruk BR, Whipple B, Crawford A, et al. Brain activation during vagina cervical self-stimulation and orgasm in women with complete spinal cord injury: fMRI evidence of mediation of the vagus nerves. Brain Res 1024:77, 2004.

10. Komisaruk JB, Beyar-Flores C, Whipple B, eds. The Science of Orgasm. Baltimore: Johns Hopkins University Press, 2006.

11. Gravina GL, Brandetti F, Martini P, et al. Measurement of the thickness of the urethra-vaginal space in women with or without vaginal orgasm. J Sex Med 5:601, 2008.

12. Komisaruk BR, Whipple B, Nauerzadeh S, et al, eds. The Orgasm Answer Guide, ed 2. Baltimore: Johns Hopkins University Press.

13. Battaglia C, Nappi RE, Mancini F, etal. 3-D volumetric and vascular analysis of the urethra-vaginal space in young women with and without vaginal orgasm. J Sex Med 7(4 Pt 1):1445, 2010.

14. Rees MA, O'Connell HE, Plenter RJ, et al. The suspensory ligament of the clitoris: connective tissue supports the erectile tissues of the female urogenital region. Clin Anat 13:397, 2000.

15. Ostrzenski A. G-spot anatomy: a discovery. JSex Med 9:1355, 2102.

16. Gress S. Form- und funktionsverbessernde Eingriffe im weiblichen Genitalbereich. *Ästhetische Chirurgie von Heimburg Lemperle.* 2012:25. [Google Scholar]

17. Herold C, Ueberreiter K, Cromme F, Busche MN, Vogt PM. The use of mamma MRI volumetry to evaluate the rate of fat survival after autologous lipotransfer. *Handchir Mikrochir Plast Chir.* 2010;42:129–34. http://dx.doi.org/10.1055/s-0029-1243204. [PubMed] [Google Scholar]

18. Herold C, Motamedi M, Hartmann U, Allert S. G-spot augmentation with autologous fat transplantation. J Turk Ger Gynecol Assoc. 2015; 16(3): 187-188

19. Hamori C., Banwell P, Alinsod R. Female Cosmetic Genital Surgery. Concepts, Classification, and Techniques. P228.

MODULE 4

SURGICAL ASPECT

HYMENOPLASTY

Garima Srivastav

What is it?

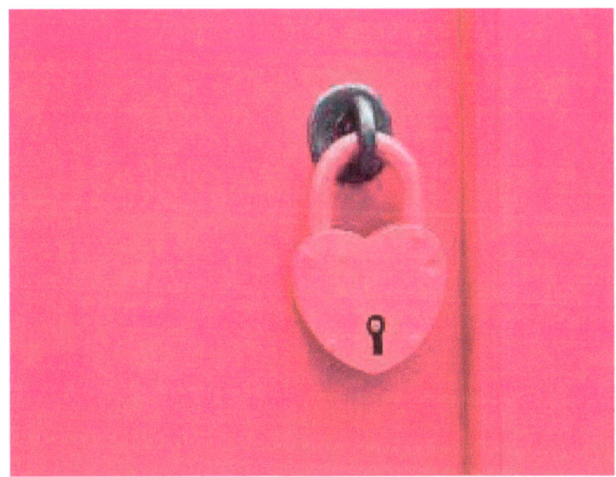

Hymenoplasty, also known as hymen restoration surgery, is a surgical procedure that aims to reconstruct the skin membrane, known as the hymen, located in the lower half of the vagina.

- This fibrous and elastic tissue is usually torn with the first sexual penetration of women, but it can also break after a physical accident, sudden movements or even using tampons.
- Hymen repair is a simple procedure that involves stitching the torn edges together with dissolvable stitches.
- Generally, it is performed with just local anesthesia and performed as a day-case procedure.
   Why is it done?
- Generally, patients who request this type of operation wish to recover the original status of the hymen for cultural or religious reasons.
- This is because, in some cultures, the hymen is seen as symbolic of virginity.
- However, it is important to note that the hymen can tear from nonsexual causes, such as tampon use or certain sports activities (e.g. horseback riding).
- Nowadays hymenoplasty is also requested by some females at their 25th anniversary to be enjoyed as re-virgin.

HYMENOPLASTY, HYMENORRHAPHY, HYMEN REPAIR

- The procedure of repairing back hymen is very controversial. Yet in the subcontinent, it is one of the most commonly performed procedures due to cultural indications.
- As a practitioner, are we justified to do it? Well, the author believes that as long as we follow the 4 ethical principles as discussed earlier, we are justified to do so.
- Sometimes the woman's future hangs by the membrane and as practitioners, our responsibility lies towards our women.

ETHICAL AND CULTURAL CONSIDERATIONS

The celebration of the bloody sheet, portrayed in popular cinema, is based on strong religious and cultural beliefs.

- Many cultures believe that the bride has to be a virgin, and according to the custom a woman found on her wedding night to have been
- "Touched" brings shame to her family. Consequences include divorce to death. Consequently, young women go to great lengths to get their hymen repaired.
- However, it is illegal in most Arab countries.
- The role and need of hymenoplasty is debatable.
- However, it is justifiable in certain circumstances, when the woman would otherwise suffer disgrace or worse.
- More importantly, however, young women and more particularly males and their families require appropriate sexual education about their adherence to the "Bloody sheet theory".
- Irrespective of the scientific and ethical controversies, demand for hymenoplasty is ever increasing.
- Hundreds of doctors advertise their hymenoplasty services over the internet.
- Unfortunately, none of them ever show the results of the procedure.

INDICATION

- No valid scintific indication
- Cultural indications
- Anyone with realistic expectations and sufficient hymenal tissue can get it done

CONTRAINDICATIONS

- Confusion with vaginal tightening
- Active vulvovaginal infections

Hymen tissue appearance may greatly vary, hence no standard hymenal appearance to reproduce

PREOPERATIVELY

- Counselling is a must before the procedure.
- Explian: No medical benefit.
- Absence of hymen or failure to bleed is not a sign of previous intercourse.
- Less than half of women say they bled with initial sexual penetration (34% of women).
- Determining on examination if the woman had sexual activity is not always possible.

SURGICAL TECHNIQUES

- Vaguely described
- 67% success rate
- For patients who want structural integrity and need the hymen to be intact on physical examination: perform hymenoplasty 3 months before the marriage.
- If bleeding is desired: Perform hymenoplasty for 3 weeks for the results.

We will be discussing the following 3 techniques in the chapter subsequently
- FLAP TECHNIQUE
- CERCLAGE TECHNIQUE
- VESTIBULO-INTROITAL TIGHTENING TECHNIQUE (VITT)

FLAP TECHNIQUE

- The patient is placed in a lithotomy position.
- 2.5 cm long and 1 cm wide rectangular flaps are marked at 2, 5, 8, and 11 o'clock positions on the anterior vaginal wall.
- Flaps at 2 and 5 o'clock positions are kept proximally based, and flaps at 8 and 11 o'clock positions are kept distally based or vice versa.
- Flaps are raised at the level of loose connective tissue below the mucosa. Donor areas are closed primarily.

- Opposing flaps are overlapped in a crisscross manner and sutured with
- 5/0 Polyglactin (Vicryl®) sutures leaving no raw area.

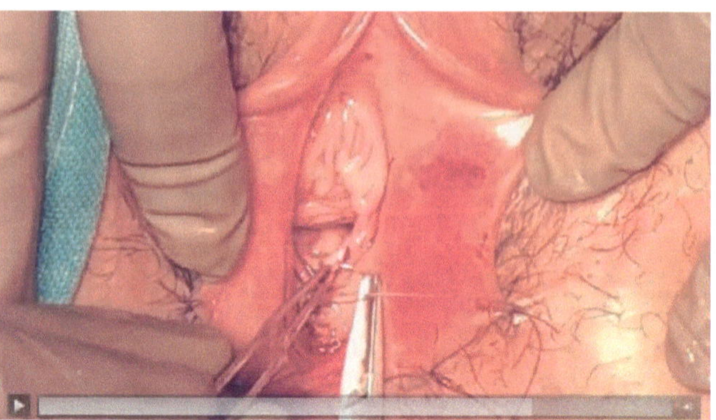

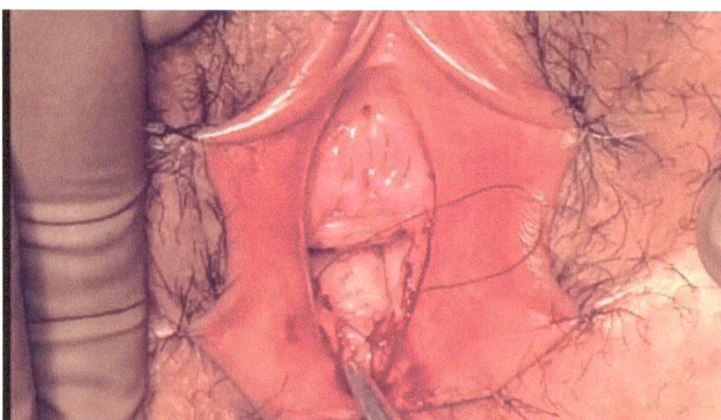

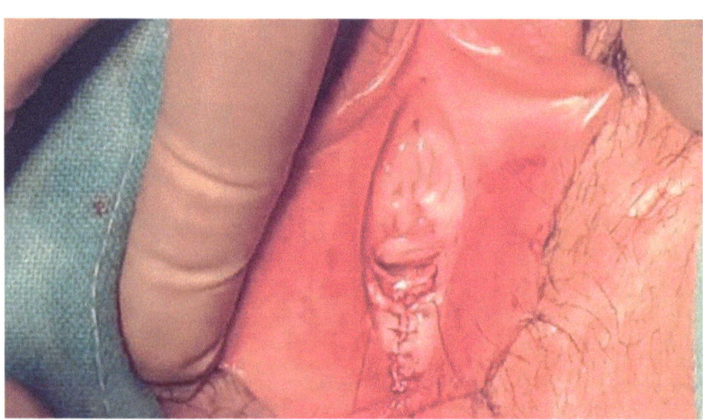

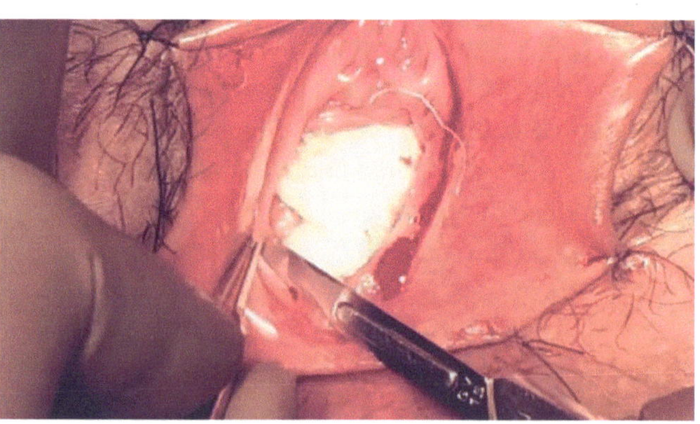

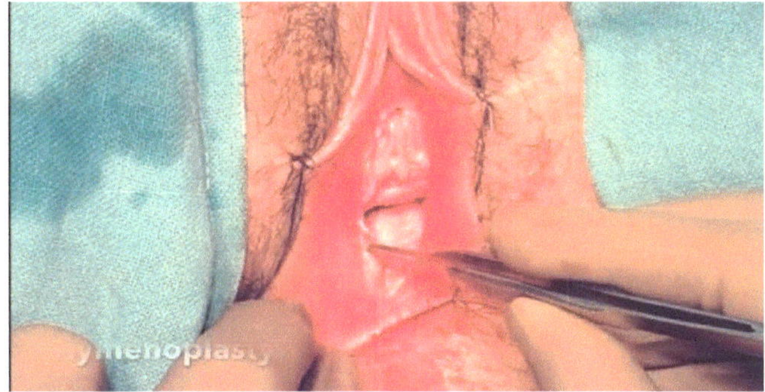

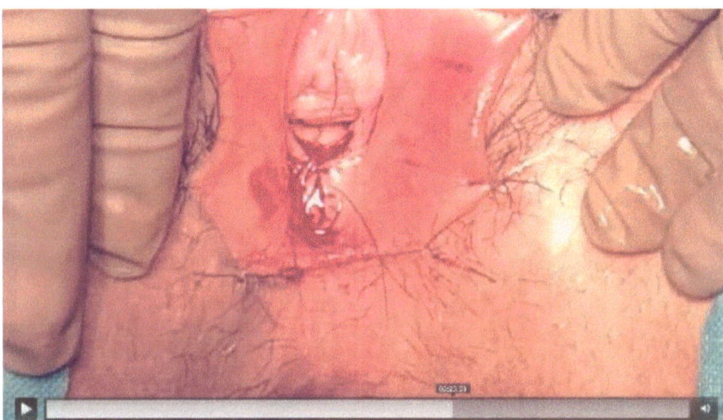

In the above patient, the hymenal tags were identified. Since the patient was done under GA, even then, long-acting anesthesia was injected into the hymenal tags for two purposes. One for long-term comfort from pain and secondly the mere act of injecting local anesthesia makes the hymenal fragments bigger and easier to work with.

The hymenal flaps were then raised – anterior and posterior, throughout the length, since they could be identified throughout.

The flaps could be made at the level of the hymen or even deeper involving vaginal mucosa if vaginal laxity is an issue too. Making the flap with vaginal mucosa had another advantage too, that it being more vascular will give more strength and increased chances of bleeding at the time of intercourse.

The posterior flaps were then sutured together, the suture used can be monocryl 5,0 or vicryl rapide 5,0 depending upon the time in hand before marriage.

The anterior flaps were then sutured together. In the author's opinion, it makes more sense to keep the knot posteriorly for future concerns.

BEFORE AND AFTER

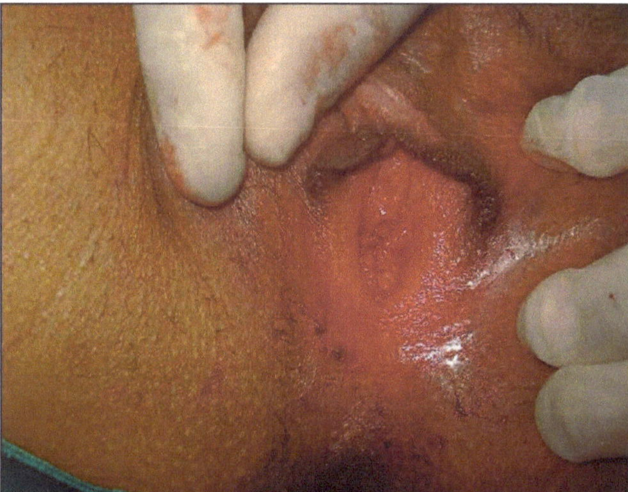

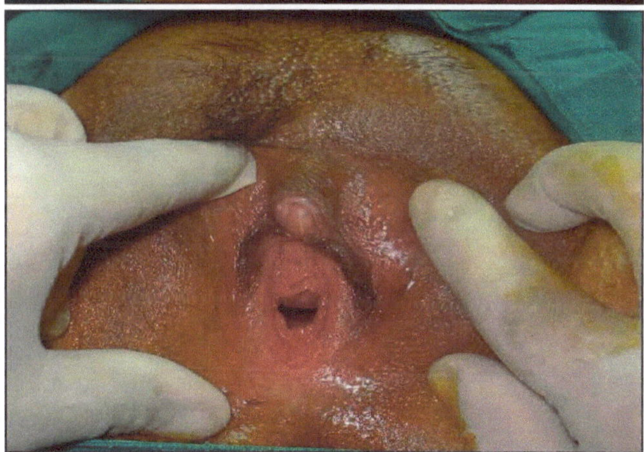

CERCLAGE TECHNIQUE

- When hymen tissue is less, then this technique is preferred.
- Labia minora is retracted.
- An entry wound is made at 6' 0 clock position with scissors.
- Entry wound dilated.
- Suture placement begins at 6 o'clock position.
- 4,0 chromic catgut is passed, through the submucosa in a clockwise fashion with exiting and re-entry into each sequential puncture wound.
- Additional tension is applied to show the decreased size of introitus.
- Suturing ends with a knot at 6'o clock position.

VITT TECHNIQUE

- Allis clamps grasped bilaterally in the vestibular area
- Diamond-shaped incision including hymen caruncles, vestibulum, and vaginal introitus given.
- The lowest point is located in the posterior midline vestibule at 6 o'clock just above the fourchette.

- The superior apex was extended 2-3 cm above the hymenal ring.
- If allis is at 4 and 8 o clock- tighten vaginal opening in comparison to 5 and 7 o 'clock
- Mucosa removed.
- Closed mucosal and submucosal layer by 4,0 vicryl rapide sutures-continuously.
- Involving vaginal mucosa enabled tightening of introitus and decreases tension on hymenal mucosa, critical in the success of the surgery.
- Hymenal edges repaired by 4-0 vicryl rapide.
- Vestibulum repaired continuously.

POST OP CARE

Icing for 24-48 hours.

Gentle irrigation after urine and motions.

Should not use public pools, hot tubs, and saunas for 4 weeks.

Limited physical activity with no exercise for 4 weeks.

Do not use tampons, cups.

Do not self-inspect the wound.

REFERENCES

1. Goodman MP. Female cosmetic genital surgery. Obstet Gynecol. 2009;113:154-9.

2. Saraiya HA. Surgical revirgination: four vagi- nal mucosal flaps for reconstruction of a hymen. Indian J Plast Surg. 2015;48(2):192-5. https://doi.org/10.4103/0970-0358.163060.

3. Ahmadi A. Ethical issues in hymenoplasty: views from Tehran's physicians. J Med Ethics. 2014;40:429-30.

4. Heger A, Jean ES, David M. Evaluation of the sexually abused child: a medical textbook and photographic atlas. 2nd ed. New York: Oxford University Press; 2000. p. 116.

5. Kimberley N, Hutson JM, Southwell BR, Grover SR. Vaginal agenesis, the hymen, and associated anomalies. J Pediatr Adolesc Gynecol 2012;25:54-8

6. Mor N Merlob P Congenital absence of 1988:82:679-80. 6. Mor N, Merlob P. only a rumor? Pediatric 1988;82679-80

7. Allinsod, Hamori, Banwell: Female Genital Cosmetic Surgery.Hymenoplasty

8. Esendag Suleyman: VITT technique of hymenoplasty

LABIOPLASTY

Sibel Ustunel

INTRODUCTION

The demand for cosmetic gynecology has exhibited a sharp rise globally in recent years. In particular, surgical procedures on the labia have become the most sought-after surgeries in this domain. According to United Nations statistics, since 2013 labiaplasty has been ranked as the fourth most prevalent aesthetic operation worldwide after liposuction, breast aesthetics, and rhinoplasty (1). While labiaplasty appears to be exclusive to a modern society with high socio-economic status, François Mauricceau drew attention to labial hypertrophy as a compelling motive for women to seek the procedure back in 1861 (2). Meissner (3) and Treub (4) similarly described labial hypertrophy and labiaplasty in the same era. The surgical approach towards labial aesthetics emerged in the 1970s (5).

While labiaplasty is typically defined as the surgical reduction of the labia minora, it should be noted that interventions involving the labia majora and clitoral hood may also be included in this definition. The evolution of labiaplasty over the years has led to a significant rise in demand for cosmetic gynecology (6, 7).

Overview of Vulvar Anatomy
Vulva

The female external genitalia, commonly referred to as the vulva, is situated above the pubic bones and extends posteriorly below the pubic arch. To ensure clarity, all technical terms will be explained upon first use. It comprises the mons pubis, labia majora, labia minora, clitoris, vestibule, vestibular bulb, Bartholin glands (large vestibular glands), small vestibular glands, Skene (paraurethral) glands, urethral and vaginal ostia.

Mons Pubis and Labia Majora

The mons pubis forms a rounded prominence anterior to the symphysis pubis, while the labia majora extends from the symphysis pubis to the perineal body. Both structures possess a subcutaneous layer similar to that of the anterior abdominal wall, composed of a superficial adipose layer and a deep membranous layer.

Labia Minor

The labia minora are two folds of skin located between the labia majora. Each labia minora is divided into two, creating two folds that enclose the glans of the clitoris. The prepuce is the anterior fold above the glans, while the frenulum is the inferior fold that passes beneath the clitoris. Both labia minora terminate in the furuncle. In contrast to the skin covering the labia majora, the skin of the labia minora is hairless. The subcutaneous skin, comprised of fragile connective tissue, lacks adipose tissue, allowing for mobility during intercourse. While the labia minora tend to display symmetry, their size and shape can be quite diverse.

Clitoris

The clitoris is the main erectile structure found in women and is comprised of the glans, corpus, and two crura. The glans of the clitoris, are rich in neural nerve endings. The corpus is roughly 2 cm in length and is connected to the pubic ramus through the crura.

Ideal Vulva Perception

While the perception of "normal" is changing rapidly due to the widespread use of the internet and constantly evolving social media trends, it is important to acknowledge that female external genital structures can vary in terms of shape, size, and volume in the context of vulvar anatomy, as in every field of human anatomy (8). Considering the anatomical variations in length, width, and color of labia minora among individuals, it is impossible to establish definitive boundaries for the concept of "normal." Several studies have been conducted on the biological diversities of labia minor width (Table 1.1). Lloyd et al. conducted a study examining 50 premenopausal women who underwent routine hysterectomy or diagnostic laparoscopy under anesthesia. The results showed no statistically significant correlation between labia minora width and age, parity, ethnicity, hormone use, or sexual activity (9). In contrast, Başaran et al. reported that postmenopausal women had considerably narrower labia minora based on their research on 50 premenopausal and 50 postmenopausal women (10). The cause of the disparity between premenopausal and postmenopausal women is ambiguous, potentially as a consequence of limited participant numbers during the study.The perception of "normal" and the variability in the concept of "ideal labia minora" vary across different societies. Women of high socio-economic status in the Western world have more access to perception-forming images in various media. Schick et al. (2008) conducted an analysis and found that just 2.7% of Playboy magazines' worldwide sales in 2007 and 2008 contained photographs with protruded labia minora beyond the labia majora. Moreover, 82.2% of the photographs shown in such magazines and media outlets only display the labia majora, completely obscuring the labia minora within them (11). With a growing variety of epilation methods, demand for which is increasing, women are prompted to inspect their genitalia more closely and contrast them with the media images they have viewed. A 2011 study conducted by Michala et al. discovered that adolescents commonly self-examine their genitalia, with 95% of those desiring labiaplasty in this group believing that their labia minora were "large" due to the influence of social media (12). Avoiding subjective evaluations, the study provides important insights into the impact of social media on adolescent body image perceptions.

Table 1: Mean labia minora width in women

Participants	Method	Mean Age±SD	Mean Labial Width±SD
50 premenopausal women	anaesthesia (+)	35,6±8,7 (18-50)	21,8±9,4 (7,0-50,,0)[1]
50 premenopausal women	anaesthesia (-)	30,2±4,2 (2-39)	17,9±4,1 (11,0-30,0)[2]
50 postmenopausal women	anaesthesia (-)	55,1±301 (7-60)	15,4-4,7 (8,0-27,0)[2]

SD*: Standard deviation
[1]**Llyod et al. *"Female genital appearance'normality' under folds"* (2005)**
[2]**Başaran et al. *"Characteristics of external genitalia in pre-and postmenopausal women"* (2008)**

In certain cultures, labial largeness and voluminosity are associated with female sexual maturity and attainment of "full" adulthood. This is particularly true in Zambian cultures where labial size is thought to be directly proportional to a woman's sexual desire and gratification. Consequently, Zambian women resort to hanging weights on their labia minora to increase the size and length of this body part (13).

Whilst literature data is still lacking, generally it is believed that Western societies have a higher demand for labiaplasty, which may be influenced by media exposure. According to Moran et al's 2014 study, Australian women who typically do not have external genitalia appearance concerns were positively affected by photographs of labia minor reduction surgery results (15). In 2017, Laan et al. conducted a study utilizing the Female Genital Self-Image Scale, which showed that German women experienced more positive thoughts regarding their genitalia after viewing numerous photographs depicting various biological variations of the vulva (16). The results of these two studies illustrate the impact of media in shaping perceptions of "normal" and emphasize the significance of receiving medical advice before undergoing cosmetic gynecological surgery. A study conducted on this topic revealed that 35% of patients who requested labiaplasty discontinued the operation after receiving comprehensive information on the functions of the vulva, vagina, and pelvic floor, various biological variations of the external genitalia, and surgical techniques employed, as well as the potential outcomes and complications that may occur (17).

Definition of Labial Hypertrophy and Overview of Classifications

Labia minora hypertrophy is a concept with varying interpretations. Interest in the subject has gained importance as a result of labial hypertrophy (LH) causing vulvar discomfort and functional symptoms or aesthetic concerns. Hypertrophy in one or both labia minora can lead to irritation, chronic infections, decreased hygiene, and pain during physical activities. Furthermore, in severe cases, hypertrophy can cause dyspareunia as the labia minora may protrude into the vagina during coitus.

Concerns regarding the external genitalia's appearance can lead to emotional and psychological distress. Patients often report feeling self-conscious about a *visible bulge, a fullness, or a hump*, especially when wearing tight clothing. Adolescents in particular, given their susceptibility to mood changes during puberty, can be acutely sensitive to the appearance of their external genitalia. Therefore, both the American Society of Gynaecology and Obstetrics and the North American Association of Paediatrics and Adolescent Gynaecology propose that all patients, particularly adolescents, who wish to undergo labiaplasty should consult a specialist to exclude the possibility of body dysmorphic disorder (18). The study by Veale D. et al. examining psychosexual variables in labiaplasty found that 9 out of 49 patients who had undergone labia minor reduction met the criteria for a body dysmorphic disorder diagnosis (19).

Although labia minora hypertrophy is usually described as "labial tissue protruding beyond the labia majora," there is no agreement on objective criteria for this definition. The physical exam involves measuring the longest distance in millimeters (mm) between the remnants of the hymen and the lateral edges of the labia after gently pulling both labia minora without excessive stretching. This method was initially introduced by Friedrich (20) and is currently used to define LH. Friedrich's classification defines labial width exceeding 5 cm as labia minor hypertrophy. According to subsequent research, normal labial width is considered to be less than 3-4 cm (18). Franco classification categorizes labia minor hypertrophy based on severity (Figure 1). Franco classification comprises 4 groups based on labia minor width: <2 cm, 2-4cm, 4-6 cm, and >6 cm (21). Ricci and

Pardo's classification, along with Davison and West's classification, are used for categorizing LH based on its severity. These classifications are comparable to Franco's (22, 23).

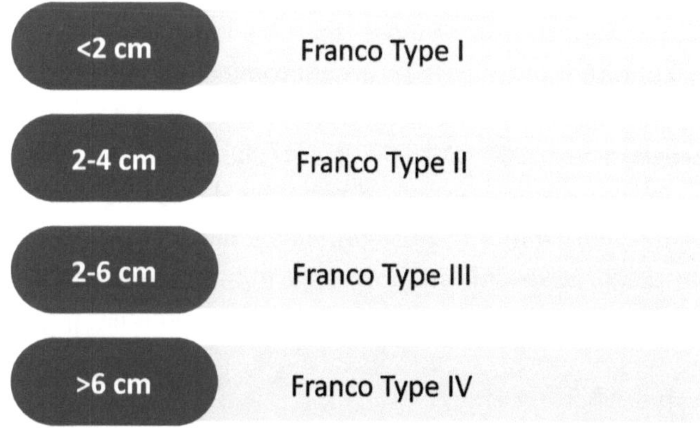

Figure 1: Franco Classification.

Other classifications based on the Franco classification or similar to it have also been published (14,24). Ellsworth and colleagues developed an algorithm that determines the surgical technique based on the Franco classification (Figure 2). For each group in the classification, the algorithm recommends a different labioplasty technique (25). In 2015, Gonzalez and colleagues modified the Franco classification and established a new system of classification (26). Labial hypertrophy in the Franco calcification system is classified based on two new dimensions: localization - anterior (A), central(B) or generalized (C) and symmetry – symmetrical (S) or asymmetrical (AS) (e.g. 2BS- Franco Type II; LH central and symmetrical).

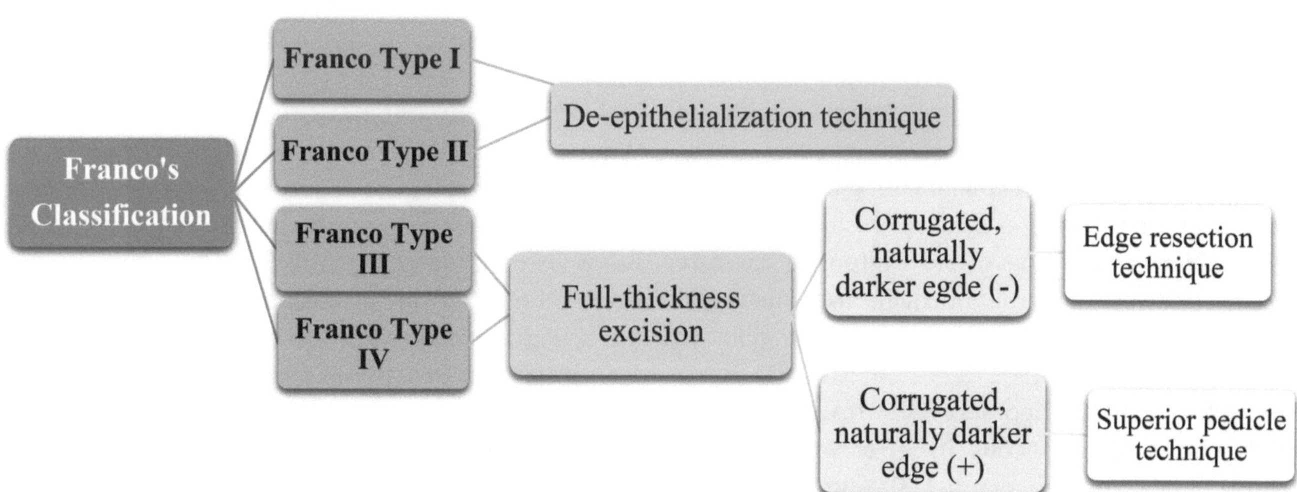

Figure 2: Ellsworth algorithm.

The cause of labia minor hypertrophy remains unclear. Despite numerous hypotheses, a definitive consensus has yet to be established. One prevailing theory suggests that hormonal lesions, such as fibroepithelial stromal polyps, may contribute to hypertrophy (27). Other hypotheses propose that LH indicates chronic lymphedema rather than an anatomical variation (28) or links it with frequent masturbation and multiple pregnancies (29). While current classifications offer a simple comprehension of the typical size and shape of the labia minora, there remains a lack of consensus on the precise definition of labia minora hypertrophy, leading to variations in its surgical management.

Labia Majoraplasty

Simultaneous observation of LH in both labia minor and labia majora is exceedingly uncommon (30, 31). Labia majora hypertrophy can stem from structural causes or excess weight gain.

Surgical interventions for labia majora are typically performed in cases of labia majora hypo- or atrophy. Research indicates that rapid weight loss, multiple births, and menopausal changes are associated with tissue loss in the labia majora (29). In these cases, there is a decrease in hyaluronic acid, dermal collagen, and adipose tissue, leading to a loss of firmness and elasticity in the labia majora, which causes it to appear loose, wrinkled, and devoid of volume. Hypertrophic labia majora may not adequately cover the labia minora, resulting in an enlarged appearance. Vulvar atrophy, particularly during menopause, may lead to complete exclusion of the labia minora and vulvovaginal dryness (32).

Augmentation methods are commonly employed for labia majora hypotrophy and atrophy which are the most prevalent reasons for labia majora surgery. Augmentation of the labia majora using autologous fat tissue transfer is highly effective in restoring volume, shape, symmetry, firmness, and contour in cases of atrophy or hypotrophy. Additionally, hyaluronic acid filling applications are a successful alternative to lipid filling. It is important to note that all the above alternatives have yielded successful results. Another viable option for correcting hypo- or atrophic labia majora is labia majora plasty (33). Surgical removal of excess tissue from the labia majora to address lost volume and sagging can result in a smoother appearance.

Clitoral Hoodoplasty

The preputium clitoris, known as the clitoral hood, is a fold of skin created by the labia minora meeting at the outer edges of the clitoral glans. This excess tissue can appear horizontally and/or vertically. The most prevalent kind is horizontal redundancy, which shows itself as additional skin folds running parallel and lateral to the central portion of the clitoral glans (34).

The folds of the clitoral hood can be unilateral, bilateral, multiple, and/or asymmetrical. In cases of vertical redundancy, the skin folds of the clitoris take on a lengthened and drooping aspect. In cases of vertical redundancy, the skin folds of the clitoris take on a lengthened and drooping aspect. In cases of vertical redundancy, the skin folds of the clitoris take on a lengthened and drooping aspect. This can lead to a lax and drooping appearance of the vulva.

Clitoral hood reduction - clitoral cordectomy or hoodoplasty involves the removal of excess tissue that covers the clitoris. The primary aim is to reduce enlarged and sagging clitoral hoods. Similar to labial tissues, the preputium tissue that covers the clitoris varies in size and volume across individuals. Consequently, it is challenging to provide a clear definition of preputial hypertrophy (34, 35). Patients usually opt for hudoplasty to enhance their vulvar appearance. Some patients may seek out hudoplasty procedures to increase their sexual satisfaction by exposing a larger surface area of the clitoris (36).

Reduction of the clitoral hood, both horizontal and vertical, should only be performed superficially. Excessive removal of neural-rich clitoral tissue can lead to unpredictable and undesirable loss of sensation.

EVALUATION OF THE REQUEST FOR LABIAPLASTY

When assessing the rationale behind the desire for cosmetic gynecological procedures, it is evident that LH and labiaplasty are the most frequently cited reasons for undergoing surgery. While this applies across the spectrum of cosmetic gynecology, there are specific, unique factors that lead patients to opt for surgery, particularly in cases of LH. The reasons for the significant surge in demand for labiaplasty procedures can be categorized into three primary categories: aesthetic, functional, and psychological reasons (Table 2).

Aesthetic Reasons

Given the cosmetic nature of labiaplasty, it's unsurprising that patient motivation typically hinges on aesthetic concerns. A study by Miklos JR et al. explored this further and found that 37% of patients were solely motivated by aesthetic reasons, while 31% cited both aesthetic and functional reasons (31). While the basis of aesthetic reasons is the patient's perception of the labium(s) as "abnormal", the most common aesthetic concerns are the size of the labium (most frequently), asymmetry and/or color changes in the labium (22, 23, 37, 38).

Functional Causes

Data from a limited number of studies indicate that the enlarged size of the labia is directly linked to functional reasons (25, 31, 39, 40).

Hygienic Concerns

The enlargement of labia minora and labial tissues, which become curved with LH, can result in a sensation of decreased hygiene, notably during menstruation (41). Moreover, in severe cases, the accumulation of physiological or pathological vaginal discharge and toilet paper residues between the hypertrophied and enlarged labial or clitoral folds can be distressing for the patient. It is therefore crucial to seek medical advice for effective management. In such cases, obsessive genital hygiene and frequent cleaning of the vulva may lead to irritation, dermatosis, and vulvovaginal dryness.

Table 2: Patient motivation in labiaplasty

Aesthetic Causes	Functional Causes	Psychological Causes
Size	Hygienic concerns	Embarrassment of the image
Asymmetry	Pain and discomfort	Loss of self-confidence
Colour change	Sexual dysfunction	Anxiety/depression
		Mood changes

Pain and Discomfort

Enlarged labia can cause discomfort and pain, particularly when wearing tight clothing (22, 25, 42). Tight undergarments, trousers, and swimsuits may lead to compression of the labia minora, causing pain and restricting daily activities. Patients have reported discomfort while closing zippers or sitting (41, 43).

Furthermore, physical activities like walking, swimming, cycling, and horse riding have been found to induce extensive discomfort and pain (43, 44, 45).

Sexual Dysfunction

Enlarged labia minora with increased size and volume can lead to pain during sexual intercourse (15, 37, 41, 43, 44, 46). Furthermore, in severe cases of hypertrophy, protruding labial and/or clitoral tissues may become inverted into the vagina during coitus, resulting in severe dyspareunia (46).

Psychological Reasons

Psychological factors are often cited among the reasons prompting patients to undergo labiaplasty. Distinguishing between psychological and aesthetic motives can be challenging due to their intertwined nature. It is important to acknowledge and address these factors inpatient consultations and treatment plans. The most frequently encountered psychological reasons in women seeking labiaplasty are embarrassment regarding the appearance of the labia and clitoris (15, 37, 38, 41, 45), anxiety and depression (39, 44), lack of self-confidence (39, 41, 44, 47), and mood changes (22). The findings of Bramwell R. et al.'s qualitative research indicate that patients who underwent labiaplasty experienced anxious insecurity regarding their labia in the preoperative stage. They also expressed fear of their partners seeing or touching their external genitalia and faced difficulty initiating new relationships (48).

RISKS AND COMPLICATIONS

Labiaplasty is a cosmetic gynecological surgery with rare complications and high patient satisfaction. However, it carries numerous general and specific surgical risks and complications. As such, the common perception of labiaplasty as a "low-risk and painless" procedure is inaccurate and needs to be corrected. The findings of a study carried out by Zuckerman D. et al. indicate that patients typically anticipate their surgical procedure to be both pain-free and risk-free (49).

Insufficient data exists on the lasting effects of labiaplasty on sexual function. The correlation between the volume increase of the labia minora and sexual stimulation and pleasure has not yet been elucidated. Thus, predictions regarding the effects of labia minor reduction on sexual pleasure are inadequate (37). Tissue loss, particularly in cases with extensive resection, may contribute to a reduction in sexual arousal and the loss of sensation (43, 50). Cases, where hymenoplasty is not performed superficially, may lead to insufficient arousal and orgasm disorders due to impaired innervation (42, 51). Therefore, careful attention should be paid to cases in the adolescent group who have not yet completed their biological, physiological, and psychological development. Unnecessary resections performed in patients with incomplete pubertal development may cause nerve damage and loss of sensation

In addition to the possible loss of sensation, labiaplasty carries a range of common risks and complications. These include bleeding, infection, hematoma, necrosis and scar formation, permanent discoloration of the tissues, postoperative asymmetry and inequality in tissue volume, dyspareunia, and dehiscence (Table 3).

Complications, such as subcutaneous ecchymosis, edema, and pain, frequently occur after labiaplasty; however, they are self-limiting within the first two weeks postoperatively, generally without the need for additional intervention (55, 56). Scar formation in excised labia minora is an extremely rare complication and remains the most frequent reason for patient-based revision requests, together with postoperative asymmetry (55). Undoubtedly, partial or total resection of the labia minora (57) is the most dramatic complication seen in labiaplasty cases. When accompanied by hudoplasty procedures not performed with the correct techniques, these cases may result in penalisation of the clitoris. This is the second most common reason for the need for revision after scar formation (56, 57, 58).

Table 3: Risks and complications in labiaplasty.

1. Anaesthesia-related risks[52]
2. General surgical complications (bleeding, infection)[52]
3. Scar formation[52'53]
4. Permanent discoloration of tissues[52]
5. Serration of labial margins[52]
6. Necrosis[52]
7. Dyspareunia[39'52]
8. Haematoma[39'53]
9. Dehiscence[40]

The main complications in labiaplasty are the formation of hematoma and dehiscence. Hence, it is necessary to conduct a thorough assessment of high-risk patients and predisposing factors during the preoperative period.

Anticoagulant usage and coagulation disorders are both significant risk factors for hematoma formation. The primary predisposing factors for hematoma formation following labiaplasty can be summarised as inadequate intraoperative hemostasis, insufficient use of epinephrine during interventions carried out under local anesthesia, the presence of dead space in the wound, and post-operative trauma (refer to Table 4). The prevention of hematoma formation requires careful perioperative bleeding control and suturing techniques that leave no dead space. Additionally, successful outcomes have been demonstrated with the application of tight dressing methods within the first 24-48 hours postoperatively for at-risk patients (source 60). Small, stable hematomas less than 2 cm can be monitored without additional intervention. Hematomas that are larger or cause significant tension on the suture line based on their location should be evacuated (60).

Table 4: Risk factors for hematoma

Patients in the risk group
Anticoagulant users and those with coagulation disorders
Predisposing factors
Intraoperative inadequate haemostasis
Not using Epinephrine in local anesthesia
Dead space in the wound
Postoperative trauma
Failure of the patient to follow postoperative instructions

Wound dehiscence typically occurs during the first week after surgery, although it may develop later in patients who are at risk for impaired wound healing. Increased tension at the suture line, tissue atrophy, inadequate wound care, patient non-compliance with postoperative instructions, systemic corticosteroid use, poor wound tissue perfusion (as in diabetes, obesity, and anemia), and infection are the main contributing factors leading to dehiscence. Dehiscence cases that occur during the early postoperative period are typically the result of technical errors related to suturing. If detected within the first 48 hours, repair can be primarily performed, provided that no signs of infection are present at the wound site.

Superficial dehiscences are more commonly reported with edge resections in labioplasties (55, 61).

In cases of superficial dehiscence, it is advisable to wash the wound daily with antiseptic and antimicrobial agents and allow for secondary healing (60). If there are indications of infection at the wound site, systemic or topical antibiotherapy may be initiated. The wound healing process is more complex with deep dehiscences. Open wounds resulting from the surgical incision of large hematomas can also fall under this classification. In such cases, the wound site is typically infected and requires time for healing before secondary suturing can take place. Wedge resection labioplasties are often associated with deep dehiscences that require secondary suturing (61). However, there is no consensus on the appropriate timing for revision (60). It is commonly recommended that wounds be left to heal secondarily and systemic treatment with broad-spectrum antibiotics should be initiated (60, 61). It is advised to closely monitor the wound and conduct surgical debridement when necessary. Secondary suturing may be considered once the wound is free from infection and necrotic tissue.

Although very rarely, cellulitis may be observed in the vulva and in the area where fat augmentation is performed in patients undergoing labia major augmentation. Symptoms of the condition typically include fever, pain, and tenderness between the 5th and 10th days (62). In the presence of required indications, hospitalization and antibiotherapy with Gram (+), Gram (-), and anaerobic broad-spectrum agents are recommended.

WHO SHOULD DO IT?

The rising popularity of labiaplasty and other vulvar cosmetic procedures often leads to the question of which medical professionals should carry out such operations. Cosmetic gynecological surgery is typically performed by gynecologists, obstetricians, as well as plastic and reconstructive surgery experts worldwide. However, there have also been instances of urologists and other specialists performing labiaplasty (37). Furthermore, it has been documented that specialized doctors, including general practitioners, are authorized to carry out cosmetic surgery on the vulva in the United States, regardless of their specialty (63).

It is a universally accepted notion that the mastery of pelvic anatomy of gynecologists and obstetricians gives them a more objective evaluation of the size, volume, and symmetry of vulvar structures (63). Additionally, their extensive experience in pelvic operations could be an asset in predicting and preventing complications unique to this area.

LABIAPLASTY IN COSMETIC GYNECOLOGICAL SURGERY

The term *labioplasty* is commonly used to describe the surgical reduction of the labia - *labial reduction*. Despite the development of numerous techniques for labial reduction in recent years, edge resection (trim technique) and wedge resection remain the most commonly employed methods (64).

Edge Resection

The edge resection technique, also known as the *trim or direct incision technique*, is considered to be the first method for reducing labia minora in the literature (65). This procedure involves the simple longitudinal excision of excessive, sagging, or hyperpigmented edges of both labia minora (Figure 3). During a labiaplasty performed with the "trim" technique, the surgeon trims away any excess tissue from the labia minora, essentially reducing the size of the labia (Figure 4). The edges are then repositioned and sutured together to create a symmetrical appearance.

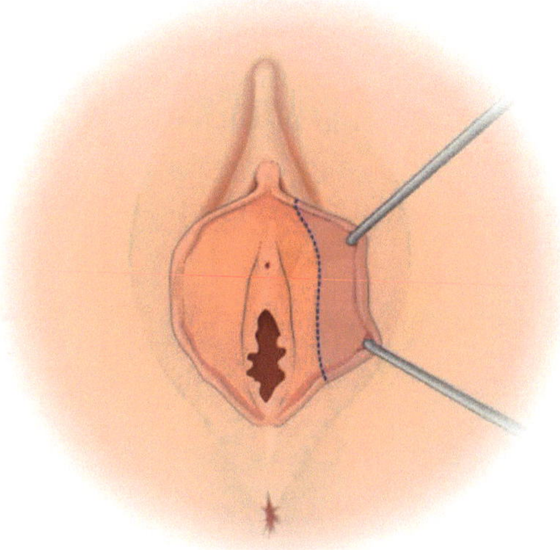

Figure 3: Edge resection technique.

** Lina Triana. Aesthetic Vaginal Plastic Surgery A Practical Guide, 2020*

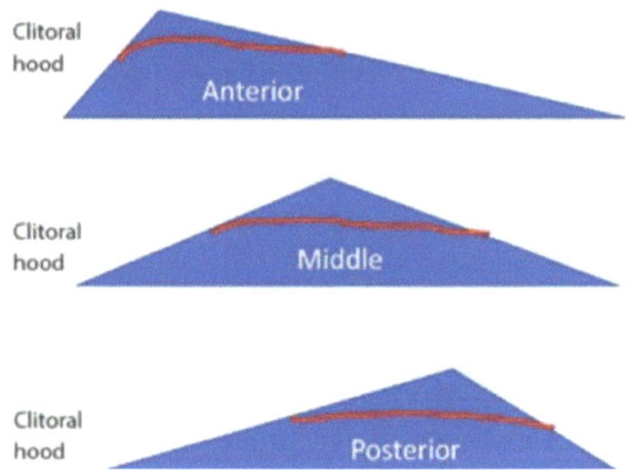

Figure 4: Edge resection (trim technique).

Ewa Majdak-Paredes, GENERAL PLASTIC SURGERY, CPD - THE PMFA JOURNAL, *2019*

Numerous studies conducted from 1976 to 2014 have favored the edge resection technique in terms of patient satisfaction and mobility rates (64). The low risk of dehiscence, technical convenience in cases to be combined with hoodoplasty, and the fact that it is the most suitable option for patients whose primary complaint is hyperpigmentation on the labia minora margins are the most important reasons for the technique to maintain its popularity today.

The most commonly documented complications associated with the trim technique are scarring and uneven labial margins, as well as thickening, sensory alteration, and scar retraction (34). These complications are predisposed by locating the suture line along the free edge of the labia minora in the edge resection technique. Performing the resection inclined by the anatomical slope of the labia minora, leaving the outer edge of the incision line a few millimeters longer than the inner edge, and not making the suturing too taut will be useful in preventing these complications (Image 1).

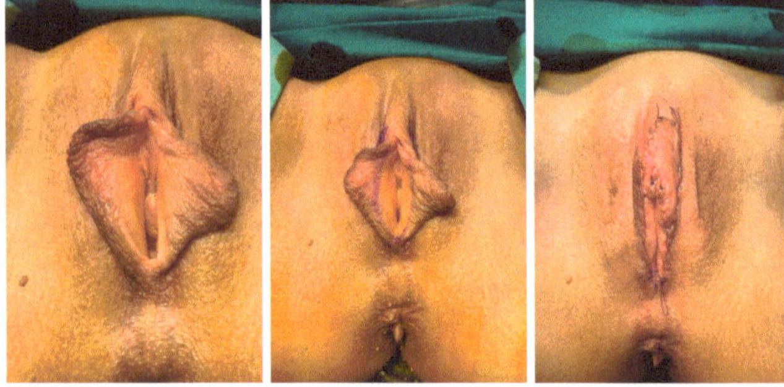

Image 1. Edge resection (trim technique).

The most dramatic complication of edge resection is undoubtedly the near-total resection of the labia minora. Complete amputation of the labial margins,

especially in cases not accompanied by hudoplasty, may cause the prepuce to appear as a protrusion-clitoral *penisation* (58,58) (Image 2). Failure to make the incision in a straight and smooth line and excessive removal of tissue from the labial margins, especially from the central region, may cause scar formation called "dog ear" (superiorly and inferiorly). Clitoral penisation and dog ear scar formation are the most common reasons for patient dissatisfaction and revision requests after labiaplasty operations performed with the edge resection technique (58). Especially in cases of clitoral penisation, revision of these deformities is very difficult because there is not enough labial tissue left behind. To avoid these complications, marking of the tissue planned to be removed should be done carefully and excessive pulling (stretching) of the labial tissue should be avoided during the incision.

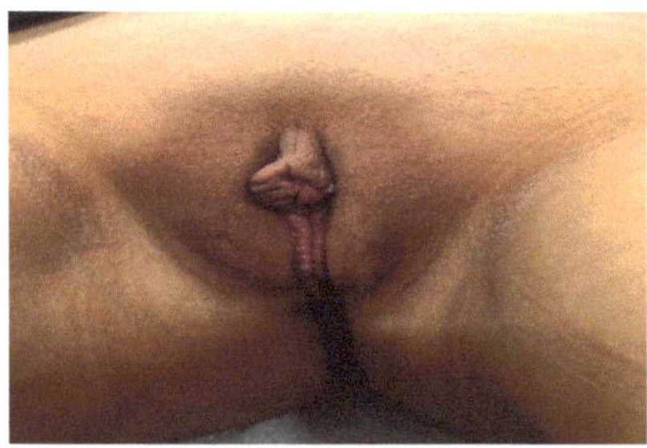

Image 2. Clitoral penisatin after trim technique.

Wedge Resection

The wedge resection technique was initially reported by Gary Alter in 1998 (66). One of the main benefits of this approach compared to the edge resection technique is the preservation of the labia minora's free edge anatomy, which results in a more natural reduction image. The technique involves removing a V-shaped tissue from the most protruding part of the labial margin via wedge resection (Figure 4).

As pigmentation changes in the labia minora generally arise at the free labial margins, the application of this technique may not be appropriate for patients whose primary concern is hyperpigmentation. Another disadvantage is that it requires a separate incision for hudoplasty in patients in whom composite reductions are planned.

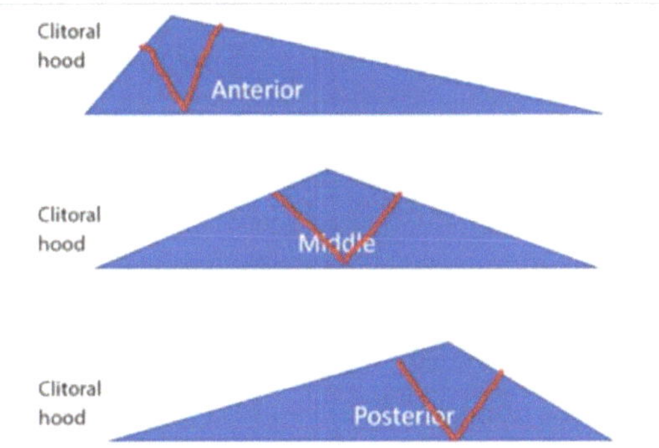

Figure 5: Wedge resection.

Ewa Majdak-Paredes, GENERAL PLASTIC SURGERY, CPD - THE PMFA JOURNAL, 2019

Over the years, different modifications of the technique have been developed both by Alter himself and by other research surgeons (see Figure 5). The high patient satisfaction rates and extremely low complication and revision requirement rates make the wedge resection technique and its modifications one of the two most popular techniques of labia minor plasty (58, 66, 67, 68, 69).

The most common complication encountered in labial reductions performed with the wedge resection technique is dehiscence and deep dehiscences requiring secondary suturing have been reported (61). To mitigate these complications, the tissue to be excised ought not to be excessively stretched during the resection process and vigilance must be maintained to ensure that the margins of resection are vertical and non-curvilinear. Curvilinear incisions may heighten the likelihood of dehiscence by intensifying tension along the suture line.

Suturing the edges of the incision every day can improve healing at the suture line and enhance the final appearance aesthetically. To minimize scar formation, it is advisable to suture the external and internal sides of the labia minora separately. It is also recommended to ensure that the free distal ends of the resection are end-to-end.

Şekil 6. Wedge rezeksiyon tekniği ve modifikasyonları: A. The wedge resection technique, G. Alter 1998 (66). **B.** The extended central wedge resection technique, G. Alter 2008 (58). **C.** The posterior wedge resection technique, Kelishadi et al 2013 (67). **D.** The inferior wedge resection technique, Rouzier et al 2000 (68). **E.** The W-shaped resection, Mass and Hage 2000 (69).

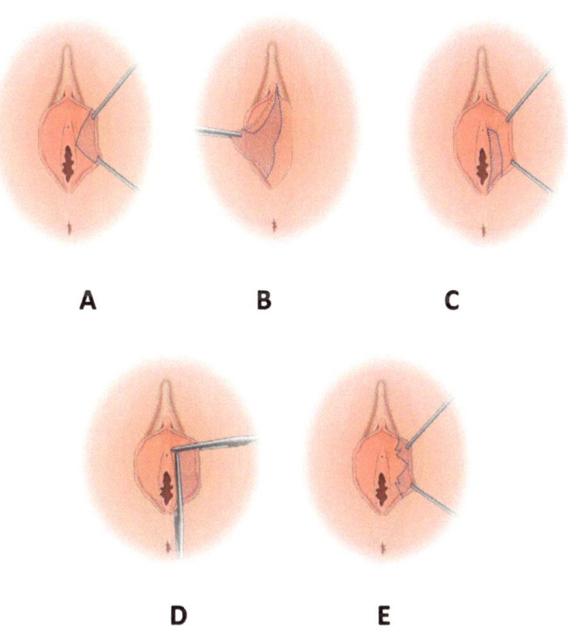

** Lina Triana. Aesthetic Vaginal Plastic Surgery A Practical Guide, 2020*

REFERENCES

1. CME review article 12. Gianna W. et all. Vaginal Rejuvenation: A Review of Female Genital Cosmetic Surgery,2018

2. Mauriceau F. *Traite des Maladies des Femmes Grosses et de Cellesqui sont Accouchees* (FRENCH) 3rd edn (Par la Compagnie des libraires, Paris, 1681)

3. Meissner, F.L. *Die Frauenzimanerkrankheiten nch den neuesten Ansichten und Bandes erste Abtheilung (GERMAN) (Otto Wigand, Leipzig, 1842)*

4. Treub, H. *Leerboek der Gynaecologie* (van Doesburgh, Leiden,1892)

5. LH Honoré, KE O'Hara. Benign enlargement of the labia minora: report of two cases. Eur J Obstet Gynecol Reprod Biol 1978 Apr;8(2):61-4.

6. Felicio Yde A. Labial Surgery. *Aesthet Sung J.* 2007;27;322-328

7. Mc Gregor JC. Labial Surgery: A new phenomenon? March 2009 Journal of Plastic Reconstructive & Aesthetic Surgery 62(3):289

8. British Association of Aesthetic Plastic Surgeons (BAAPS). Aesthetic genital surgery: female genital aesthetic surgery (aesthetic genital surgery, designer vaginas). London: British Association of Aesthetic Plastic Surgeons (BAAPS); [2011].

9. Lloyd, J. N. S. C., Minto, C. l., Liao, L. M. & Creighton, S. M. Female genital appearance: 'normality' unfolds*. BJOG 112, 643–646 (2005)

10. Basaran, M., Bayar, U. & Civelek, B. Characteristics of external genitalia in pre-and postmenopausal women. Climacteric 11, 416–421 (2008)

11. Schick, V. R., Rima, B. N. & Calabrese, S. K. Evulvalution: the portrayal of women's external genitalia and physique across time and the current Barbie Doll ideals. J. Sex. Res. 48, 74–81 (2011).

12. Michala, L., Koliantzaki, S. & Antsaklis, A. Protruding labia minora: abnormal or just uncool? J. Psychosom. Obstet. Gynaecol. 32, 154–156 (2011)

13. Pérez, G. M., Mubanga, M., Aznar, C. T. & Bagnol, B. Zambian women in South Africa: Insights into health experiences of labia elongation. J. Sex. Res. 52, 857– 867 (2015).

14. Müjde Ö, Indiana M, Elise P. J, Margriet G. M. Labiaplasty: motivation, techniques, and ethics. NATURE REVIEWS | UROLOGY, 2018

15. Moran, C. & Lee, C. What's normal? Influencing women's perceptions of normal genitalia: an experiment involving exposure to modified and nonmodified images. BJOG 121, 761–766 (2014)

16. Laan, E., Hesselink, S., Snijders, N. & van Lunsen, R. H. W. Young women's genital self-image and effects of exposure to pictures of natural vulva. J. Psychosom. Obstet. Gynaecol. 38, 249–255 (2017).

17. Ozer, M., Laan, E. T. M. & van Lunsen, R. H. W. Read my lips: het effect van counseling van vrouwen met een verzoek tot labiareductie [DUTCH]. Reproductieve geneeskunde, gynaecologie en obstetrie 646–650 (2009).

18. Marc R Laufer, MDJhansi Reddy, MD, FACOG. Labia minora hypertrophy. UpToDate, 2020

19. Veale D, Naismith I, Eshkevari E, et al. Psychosexual outcome after labiaplasty: a prospective case-comparison study. Int Urogynecol J 2014; 25:831.

20. Freidrich EG. Vulvar Disease, 2nd ed, WB Saunders, Philadelphia 1983.

21. Franco, T. & Diogo, F. Nympha hypertrophy. J. Bras. Gynecol. 103, 163–168 (1993).

22. Pardo J, Ricci P, Solà V. Comment on Pauls: "Nip, tuck and rejuvenate: the latest frontier for the gynecologic surgeon". International Urogynecology Journal And Pelvic Floor Dysfunction. 2008;19(6):889-90.

23. Davison SP, de la Torre JI. Labiaplasty and labia minora reduction. Medscape Reference. 2011(Article 1372175 (Nov. 28)):1-5.

24. Women's Health Issue Paper No. 9. Women and Genital Cosmetic Surgery. Women's Health Victoria, 2018

25. Ellsworth, W. A. et al. Techniques for labia minora reduction: an algorithmic approach. Aesthet. Plast. Surg. 34, 105–110 (2010).

26. Gonzalez, P. I. Classification of hypertrophy of labia minora: consideration of a multiple component approach. Surg. Technol. Int. 27, 191–194 (2015).

27. Heller DS, Kuye OO. Recurrent hypertrophy of the labia minora: a hormonally related lesion possibly related to fibroepithelial stromal polyps of the vulva. J Lower Genit Tract Dis. 2011;15:69-70.

28. Barrett MM, Carlson JA. A clinicopathologic study of labia minora hypertrophy: signs of localized lymphedema were universal. J Lower Genit Tract Dis. 2014;18:13-20

29. Carlo Maria Oranges, MD; Andrea Sisti, MD; and Giovanni Sisti, MD. Labia minora reduction techniques: a comprehensive literature review. Aesthet Surg J 2015 May;35(4):419-31.

30. Di Saia JP. An unusual staged labial rejuvenation. J Sex Med. 2008;5:1263-1267. [discussion].

31. Miklos JR, Moore RD. Labiaplasty of the labia minora: patients' indications for pursuing surgery. The Journal Of Sexual Medicine. 2008;5(6):1492-5.

32. Salgado CJ, Tang JC, Desrosiers AE 3rd (2012) Use of dermal fat graft for augmentation of the labia majora. J Plast Reconstr Aesthet Surg 65(2):267–270

33. Alinsod R (2006) Overview of vaginal rejuvenation, new frontiers in pelvic surgery. NSOCP/AAOCG, Las Vegas

34. Lina Triana. Aesthetic Vaginal Plastic Surgery A Practical Guide. ISBN 978-3-030-24818-5 ISBN 978-3-030-24819-2 (eBook) https://doi.org/10.1007/978-3-030-24819-2

35. Cheryl B Iglesia. Ladin Yurteri-Kaplan. Red Alison. Female genital cosmetic surgery: a review of techniques and outcomes. Int Urogynecol J 2013 Dec;24(12):1997-2009.doi:10.1007/s00192-013-2117-8. Epub 2013 May 22.

36. Goodman MP (2009) Female cosmetic genital surgery. Obstet Gynecol 113(1):154–159

37. Braun V. Female genital cosmetic surgery: a critical review of current knowledge and contemporary debates. Journal of Women's Health. 2010;19(7):1393-407.

38. Benadiba L. [Labiaplasty: plastic or cosmetic surgery?: indications, techniques, results, and complications]. Annales De Chirurgie Plastique Et Esthétique. 2010;55(2):147-52.

39. Ostrzenski A. Cosmetic gynecology in the view of evidence-based medicine and ACOG recommendations: a review. Archives Of Gynecology And Obstetrics. 2011;284(3):617-30.

40. Tepper OM, Wulkan M, Matarasso A. Labioplasty: anatomy, etiology, and a new surgical approach. Aesthetic Surgery Journal / The American Society For Aesthetic Plastic Surgery. 2011;31(5):511-8.

41. Lynch A, Marulaiah M, Samarakkody U. Reduction labioplasty in adolescents. Journal Of Pediatric And Adolescent Gynecology. 2008;21(3):147-9

42. Liao LM, Creighton SM. Requests for cosmetic genitoplasty: how should healthcare providers respond? BMJ: British Medical Journal. 2007;334(7603):1090-2.

43. Davison SP, de la Torre JI. Labiaplasty and labia minora reduction. Medscape Reference. 2011(Article 1372175 (Nov. 28)):1-5.

44. Berer M. Labia reduction for non-therapeutic reasons vs. female genital mutilation: contradictions in law and practice in Britain. Reproductive Health Matters. 2010;18(35):106-10.

45. Deans R, Liao L-M, Crouch NS, Creighton SM. Why are women referred for female genital cosmetic surgery? The Medical Journal Of Australia. 2011;195(2):99-. Available from:

46. Bramwell R, Morland C. Genital appearance satisfaction in women: the development of a questionnaire and exploration of correlates. Journal of Reproductive and Infant Psychology. 2009;27(1):15-27.

47. Crouch N, Deans R, Michala L, Liao L, Creighton SM. Clinical characteristics of good women seeking labial reduction surgery: a prospective study. BJOG: An International Journal Of Obstetrics And Gynaecology. 2011;10:1-4.

48. Bramwell R, Morland C, Garden AS. Expectations and experience of labial reduction: a qualitative study. BJOG an International Journal of Obstetrics and Gynaecology. 2007;114(12):1493-9.

49. Zuckerman D. Reasonably safe?: breast implants and informed consent. Reproductive Health Matters. 2010;18(35):94-102.

50. Schober J, Cooney T, Pfaff D, Mayoglou L, Martin-Alucil N. Innervation of the labia minora of prepubertal girls. Journal Of Pediatric And Adolescent Gynecology. 2010;23(6):352-7.

51. Zielinski RE. Private places- private shame: women's genital body image and sexual health [Thesis]. Ann Arbor, Michigan: University of Michigan; 2009.

52. Australian Society of Plastic Surgeons (ASPS). Cosmetic genital surgery: labiaplasty and phalloplasty. Melbourne: Victoria. Department of Health; 2011 - (Better Health Channel Factsheet).

53. Goodman MP. Female genital cosmetic and plastic surgery: a review. The Journal Of Sexual Medicine. 2011;8(6):1813-25.

54. Green FJ. From clitoridectomies to 'designer vaginas': the medical construction of heteronormative female bodies and sexuality through female genital cutting. Sexualities, Evolution and Gender. 2005;7(2):153-87.

55. Liasta F. et al. The Safety of Aesthetic Labioplasty. Aesthet Surg J. 2015

56. Hunter JG et. al. Cosmetic Surgery of the Female External Genitalia. Current Cosmetic Surgery,2010

57. Ckoi HY et al. *A new Method of aesthetic reduction of labia minora.* Plast Reconstr Surg, 2000

58. Alter GJ et al. *Aesthetc Labia Minora and Clitoraql Hood Reduction.* Plast Reconstr Surg, 2008

59. Oranges CM et al. *Labis Minora Reduction Techniques.* Aesthetic Surg J. 2015

60. Uptodate. Basic principles of wound healing. Prevention and treatment of complications. 2020

61. John G et al. Labia minaora, Labia majora and Clitoral Hood Alteration,2015

62. Marc P. Lachiewicz et al. Pelvic surgical site infections in gynecologic surgery, 2015.

63. Keil A. Genital anxiety and the quest for the perfect vulva: a feminist analysis of female genital cosmetic surgery. Irvine, CA: Unpublished paper, submitted to University of California Irvine. Department of Anthropology. Women and the Body Subject; 2010.

64. Carlo Maria Oranges, MD; Andrea Sisti, MD; and Giovanni Sisti, MD. Labia Minora Reduction Techniques: A Comprehensive Literature Review. Aesthetic Surgery Journal 2015, Vol 35(4) 419–431 © 2015 The American Society for Aesthetic Plastic Surgery, Inc.

65. Capraro VJ. Congenital anomalies. Clin Obstet Gynecol. 1971;14:988-1012.

66. Alter GJ. A new technique for aesthetic labia minora reduction. Ann Plast Surg. 1998;40:287-290.

67. Kelishadi SS, Elston JB, Rao AJ, Tutela JP, Mizuguchi NN. Posterior wedge resection: a more aesthetic labiaplasty. Aesthet Surg J. 2013;33:847-853.

68. Rouzier R, Louis-Sylvestre C, Paniel BJ, Haddad B. Hypertrophy of labia minora: experience with 163 reductions. Am J Obstet Gynecol. 2000;182:35-40.

69. Maas SM, Hage JJ. Functional and aesthetic labia minora reduction. Plast Reconstr Surg. 2000;105:1453-1456.

CLITORAL HOOD REDUCTION

Garima Srivastav

- Clitoral hood reduction (CHR) is rarely done as an isolated procedure.
- Most commonly performed with labia minora reduction.
- Functional outcome is poorly understood, and the effect on sexual function has not been established.
- More of an aesthetic procedure.
- Distinguished from other clitoral procedures.
- Clitoral hood resection, also termed clitoral cordectomy, clitoral unhooding, clitoridectomy, or partial hoodectomy is a procedure for reducing the size and area of Clitoral hood (prepuce) in order to further expose clitoral glans.
- Therapeutic goals are to improve sexual gratification and aesthetic refinement of the vulva.
- The upper part of labia minora diverges into 2 branches. the superior branch of labia minora is termed as clitoral prepuce and inferior branch as clitoral frenulum.

ANATOMY

- Poorly defined in literature.
- Some authors write it as a superior division of labia minora.
- Most refer to the free edge of the prepuce to the clitoral hood.
- Aesthetic surgeons consider it as extending anteriorly and superiorly to the anterior labial commissure, the inferior border is the free edge of the prepuce and extends down to the junction of labia minora.
- Frenulum – portion of labia minora that extends to the clitoris and begins medial to the attachment of clitoral hood.
- Laterally bounded by interlabial sulcus.
- The layers of the midportion of the hood from superficial to deep are skin, subcutaneous tissue, dartos fascia, buck fascia and suspensory ligament, neurovascular bundle, tunica albuginea, and clitoris.
- An ideal configuration of glans to prepuce has not been established.
- Typically, glans will protrude slightly beyond the hood with varying degrees of visibility.
- Innervation by dorsal nerve of clitoris.

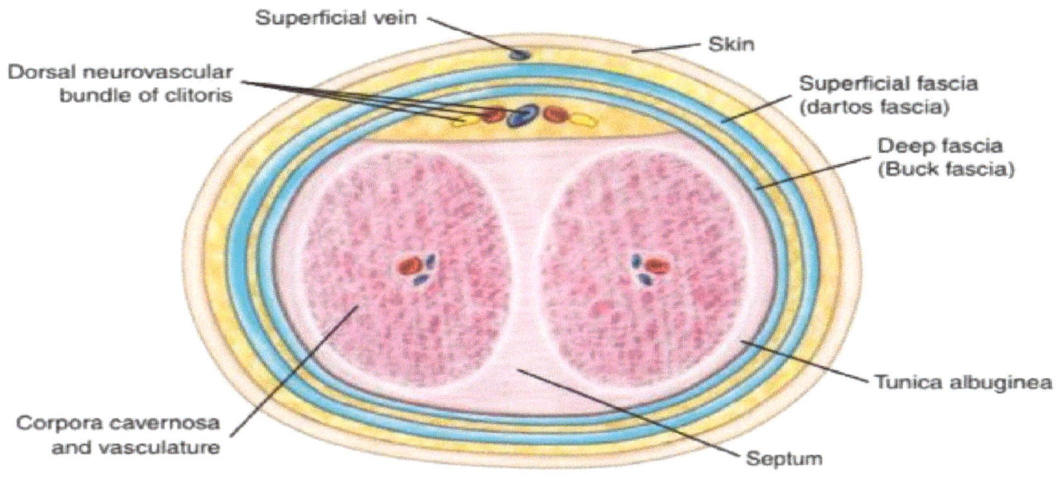

A Transverse section through the body of clitoris.

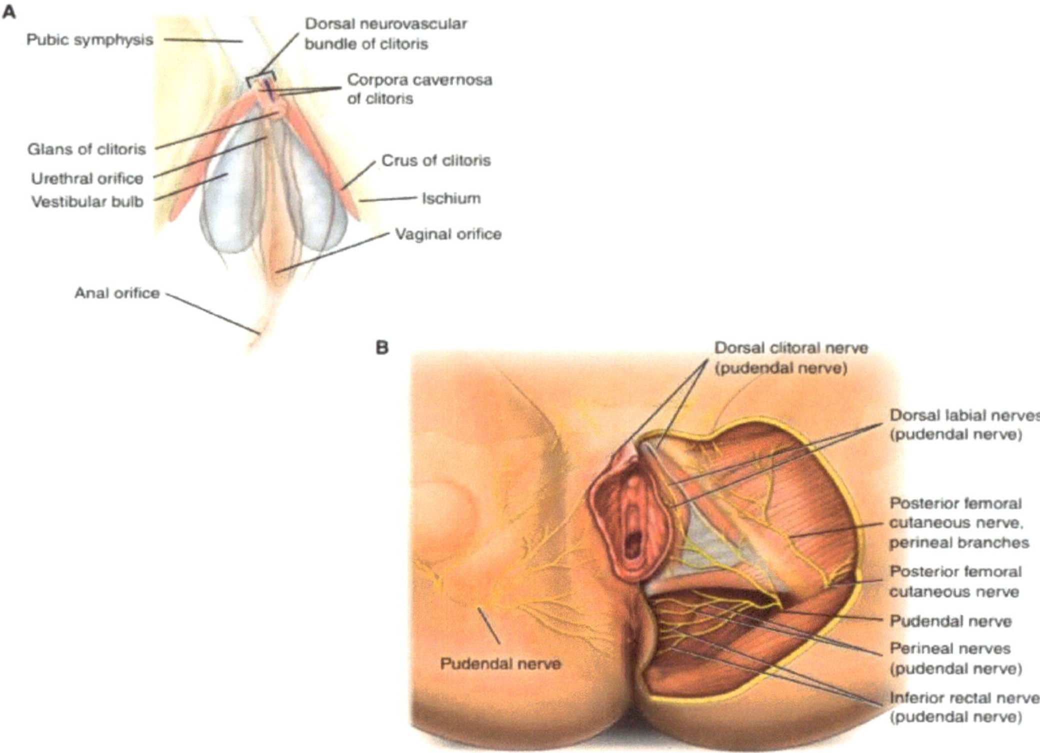

A. Clitoral structures and relationshio to pubic bone with pudendal nerve and sensory branches of the clitoris

B. Sensory nerves of the vulva with relationship to pelvic floor muscles.

Ostrzenski clitoris hood abnormalities classification

Description	Anatomic Presentation
Type 1: occluded	The clitoris is buried under a partially or completely closed clitoral hood opening
Type 2: hypertrophic-gaping	The clitoral hood skin is elongated or thick
Type 3: hypertrophic with subdermal asymmetry	The thickness of the clitoral hood skin is uneven

INDICATIONS

- The goal of surgery is to debulk and reduce excess or redundant clitoral prepuce.
- However specific indications are less clear.
- Goodman noted that CHR is intended to produce more exposure of the clitoral body, theoretically providing improved sexual stimulation but did not substantiate the claim, he restated aesthetic indications.
- Removal of unsightly lateral hood.
- Hunter suggested surgeons must never expose/ further expose the clitoris.

Evaluation

- No established tools for evaluating CHR patients have been established.
- Evaluation at both lying down and standing level.
- Gress advised measuring the distance from the glans clitoris to the urethral meatus and stated that it must be a minimum of 1.5 cm
- Ostrazenski proposed clitoral hood classification which is not widely accepted but related to his surgical approaches

CLITORAL HOOD REDUCTION

Cannot be performed in patients whose clitoral hood opening is occluded. (Ostrzenski Type 1). Used in patients with Ostrzenski type 2 hypertrophic- gaping deformities of the clitoral hood.

Resection of an extended central wedge reduces tissue at the clitoral hood using the anterior hockey stick–shaped resection.

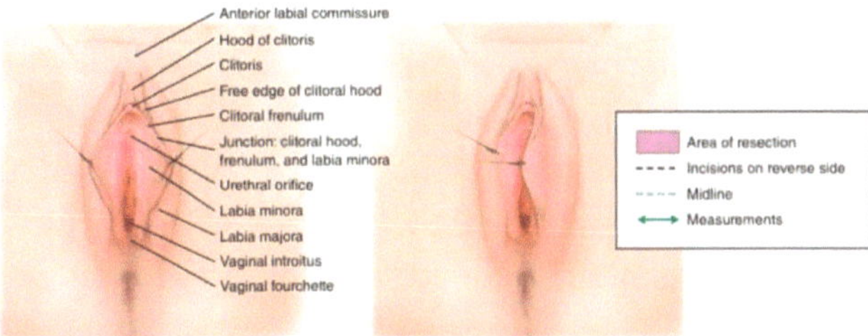

Fig. 7-4 Female vulvar anatomy.

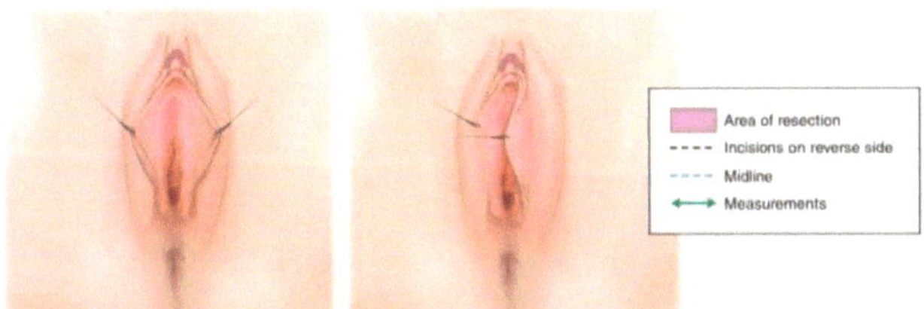

Fig. 7-5 CHR described by Graves et al[1] as an integral part of clitoromegaly surgery.

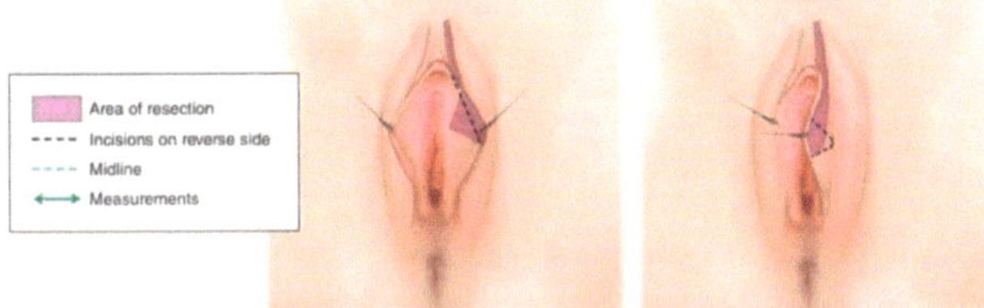

Fig. 7-6 CHR described by Alter[24] as an addition to labia minora wedge resection.

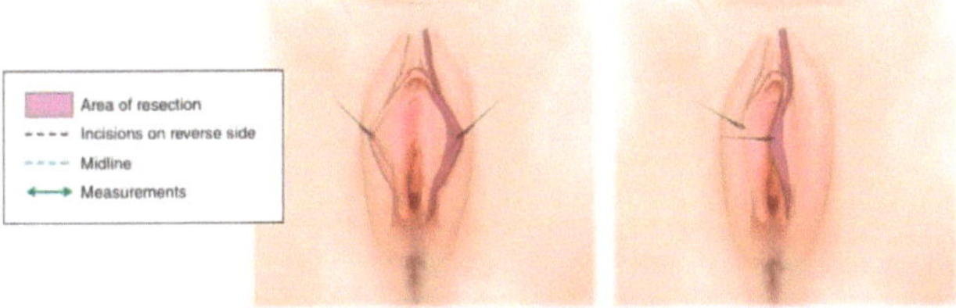

Fig. 7-7 CHR initially described by Gress[26] as part of a composite reduction labiaplasty.

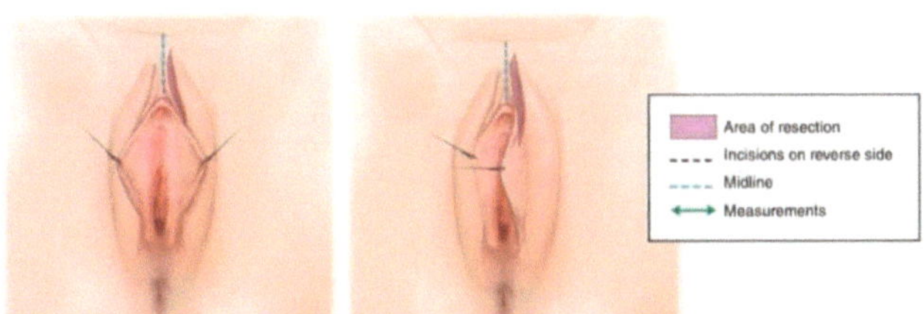

Fig. 7-8 Isolated CHR described by de Alencar Felicio.[6]

Clitoral Hood Reduction

Clitoral hood may be excessive tissue in the horizontal or vertical plane.

Vertical excess

Vertical hood excess is addressed by transverse excision of a portion of the hood, usually by an inverted V wedge across its full width.

Clitoral Hood longitudinal resection

- Mild to moderate excess of the clitoral hood can be treated by longitudinal resection and reapproximation of the edges.
- This approach involves amputation of the clitoral hood border and positions the scar in the skin-mucosa transition.

To perform this procedure, the clitoral hood is lifted, and the excess skin is resected with scissors.

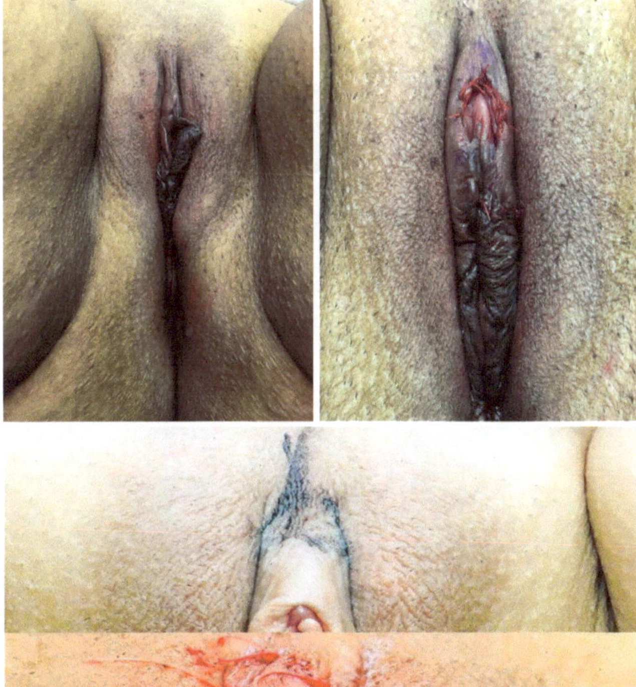

Horizontal excess

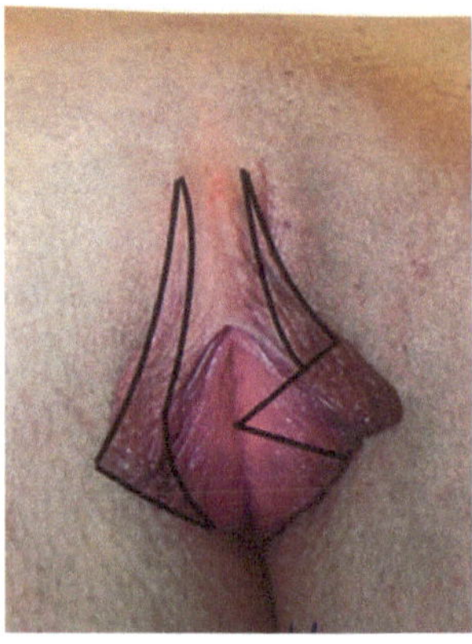

Horizontal excess in the form of extra hood folds parallel and lateral to the portion of the central portion of the clitoral hood and is most commonly observed.

Clitoral Hood horseshoe resection

- Excess tissue at the clitoral hood can be resected in a horseshoe design with the incision at the base of the hood.
- This technique can be performed in patients who have severe tissue excess, but care must be taken to avoid overresection and exposure of the clitoris.
- The horseshoe resection may be extended beyond the limits of the clitoral hood to treat hypertrophy of the labia minora.

Clitoral Hood Reduction

- A crescent shape is marked, with the U oriented upside down.
- The redundant clitoral hood tissue is grasped to determine the width of the crescentic resection.
- Local anesthetic is injected and the clitoral skin excised.
- No fat is resected.
- Closure is done in two layers with interrupted 5-0 Monocryl suture in the deep dermis and 5-0 Vicryl Rapide.

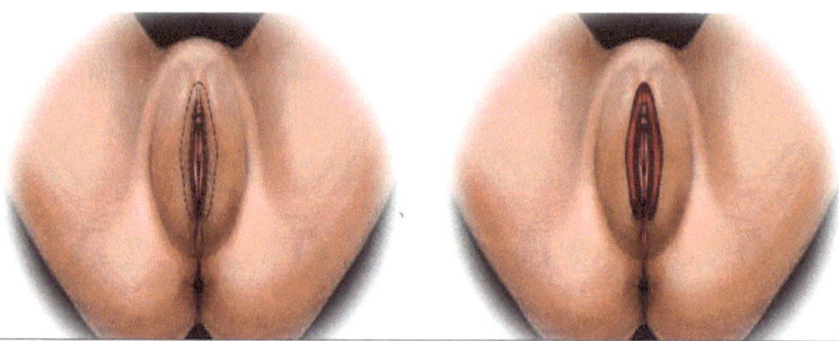

Results

Difficult to assess as we don't have enough data. Most practitioners advise conservative surgery as the positive effects are still not clear.

REFERENCES

1. Hunter JG, Commentary ON post-operative clitoral hood deformity after labioplasty. Aesth Surg Journal 2013; 30(7)1030-1036

2. Ostrzenski A. A new hydro dissection with reverse V-plasty technique for the buried clitoris as-associated with lichen sclerosis. J Gynecol Surg 26:41, 2010.

3. Tepper OM, Wulkan M, Matarasso A. Labioplasty: anatomy, etiology, and a new surgical approach. Aesthet Surg J 31:511, 2011.

4. Alter GJ. Labia minora reconstruction using clitoral hood flaps, wedge excisions, and YV advancement flaps. Plast Reconstr Surg 127:2356, 2011.

5. Hamori CA. Postoperative clitoral hood deformity after labiaplasty. Aesthet Surg J 33:1030, 2013.

6. de Alencar Felicio Y. Labial surgery. Aesthet Surg J 27:322, 2007.

7. Yavagal S, de Farias TF, Medina CA, et al. Normal vulvovagina 8. Cold CJ, McGrath KA. Anatomy and histology of the penile and clitoral prepuce in primates. In Denniston GC, Hodges FM, Milos FM, eds. Male and Female Circumcision. New York: Springer, 1999.

9. van der Putte SC, Sie-Go DM. Development and structure of the glandopreputial sulcus of the human clitoris with a special reference to glandopreputial glands. Anat Rec (Hoboken) 294:156, 2011.

10. Hodgkinson DJ, Hait G. Aesthetic vaginal labioplasty. Plast Reconstr Surg 74:414, 1984.

11. Alter GJ. Aesthetic labia minora and clitoral hood reduction using extended central wedge resettion. Plast Reconstr Surg 122:1780, 2008.

12. Alter GJ. Aesthetic labia minora reduction with inferior wedge resection and superior pedicle flap reconstruction. Plast Reconstr Surg 120:358, 2007.

13. Gress S. Composite reduction labiaplasty. Aesthetic Plast Surg 37:674, 2013.

14. Goodman MP. Female cosmetic genital surgery. Obstet Gynecol 113:154, 2009.

15. Hunter JG. Considerations in female external genital aesthetic surgery techniques. Aesthet Surg J 28:106, 2008.

16. Hamori CA. Aesthetic surgery of the female genitalia: labiaplasty and beyond. Plast Reconstr Surg 134:661, 2014.
https://t.me/Free_Plastic_Reconstruction_Book

17. Ostrzenski A. Clitoral subdermal hoodoplasty for medical indications and aesthetic motives. A new technique. J Reprod Med 58:149, 2012.

18. Benson R. Clitoral hood reduction. Presented at the Seventh Annual Congress for Aesthetic Vagi- nal Surgery, Tucson, AZ, Jan 2012.

19. Lloyd J, Crouch NS, Minto CL, et al. Female genital appearance: "normality" unfolds. BJOG 112:643, 2005.

20. Ostrzenski A. Selecting aesthetic gynecologic procedures for plastic surgeons: a review of target methodology. Aesthetic Plast Surg 37:256, 2013.

21. Shaw D, Lefebvre G, Bouchard C, et al; Society of Obstetricians and Gynaecologists of Canada. Female genital cosmetic surgery. J Obstet Gynaecol Can 35:1108, 2013.

22. Foldès P, Droupy S, Cuzin B. [Cosmetic surgery of the female genitalia] Prog Urol 23:601, 2013.

23. Lean WL, Hutson JM, Deshpande AV, et al. Clitoroplasty: past, present and future. Pediatr Surg Int 23:289, 2007.

24. Alter GJ. Central wedge nymphectomy with a 90-degree Z-plasty for aesthetic reduction of the labia minora. Plast Reconstr Surg 115:2144, 2005.

25. Alter GJ. A new technique for aesthetic labia minora reduction. Ann Plast Surg 40:287, 1998.

26. Gress S. [Aesthetic and functional corrections of the female genital area] Gynakol Geburtshilfliche Rundsch 47:23, 2006.

27. Apesos J, Jackson R, Miklos JR, et al, eds. Vagina Makeover & Rejuvenation. Cape Town: MWP Media, 2008.

28. Triana L, Robledo AM. Aesthetic surgery of female external genitalia. Aesthet Surg J 35:165, 2015.

29. Placik OJ, Arkins JA. A prospective evaluation of female external genitalia sensitivity to pressure following labia minora reduction and clitoral hood reduction. Plast Reconstr Surg 136:442e, 2015.

30. Minto CL, Liao LM, Woodhouse CR, et al. The effect of clitoral surgery on sexual outcome in individuals who have intersex conditions with ambiguous genitalia: a cross-sectional study. Lancet 361:1252, 2003.

31. Smith YR, Haefner HK. Vulvar lichen sclerosis. Am J Clin Dermatol 5:105, 2004.

PERINEOPLASTY AND VAGINOPLASTY

Chitra Jha

Vaginal rejuvenation procedures are elective surgeries which are meant to alter the dimensions of the vaginal canal and perineum. These surgeries are derived from classic gynecologic procedures to treat pelvic floor defects. The classic procedures aim to restore anatomic support by repairing damaged tissues and reinforcing them where necessary. Rejuvenation procedures focus mainly on tightening the lower vagina and perineum.

Definition

Vaginoplasty is a general term for any procedure that reshapes the vagina. These include cosmetic as well as therapeutic operations of both the introitus and the vaginal canal.

In Aesthetic Gynaecology, *vaginoplasty* specifically refers to procedures that narrow the vaginal introitus and the vaginal canal along with plication of the Levator ani muscles. Perineoplasty is a component of vaginoplasty.

Surgical reduction of the width of the perineum is called *perineoplasty* leading to tightening of the vaginal introitus only. *Perineorrhaphy* means suturing of the perineum and is sometimes used synonymously with perineoplasty.

Most practitioners use these words interchangeably though -rrhaphy means 'to suture,' and -plasty means 'to shape.'

In therapeutic gynecologic operations, perineoplasty is performed to enhance support of the pelvic floor at the time of pelvic reconstructive surgery. In cosmetic Gynaecology, perineoplasty is performed to narrow the vaginal hiatus. A secondary, purely aesthetic effect of perineoplasty is a convergence of the labia majora posteriorly.

History

Although surgical vaginal tightening procedures are not new, historically they have been performed for repairs after obstetrical delivery, rather than for sexual or aesthetic reasons.

As per the literature the procedure was originally invented in 1919 in Berlin, where it was used to treat patients who had difficulty coming to terms with their gender. In the 1950s, a Danish-American transgender woman underwent this gender-affirming procedure successfully.

It is difficult to know the exact history of the procedure but the credit for vaginoplasty as we know it today would probably go to a California-based Gynaecologist David Matlock who was the first to bring it into the public eye in 1990.

Some of his patients who underwent anterior and posterior colporrhaphies for medical indications reported increased sexual satisfaction postoperatively. This led him to offer variations of these procedures to women requesting it.

During the past decade, the number of physicians performing these operations has been steadily rising. As public awareness regarding treatment options for vaginal laxity has increased, vaginal tightening procedures have increased in popularity.

Indications

Vaginal delivery can result in widening of the vagina by stretching the tissues and separating adjacent muscles with disruption of the structural integrity of the rectovaginal fascia and perineal body.

Disruption of the perineal body may cause descent of the posterior vaginal wall and the lower part of the anterior rectal wall into the vaginal canal, especially during coughing and straining. Perineorrhaphy will help reinforce the perineal body and thus augment pelvic support.

Aside from prolapse repair, perineorrhaphies are performed to improve sexual function, by narrowing an enlarged introitus or excising sensitive tissue to decrease dyspareunia.

Vaginal laxity can create a gaping introitus and reduced vaginal sensation, and a generalized feeling of laxity and lack of support. Severe perineal lacerations or an incorrectly repaired episiotomy may add to the problems.

Furthermore, women commonly complain of gaping of the vaginal vestibule, which creates an aesthetic deformity and visibility of the vaginal mucosa. This may cause symptoms such as excessive vaginal discharge due to mucosa exposure and vaginal air entrapment.

Women seeking vaginal rejuvenation feel that vaginal laxity is an undesirable condition due to reduced sensitivity and tightness, compared to their sexual experiences before childbirth.

Anatomy

The main muscles involved while performing these procedures are the bulbocavernosus and the transverse perineal muscles.

The bulbocavernosus muscles are positioned deep to the labia majora, encircling the vaginal opening, and uniting posteriorly to form a part of the perineal body.

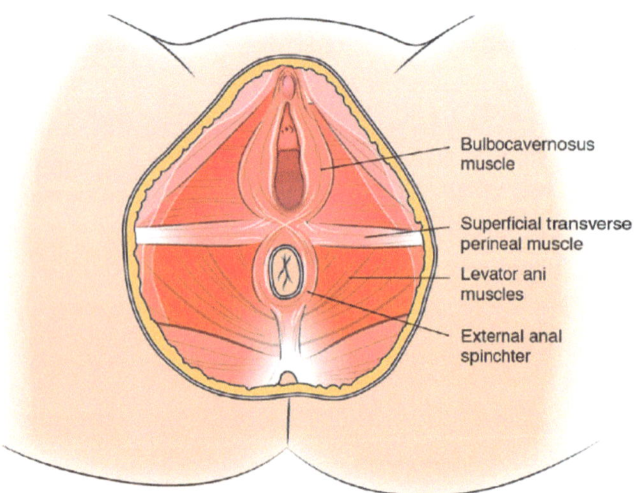

Anatomy of pelvic muscles

The transverse superficial perineal muscles which arise from the ischial tuberosities, unite in the midline and contribute to the remaining bulk of the perineal body.

The pubococcygeus, iliococcygeus, and puborectalis constitute the levator ani muscles. These broad, thin muscles that form a major part of the pelvic floor may separate with childbirth, predisposing to vaginal laxity.

Contraindications

Perineoplasty and vaginoplasty procedures should ideally be deferred for women who plan to have vaginal deliveries in the future as a vaginal delivery after the procedure is likely to disrupt the repair. Alternatively, the woman may opt for a Caesarean section in a subsequent pregnancy.

Active vaginal infections, undiagnosed skin lesions, or pathologies of the vulva and vagina which could have the potential to increase the risk of surgical injury or perioperative morbidity should be assessed and managed by appropriate means before surgery.

A history of vulvodynia, dyspareunia, or chronic pelvic pain are relative contraindications to vaginal tightening surgery.

Vaginal rejuvenation primarily involves repair of the posterior vaginal wall and perineal body. Many patients seeking this procedure have an undiagnosed and asymptomatic rectocele that may vary in extent. The correct procedure in this scenario would be rectocele repair as the first step of the vaginal rejuvenation procedure. Pelvic organ prolapse would be a contraindication for a sole vaginal rejuvenation surgery. A rectocele, enterocele, or cystocele if undiagnosed and left untreated at the time of vaginal rejuvenation surgery, would likely worsen after the procedure. Similarly, any previously undiagnosed gynecologic or urologic pathology must be addressed in advance of any cosmetic procedure.

Preoperative Evaluation

Vaginal laxity is a sensitive and highly personal issue. Consultation should take place in a private, comfortable setting and should not be rushed.

A careful review, medical history, and physical examination can help the surgeon wisely choose the right candidates and the most suitable procedure.

It is worth remembering that the tolerance for morbidity with vaginal cosmetic procedures is much lower than that for therapeutic operations. The best candidates for these operations are physically fit, non-obese, and non-smokers.

The importance of a detailed history and patient concern and motivation for the surgery cannot be over-emphasized. A complete history should be obtained including past medical and surgical history including any prior nonsurgical treatments for vaginal tightening, medications, allergies, and smoking status. A focused gynecological history should include menstrual history, contraceptive use, history of urinary incontinence, any abnormal cervical cytology, history of hemorrhoids, sexually transmitted infection, or history to suggest a pelvic pathology or malignancy. Obstetric history and mode of previous deliveries are equally important.

It is imperative to develop an understanding of the patient's concerns and motivations for seeking vaginal tightening surgery. Because sexual satisfaction is affected by multiple factors, patients should be screened and counseled so that their expectations are realistic.

There could be an incident where surgery is being used to remedy relationship issues or is being requested by the partner.

During a physical pelvic examination, the degree of vaginal laxity, perineal body length (i.e., the distance between the anus and posterior fourchette), and the presence of hemorrhoids if any should be noted. A rectovaginal examination will help assess the integrity of the posterior vaginal wall. Lax, widely separated levator ani muscles are best treated with a vaginoplasty.

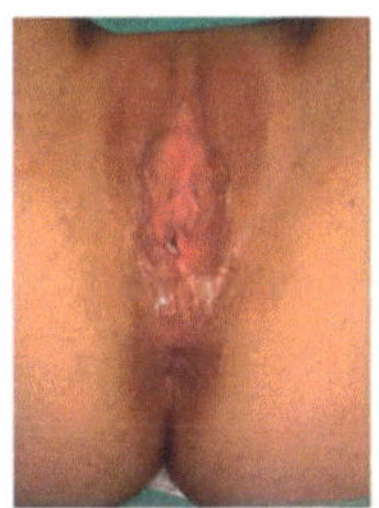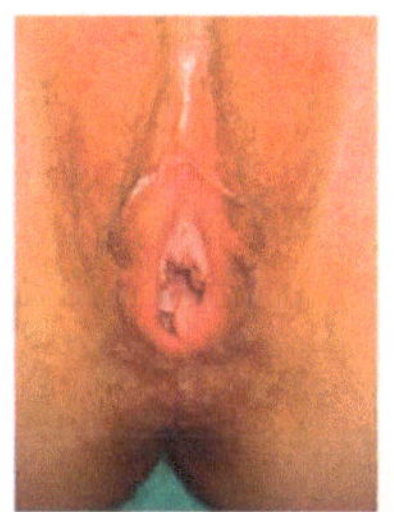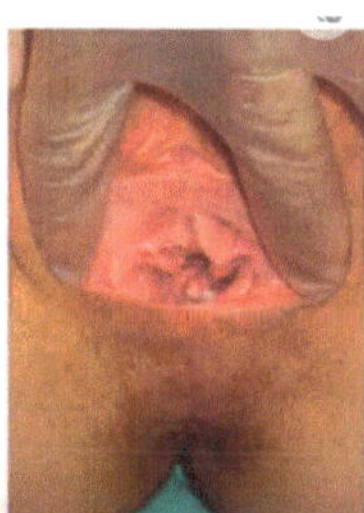

Preoperative

As discussed previously, candidates for vaginoplasty and perineoplasty should be evaluated for pelvic organ prolapse, including rectocele and cystocele.

General principles of vaginoplasty and perineoplasty procedures

A perineoplasty aims to restore the integrity of the rectovaginal fascia and perineal body and the circular structure of both bulbocavernosus muscles. Perineoplasty requires plication of the superficial and deep transverse perineal muscles and the bulbocavernosus muscles, as well as fibromuscular tissue in the midline between the vagina and the anus.

It is a component of posterior colporrhaphies for rectocele repair. This procedure is ideal for patients who are interested in improving the appearance and sexual function of a postpartum perineum.

The goals of vaginoplasty are to reunite separated muscles and narrow the vaginal canal.

A vaginoplasty includes a perineoplasty along with tightening of the proximal posterior vaginal canal. The repair involves exposure and plication of the Levator ani muscles, excess vaginal tissue is trimmed before repairing the vaginal mucosa and fortification of the perineal body.

Procedure

Vaginoplasty and Perineoplasty are performed as a day surgery procedure. Local, Regional, or General anesthesia can be used depending on patient preference.

Following administration of prophylactic antibiotics, the patient is placed in the lithotomy position in stirrups.

Preoperative photographs should be taken for documentation at this time.

Skin markings

It is always helpful to make skin markings before starting the procedure – a suggested marking could be two mirror-image triangular shapes, one pointing inside the vagina and the other on the skin pointing towards the anus.

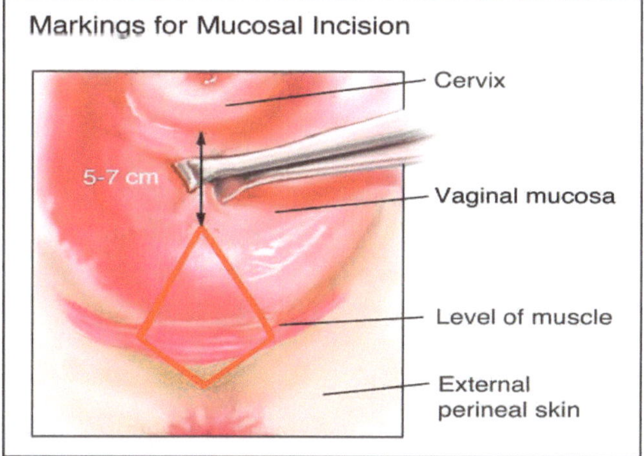

Skin markings

The two triangles meet at the level of the hymenal ring, corresponding to the widest point of planned excision. This gives the overall excision pattern a diamond shape. The tip of the internal triangle is placed about 6 centimeters inferior to the posterior fornix of the vagina.

The width of the resection can be confirmed by approximating the planned margins with tissue forceps to ensure they can be approximated with minimal tension. inferior edges of the labia majora will form the posterior fourchette of the vaginal opening.

If any doubt exists regarding the width of the planned resection, it is better to err on the side of under-resection to avoid overtightening rather than risking vaginal stenosis.

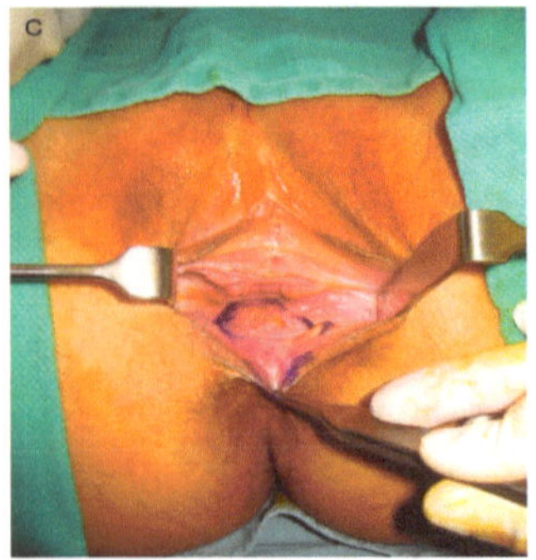 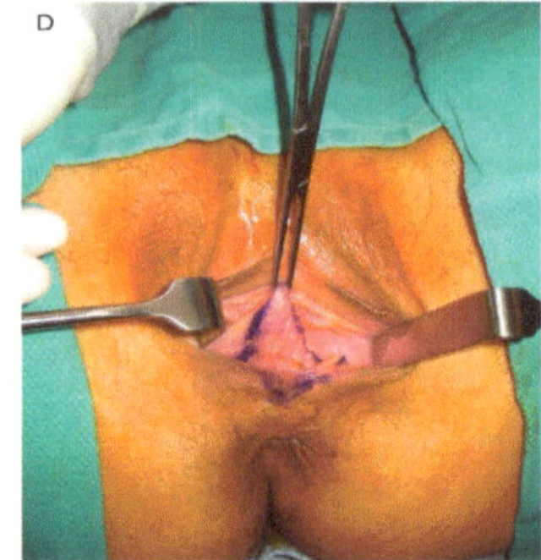

Marked area of dissection

Surgical technique

Every surgeon has his or her preferred technique, however, the general principles and steps remain the same.

Injection of diluted lignocaine in the submucosal plane provides analgesia as well as helping to create a plane of dissection between the vagina and the rectal mucosa.

Long right-angled retractors or lone star retractors help visualization and access to the posterior vaginal wall.

Posterior vaginal mucosa dissection

The posterior vaginal fourchette is elevated with clamps. Allis clamps are placed at the superior tip of the marked internal triangle and bilaterally at the border of the hymen. A transverse incision is made using a scalpel along the mucocutaneous junction to raise a mucosal flap. Blunt scissor dissection will help develop a submucosal plane, and the posterior vaginal mucosa is split along the midline to the tip of the internal triangular marking with the dissecting scissors pointing anteriorly.

Intraoperative digital rectal examination can be performed to confirm tissue thickness and a gliding plane between the vaginal and rectal surfaces.

Elevate the mucosa of the rectovaginal fascia.

Be mindful not to go too deep.

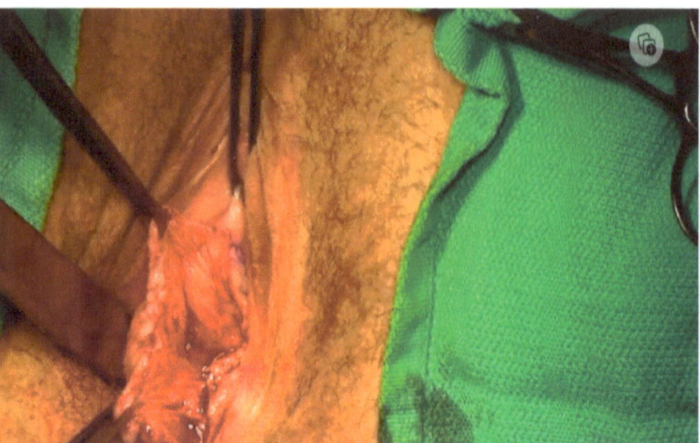

Midline dissection is performed using blunt and sharp scissor dissection. Continue to dissect till the apex. careful finger dissection and gauze can be used to sweep the mucosa of the underlying tissue more laterally.

Elevated mucosal flap

Placement of Allis clamps along the medial edge of the mucosal flap helps in retraction and dissection.

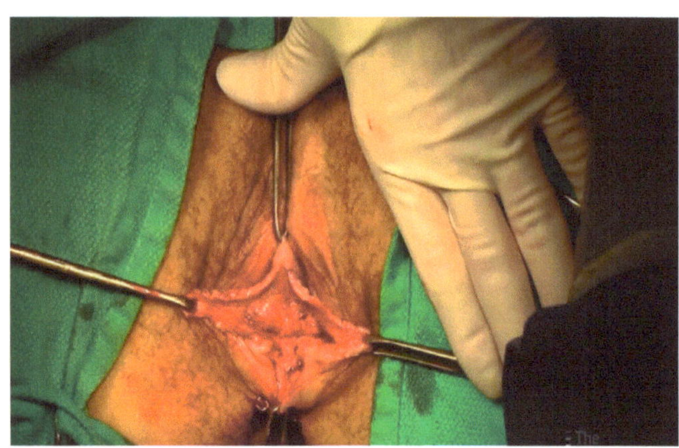

Dissected mucosal flaps on both sides.

Once both mucosal flaps have been elevated to the level of the planned resection, the excess tissue can be trimmed.

Some authors are against vaginal mucosal excision. There may be some concern that in vaginal mucosal excision procedures, fibrosis, and scar tissue may lead to decreased blood flow to the vagina resulting in vaginal dryness and dyspareunia. However, most agree that trimming excess tissue helps in narrowing the vaginal canal and has shown good results.

Proximal to the level of the hymenal ring, the perineal skin and vaginal mucosa are sharply resected along with underlying scar tissue if any. This will expose the underlying pelvic musculature ie the bulbospongiosus at the hymenal ring and the superficial transverse perineal muscle in the perineum.

The use of microsurgical scissors can help dissect the skin from underlying subcutaneous tissue without damage to the perineal musculature and provide a dissecting cleavage plane with little bleeding.

Posterior vaginal wall repair

Repair of the posterior vaginal wall proceeds from internal to external, starting at the apex. The rectovaginal fascia and elevators are plicated with interrupted 2-0 Vicryl sutures. A finger in the rectum provides counter tension to help suturing of the levators which lie more laterally. Care should be taken to avoid deep suture bites to minimize the risk of accidental injury to the rectum or the perirectal venous plexus.

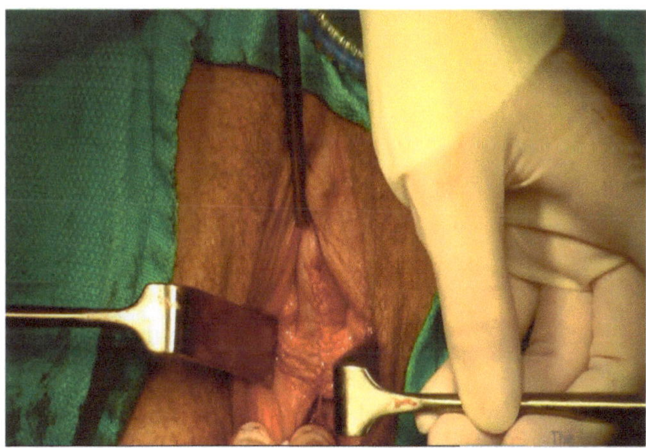

Suturing of Vaginal mucosa

The overlying mucosa is then reapproximated with running 3-0 Vicryl sutures.

Ensuring hemostasis is of utmost importance.

Perineoplasty

The separated edges of the bulbospongiosus muscle are identified at the level of the hymenal ring and reapproximated using deep interrupted 2-0 Vicryl sutures. This should create a vaginal canal diameter of about 2.5–3.5 centimeters, which will accommodate two fingers on digital examination. Overtightening should be avoided as this may result in vaginal stenosis and dyspareunia.

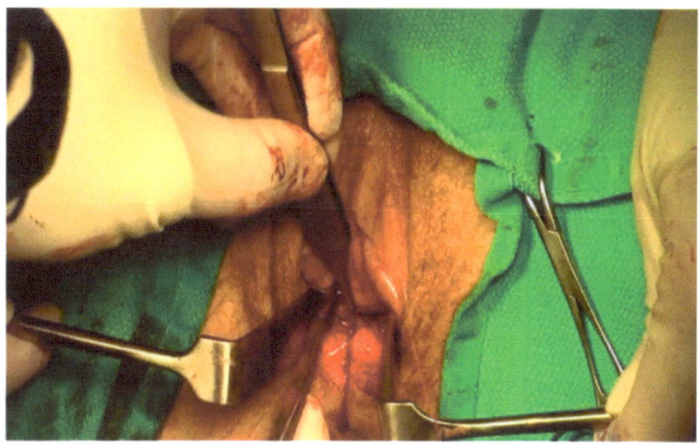

Suturing of the bulbospongiosus muscles

In the perineum, repair of the superficial transverse perineal muscles is performed similarly. The perineal repair will reconstruct and lengthen the perineal body, reconstitute the posterior fourchette, and correct the gaping of the vaginal vestibule.

Skin is repaired using Subcuticular 3-0 or 4-0 Vicryl sutures. Subcuticular sutures provide a good cosmetic appearance and are more comfortable for the patient.

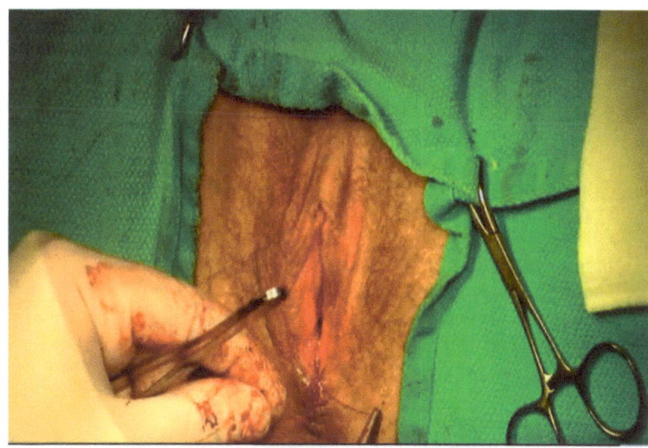

Suturing of perianal skin

Care should be taken to suture mucosa to mucosa and skin to skin to avoid a color mismatch.

Postoperative

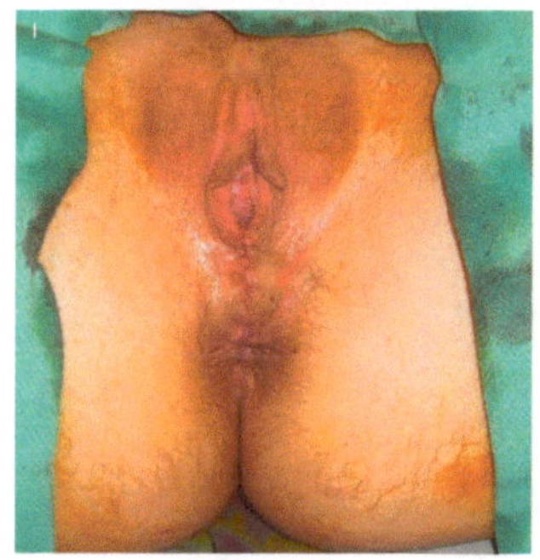 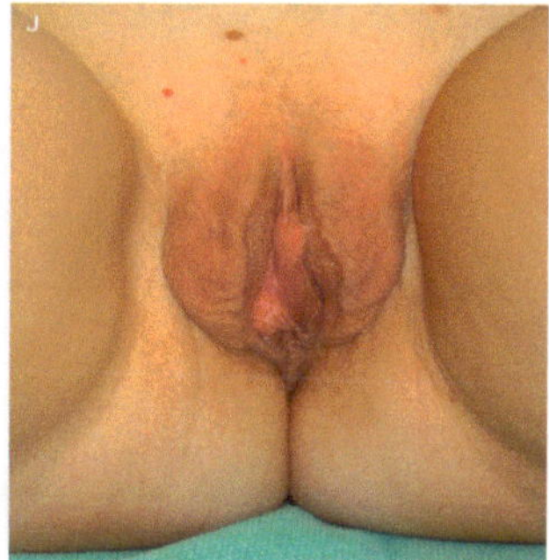

After the procedure, the vaginal canal is packed with petroleum jelly coated 1" ribbon gauze which can be removed before the woman goes home. No additional dressing is required, though patients are instructed to wear a perineal pad.

Thromboprophylaxis risk assessment and Deep vein thrombosis prevention must not be forgotten, especially in obese women, those with medical conditions, and in the perimenopausal age group. The use of intraoperative compression stockings is recommended. Advise the woman to remain well-hydrated and active.

Post-operative care

Patients are instructed to gently rinse the perineum with soapy water regularly and after every washroom visit, to keep the area clean, minimize the risk of infection, and prevent the formation of scabs on the skin.

A follow-up visit is advisable after 2 and 6 weeks. If any external perineoplasty sutures remain at the 2-week visit, these are removed.

Postoperative Instructions after vaginal Surgery

Bathing	Patients can shower right away. During the first week, sitting in a hot bath for a long time should be avoided to minimize venous pressure and vasodilation in the operated area and avoid the chance of bleeding.
Dressing	Antibiotic ointment and peri-pad can be used during the first week for oozing and padding. Some surgeons prescribe topical Estrace to place on the incisions, especially within the vaginal canal after perineal and vaginoplasty.
Pain relief	These procedures are associated with mild to moderate pain. Nonopioid pain medications including NSAIDs are usually sufficient
Exercise	To reduce the risk of bleeding, patients should take it easy for 2 weeks. Low-impact exercise may be resumed, if comfortable, at 4 weeks, and high-impact exercises after 6 weeks. No saddles (bicycle, horseback, motorcycle) for 8 weeks or longer, depending on comfort and duration.
Sexual activity	Tampons and intercourse are avoided for 6–8 weeks

Complications

Posterior vaginoplasty with perineoplasty has high patient satisfaction with minimal complications. Female genital cosmetic surgery is one of the fastest-growing areas in aesthetic plastic surgery. When performed in the appropriate patients, these procedures have high satisfaction and low complication rates.

Risks include bleeding, hematoma, injury to the bowel or bladder, rectovaginal fistula, scarring, vaginal stenosis, and dyspareunia.

Reported complication rates including inadvertent rectal entry of 2% and minor complication rates with no long-term sequelae ranging from 3.8% to 19.7% have been reported.

The Debate

In 2019 The American College of Obstetricians and Gynaecologists Committee gave an opinion that vulvovaginal surgery for appearance and sexual function reasons is not medically indicated and poses substantial risks. Hence women interested in surgery should instead be reassured of the normalcy of their anatomy.

However, the debate continues as this recommendation ignores the negative impact of not performing a cosmetic procedure that can improve quality of life.

The line between enhancement of sexual functioning and medically indicated surgical procedures is a grey area and vaginal tightening procedures are performed for both purposes. The number of vaginal rejuvenation procedures for improvement of sexual function is dramatically increasing worldwide.

Women want to feel sexually secure and attractive, and this should not exclude the vaginal area. Wellness is not just freedom from disease, and one should adopt a holistic approach.

When practiced safely vaginal surgery can improve the quality of life for many women seeking relief and patient satisfaction is also a very important measure of success.

REFERENCES

1. **Safety, Efficiency, and Outcomes of Perineoplasty: Treatment of the Sensation of a Wide Vagina**
Mustafa Ulubay, [1, *] Ugur Keskin, [1] Ulas Fidan, [1] Mustafa Ozturk, [2] Serkan Bodur, [1] Ali Yılmaz, [3] Mehmet Ferdi Kinci, [1] and Mufit Cemal Yenen [1]
Published online 2016 Aug 17. doi: 10.1155/2016/2495105

2. **Posterior Vaginoplasty With Perineoplasty: A Canadian Experience With Vaginal Tightening Surgery** Ryan E Austin, MD FRCS(C), Frank Lista, MD FRCS(C), Peter-George Vastis, Jamil Ahmad, MD FRCS(C)
Author Notes
Aesthetic Surgery Journal Open Forum, Volume 1, Issue 4, December 2019, ojz030, https://doi.org/10.1093/asjof/ojz030

3. **Vaginoplasty and Perineoplasty**
Heather J. Furnas, MD[*†] and Francisco L. Canales, MD[†]
Plast Reconstr Surg Glob Open. 2017 Nov; 5(11): e1558.
Published online 2017 Nov 9. doi: 10.1097/GOX.0000000000001558

4. **The Safe Practice of Female Genital Plastic Surgery**
Plast Reconstr Surg Glob Open 2021 Jul 6;9(7):e3660.
doi: 10.1097/GOX.0000000000003660. eCollection 2021 Jul.
Heather J Furnas [1 2], Francisco L Canales [2], Rachel A Pedreira [1], Carly Comer [3], Samuel J Lin [3], Paul E Banwell [4]

5. **Elective Female Genital Cosmetic Surgery: ACOG Committee Opinion, Number 795**
Obstet Gynecol 2020 Jan;135(1):e36-e42.
doi: 10.1097/AOG.0000000000003616.
Committee on Gynecologic Practice, American College of Obstetricians and Gynecologists

6. **ACOG Committee Opinion No. 378: Vaginal "rejuvenation" and cosmetic vaginal procedures**
Obstet Gynecol. 2007 Sep;110(3):737-8.
doi: 10.1097/01.AOG.0000263927.82639.9b.
Committee on Gynecologic Practice, American College of Obstetricians and Gynecologists

7. **Vaginal Rejuvenation: A Review of Female Genital Cosmetic Surgery**
Obstet Gynecol Surv. 2018 May;73(5):287-292.
doi: 10.1097/OGX.0000000000000559.
Gianna Wilkie [1], Deborah Bartz [2]

8. **Safety, Efficiency, and Outcomes of Perineoplasty: Treatment of the Sensation of a Wide Vagina**
Biomed Res Int. 2016; 2016: 2495105.
Published online 2016 Aug 17. doi: 10.1155/2016/2495105
Mustafa Ulubay, [1, *] Ugur Keskin, [1] Ulas Fidan, [1] Mustafa Ozturk, [2] Serkan Bodur, [1] Ali Yılmaz, [3] Mehmet Ferdi Kinci, [1] and Mufit Cemal Yenen [1]

9. **Experience of Vaginoplasty for Enhancement of Sexual Functioning in a Center in Turkey: A Before and After Study**
Cureus. 2021 Apr; 13(4): e14767.
Published online 2021 Apr 30. doi: 10.7759/cureus.14767
Monitoring Editor: Alexander Muacevic and John R Adler

10. **Vaginal Rejuvenation: An In-Depth Look at the History and Technical Procedure**
Dolores Kent, MD, FACOG, FAACS; Marco Antonio Pelosi III, MD, FACOG, FACS, FICS
The American Journal of Cosmetic Surgery Vol. 29, No. 2, 2012

11. **Female Aesthetic Genital Procedures**
CA Hamori - Clinics in Plastic Surgery, 2022 - plasticsurgery.theclinics.com

12. **Female genital cosmetic surgery: the good, the bad, and the ugly**
M Serati, S Salvatore, D Rizk - International Urogynecology Journal, 2018

Vaginal laxity results from the trauma and stretching associated with pregnancy and vaginal delivery. Vaginal laxity results from the trauma and stretching associated with pregnancy and vaginal delivery. The stretching can attenuate the tissues and separate, bulboca

THREADS IN COSMETIC GYNECOLOGY

CHAPTER 24

Garima Srivastav

WHAT ARE THREADS?

- Temporary sutures, that are used to produce a subtle but visible lift in skin.
- The thread pulls the skin in a desired direction therefore lifting and tightening the skin.
- Secondly, it provokes the body's healing mechanism and induces collagen production.

ADVANTAGES OF THREAD

- Better than surgery due to reduced recovery time.
- No anesthesia
- No bleeding
- Minimally invasive
- Better results than non-surgical skin tightening.
- Easy to do procedures.

TYPES OF THREAD

Types of threads can be divided based on
- Mode of absorption
- Texture: presence of barbs
- Length

MODE OF ABSORPTION

- PDO threads – absorb in 6 months but help to stimulate collagen in 12 months.
- Poly-l-lactic acid (PLLA) silhouette threads- life of 18 months to 2 years.
- Functions as a volumizer and can simulate collagen.
- Polycaprolactone (PCL) lasts up to 2 years or more. maximum collagen production

BASED ON TEXTURE

Barbed threads
- Bi-directional threads
- Unidirectional threads
- Cogged – mono threads

Non- barbed threads
- Monofilament Plain
- Monofilament Screw

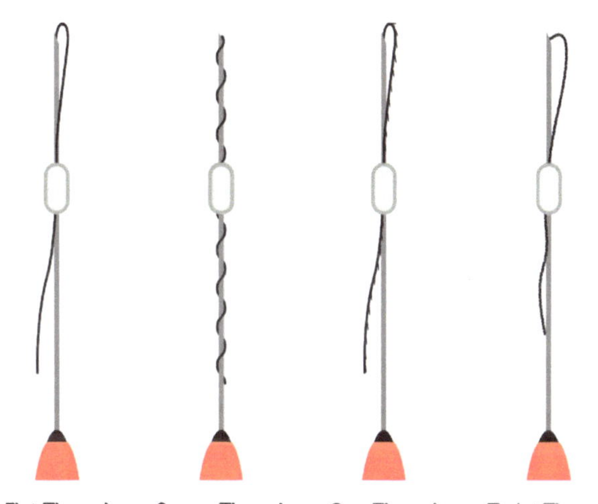

Types of PDO Threads

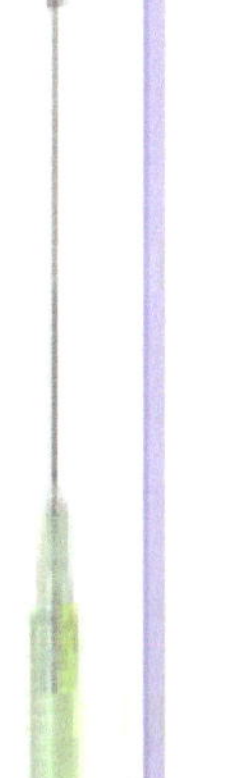
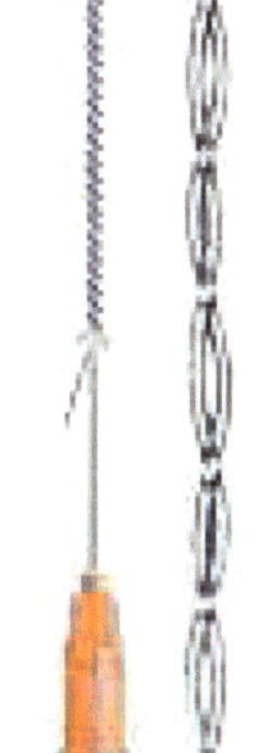
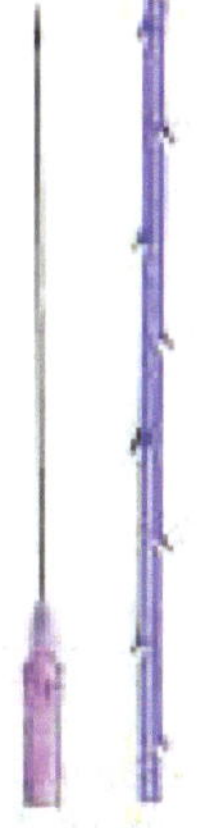
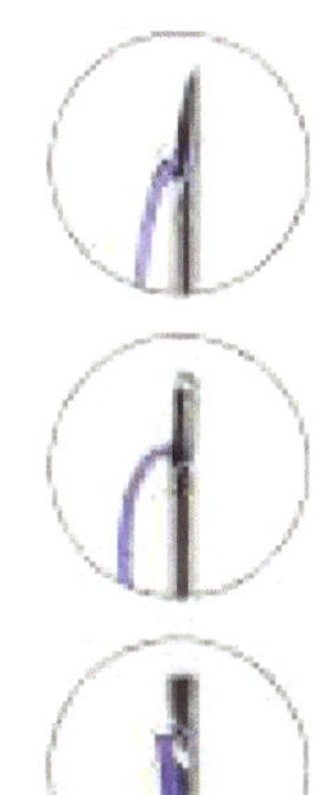

BASED ON THE LENGTH OF THE THREAD

- Short suture – less than 90 mm (PDOs are usually short)
- Long suture – more than 90 mm (usually, barbed threads)

MECHANISM OF ACTION

- By immediately, pulling the tissue by mechanical action and by generating a strong secondary fibrotic reaction that leads to the formation of the so-called "secondary vector of pull".

- The effect given by fibrosis remains even after the total absorption of the thread, ensuring a permanent and lasting result over time.

INDICATIONS

- Revirgination
- Vaginal tightening
- Perineal reconstruction after postpartum episiotomy
- Perineal reconstruction after lacerations from childbirth
- Scars due to episiotomy
- Lacerations/ tears in the skin
- Labia majora upliftment

CONTRAINDICATIONS

- Hypersensitivity to anaesthesia
- Acute and rate blood clotting disorders
- Acute inflammatory conditions of the vagina and perineum (procedure can be performed after the inflammation is healed)
- Menstruation bleeding or other types of vaginal bleeding
- Neoplastic disease of the genital organs
- Pregnancy
- Early postpartum period when physiological postpartum uterine discharge continues

BENEFITS

- Local anesthesia
- No need for hospitalization
- Enhancing the aesthetics
- Minimally invasive
- Improved comfort and functioning of the vagina and perineum
- Fast healing and short recovery after a few days of downtime
- NLong-lasting results for a few years

COMPLICATIONS

- Very rare
- Mild bleeding
- Infection
- No serious complications have been reported

PROCEDURE

The procedure can be done under short GA or local anesthesia, although the author prefers short GA.

Patient preparation is done.

The introduction of vaginal tampons and catheterization is done.

Introduction of anoscope and evaluation of anatomical layers of the urogenital and anal triangle and introduction of anal tampon.

The various entry and exit points are marked as shown in the diagram above. The vectors are drawn, which indicate the direction of tightening.

Long-acting anesthesia or topical block for lumbosacral nerve plexus is given.

The cutaneous incision is given with a dermal punch or 18 G needle.

Insertion of sutures according to the path already illustrated and then tension given on the latter as the last exit point is reached.

The threads are secured with the knot.

Skin sutured back, tampons removed and patient shifted to recovery room.

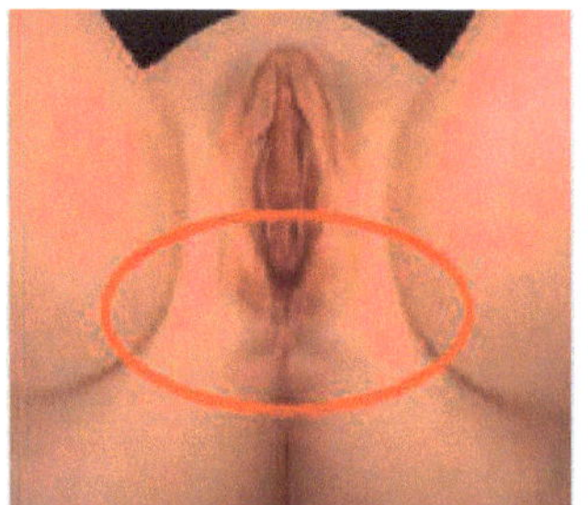
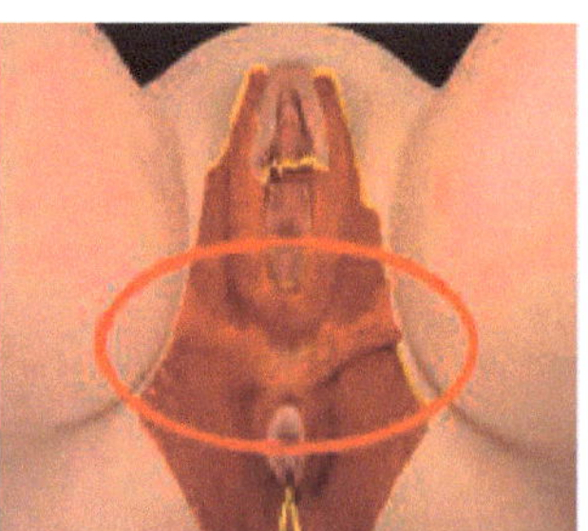

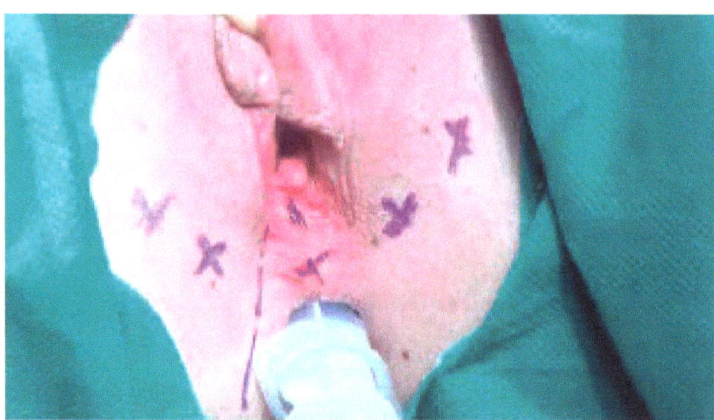

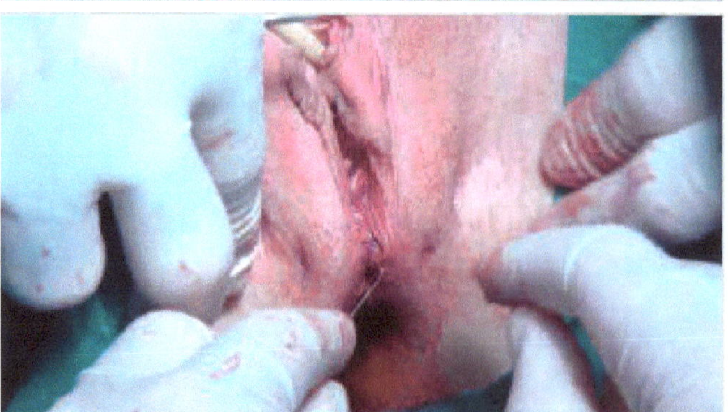

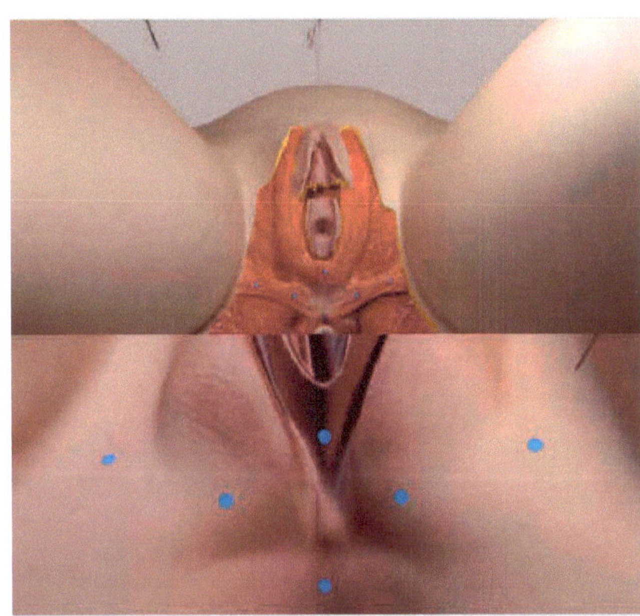

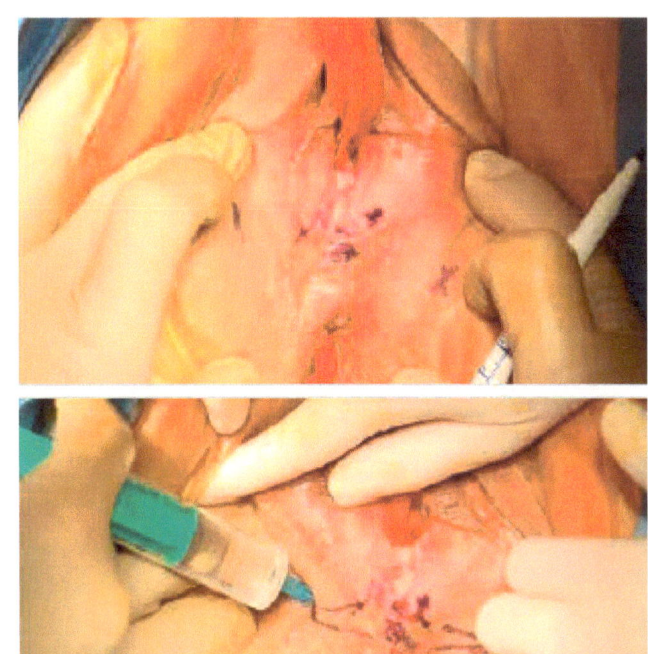

MODULE 5

RECENT ADVANCES

MANAGEMENT OF URINARY INCONTINENCE

Dr. Akhil Saxena, Dr. Chanchal Gupta

INTRODUCTION:

Urinary incontinence is a common problem amongst women in all age groups hurting women's physical, social, psychological, and sexual lives. Approximately 10% of adult women suffer from urinary incontinence. Prevalence increases with increasing age and more than 40% of the female population above 60 years is affected. However, because of social and psychological problems, many women hesitate to admit and take treatment. Therefore, healthcare professionals should make efforts to spread awareness of this problem among women and provide appropriate medical care and psychological support.

BASICS OF URINARY INCONTINENCE:

Urinary continence is maintained by
- Internal urethral sphincter
- External urethral sphincter
- Muscles of the pelvic floor

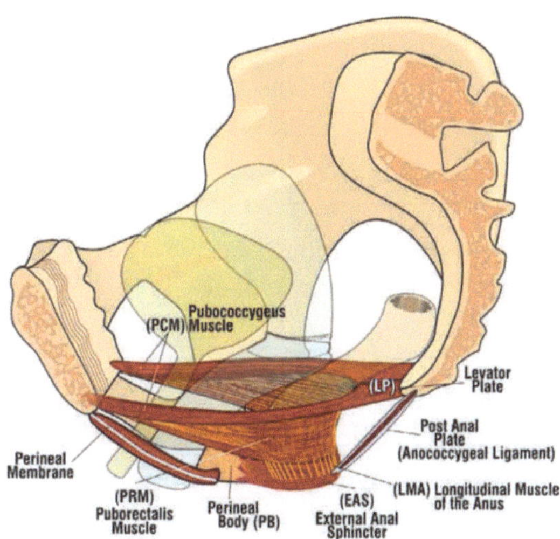

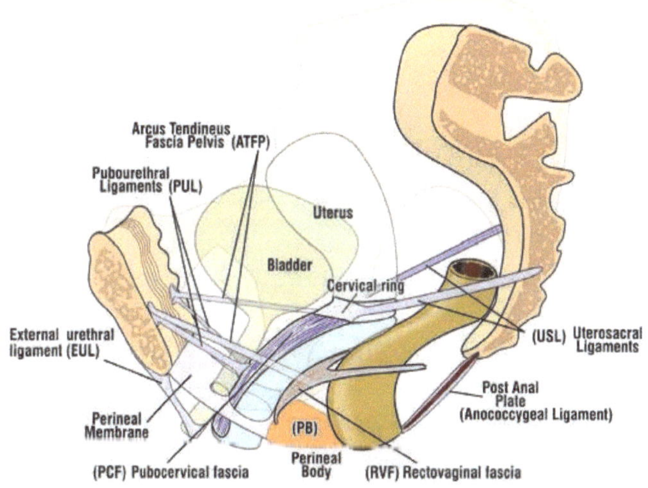

Urinary incontinence refers to:
- Involuntary loss of urine with coughing, sneezing, laughing, exercise, or intercourse
- Loss of urine before reaching the toilet
- Urgency
- Frequency > 8 voids/day
- Nocturia > 2 voids/night
- Bedwetting
- Constant wetness

Types of Urinary incontinence:
- Stress Incontinence
- Urge Incontinence
- Mixed Incontinence
- Overflow Incontinence
- Total Incontinence
- Functional Incontinence

HISTORY TAKING IN A PATIENT WITH URINARY INCONTINENCE

- How often does the patient void during the day and night and how long can she wait comfortably between urinations?

- Why does voiding occur as often as it does (urgency, convenience, attempt to prevent incontinence)?
- How severe is incontinence (e.g., a few drops, saturate outer clothing)?
- Are protective pads worn?
- Do pads become saturated?
- How often and why are pads changed?
- Is the patient aware of incontinence occurring? If so, how long can micturition be postponed?
- Does stress incontinence occur during coughing, during sneezing, while the patient rises from a sitting to a standing position, or only during heavy physical exercise?
- If the incontinence is associated with stress, is urine lost only for an instant during the stress, or is there uncontrolled voiding?
- Is there difficulty initiating the stream, requiring pushing or straining to start?
- Is the stream weak or interrupted?
- Is there postvoid dribbling?
- Has the patient ever had urinary retention?

CATEGORIZING PATIENTS OF URINARY INCONTINENCE BASED ON SYMPTOMS:

Questions	Stress UI	Urge UI	Overflow UI
1. Description of incontinent episodes	Loss of activity, cough	Sudden urgency; inability to each toilet	Continuous slow loss
2. Precipitating factors	Cough, physical activity	Full bladder, sensory triggers	None, stress may worsen
3. Urinary frequency	Normal	Increased	Hesitancy: inability to void
4. Nocturia	<1	Variable	Nocturnal enuresis
5. Volume loss	Small	Large	Continuous

STRESS URINARY INCONTINENCE:

Immediate leakage of urine on:
- Coughing
- Laughing
- Exercise
- Sneezing
- Intercourse

Mechanism of SUI:

- Poor support of the urethra or bladder neck and change of urethrovesical angle
- Improper functioning of the urethral sphincter mechanism
- Loss of urethral mucosal coaptation
- Due to laxity, the urethra becomes hypermobile and extraperitoneal. When there is a rise in intraabdominal pressure due to coughing, sneezing, etc, vesical pressure exceeds intraurethral pressure thereby causing incontinence.

Types of stress Urinary incontinence

- Type I: Mildest form. Urine loss occurs in the absence of urethral hypermobility.
- Type II: (Genuine SUI). Urine loss occurs due to urethral hypermobility.
- Type-III: (ISD). Urine leakage occurring from sphincter dysfunction

URGE URINARY INCONTINENCE:

Also known as overactive bladder. It is:
- Loss of urine before reaching the toilet
- Frequent urination of small amounts of urine
- Night-time urination greater than 2 per night
- Bedwetting

Causes:

- Detrusor Instability
- Detrusor Hyperreflexia (CNS)
  - Stroke
  - Multiple Sclerosis
  - Lumbar spine or sacral disc disease
  - Parkinson's disease
  - Dementia
  - Brain tumor

MIXED URINARY INCONTINENCE:

Combination of Stress and Urge urinary incontinence
- In 4-30% of patients
- One factor predominates
- Patients leak larger volumes of urine and more incontinence episodes per week

OVERFLOW INCONTINENCE:

- Involuntary loss of urine associated with overdistension of the bladder
- Non-contractile bladder
- Loss of normal voiding reflex

Causes:

- Outflow tract Obstruction
- Nerve injury
- Medications

TOTAL INCONTINENCE:

- Leakage that occurs constantly
- Usually associated with a hole in the urinary tract
- Fistulas can occur between the bladder, vagina, urethra, uterus, ureter
- The result of a fistula is constant leakage

FUNCTIONAL INCONTINENCE:

- Functional issues contribute significantly to the ability to stay continent
- Mobility, lack of independent care, and cognitive state are key factors contributing to incontinence

EVALUATION OF PATIENT WITH URINARY INCONTINENCE:

PHYSICAL EXAMINATION:

- **General Examination** To assess edema
- **Neurologic Abnormalities**
  - Mobility
  - Cognition
  - Dexterity
- **Abdominal Examination**
  - To detect an enlarged bladder
  - Other abdominal masses
- **Speculum examination.**
  - Examining the perineum includes a careful assessment of estrogen status and any associated genitourinary prolapse.
  - The degree of pelvic organ prolapse (POP) should be noted.
- **Bimanual examination**

SPECIFIC CLINICAL TESTS:

Pad test

- Marshall Bonney Test- If continence is improved by elevating the urethra with two fingers placed inside the vagina paraurethrally then it indicates that surgery for incontinence should be successful.
- Q-Tip Test- An abnormal upward deflection of Q tip more than 30 degrees by Valsalva maneuver/cough shows urethral hypermobility.
- Cough Stress Test
- Standing Pelvic Examination
- Voiding Diary

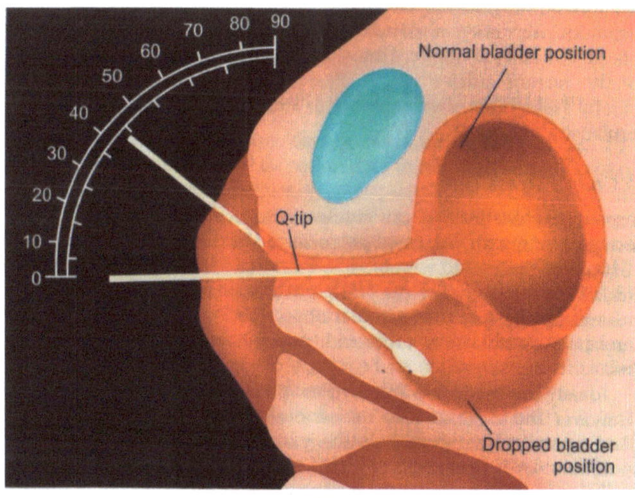

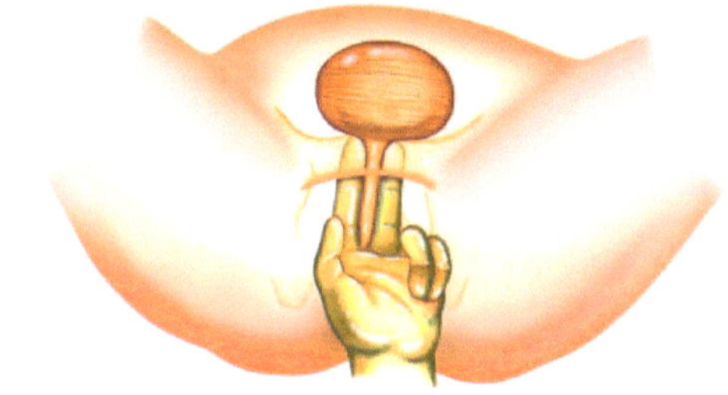

PRE-OP INVESTIGATIONS:

- Urinalysis
- Urine culture
- Urine cytology- to rule out carcinoma of the urinary bladder
- BUN and serum creatinine levels if compromised renal functions are suspected.
- USG of the urinary tract especially for PVR
- MRI and dynamic MRI
- Urodynamic studies

Diagnosis	Urodynamic picture
Normal	No leak with coughing, sneezing, exertion, and no phasic rise of detrusor pressure during the filling phase.
SUI	Involuntary leakage of urine shown during raised abdominal pressure, in the absence of detrusor contraction is referred to as urodynamic stress incontinence.
Bladder neck hypermobility	High Valsalva leak point pressure or high maximum urethral closure pressure.
Intrinsic sphincter deficiency	Low Valsalva leak point pressure or low maximum urethral closure pressure.
Urge urinary incontinence	Incontinence due to involuntary detrusor contraction, usually with the sensation of urge is called detrusor overactivity incontinence.
Mixed incontinence	**SUI + Urge incontinence**

TREATMENT

NONSURGICAL THERAPY FOR STRESS UI

- Pelvic floor muscle exercises (Kegel)
- Avoiding tea, coffee
- Timed voiding
- Biofeedback
- Electrical Stimulation
- Vaginal cones, etc

MEDICAL TREATMENT

- Anticholinergics
- Antispasmodic agents
- Tricyclic antidepressants
- Alpha-adrenergic Agonists
- Estrogens
- Antidepressants, Serotonin/ Norepinephrine Reuptake Inhibitors
- Beta 3 adrenergic receptors

Anticholinergic drugs

- First-line medicinal therapy for
  - Urge incontinence
  - Urinary frequency and urgency
  - Nocturnal enuresis
- Anticholinergics agents cause direct smooth muscle relaxation of the U.B. and have local anesthetic properties thus they increase the bladder capacity.
- Commonly used salts are Darifenacin, solifenacin, hyoscyamine sulfate, propantheline, dicyclomine hydrochloride, tolterodine, trospium, fesoterodine

Antispasmodic drugs

- These agents relax the smooth muscles of the urinary bladder by direct spasmolytic action
- Commonly used drugs are:
  - Oxybutynin chloride (also has anticholinergic effect)
  - Flavoxate

Alpha-adrenergic agonists

- Increase the bladder outlet resistance by contracting the bladder neck.
- Commonly used drugs are
  - Midodrine
  - Pseudoephedrine hydrochloride

Tricyclic antidepressants

- They facilitate urine storage by decreasing bladder contractility and increasing outlet resistance. They also have a local anesthetic effect on bladder mucosa.
- Name of salts are:
  - Imipramine hydrochloride
  - Amitriptyline hydrochloride

Estrogens

- Conjugated estrogens increase the tone of the urethral muscle, and strengthen the pelvic muscles thus increasing the urethral support.
- Mucosal turgor of the periurethral tissue from proper nourishment enhances urethral mucosal coaptation-thus improving the mucosal seal effect.
- Most effective in postmenopausal women
- Conjugated estrogen (Premarin) can be used orally, vaginal application, or both.

Beta 3 adrenergic agonist- Mirabegron

- Is the latest drug in the treatment of overactive bladder.
- It activates the beta-3 adrenergic receptor in the detrusor muscle in the bladder, which leads to muscle relaxation and an increase in bladder capacity.

MINIMALLY INVASIVE PROCEDURES

- Platelet Rich Plasma
- Platelet Poor Plasma
- Amniotic Fluid
- Autologous Fat Transfer
- Laser therapy (intra-urethral probe)
- Radiofrequency
- HIFU & Nano-Ultrasound
- Focused electromagnetic waves - HIFEM
- InterStim: implantable device
- Intravesical electric stimulation

Radiofrequency and laser therapy increase mucosal thickness by increasing the number of cell layers, vascularization, glycogenesis, collagen, elastin, small nerve fibers, and stromal density.

SURGICAL MANAGEMENT

It can be divided into abdominal and vaginal procedures.

Abdominal surgeries can be performed by laparotomy and laparoscopy/robotic. These include:

- MMK (Marshall-Marchetti-Kranz)
  - Paraurethral tissue sutured to the periosteum of the symphysis pubis and rectus muscles

- Modified MMK
- Burch colposuspension

Laparoscopic/robotic Burch colposuspension has the best results in patients with urethral hypermobility. Paraurethral tissue sutured bilaterally to the Cooper's ligament. The success rate is 69- 90%. Complications include retropubic space bleeding, hematoma, cystotomy, ureteric injury, voiding problems, de novo detrusor overactivity, and enterocele.

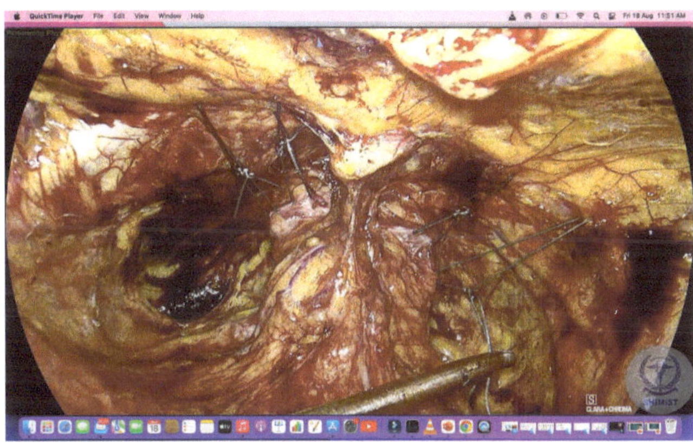

Vaginal procedures include:

- Needle urethropexies: not performed nowadays.
- Anterior Colporrhaphy with "Kelly Plication": More useful with elderly & medically unfit patients.
- Anterior Colporrhaphy
  - Anterior vaginal wall incision
  - Vesicovaginal space dissection
  - Plication of endopelvic fascia at urethrovaginal junction
  - Plication of endopelvic fascia beneath the bladder
  - Closure of anterior vaginal wall

Complications include urinary retention, narrowing of the vagina, dyspareunia, recurrent or persistent UI, urethral or bladder injury. The overall complication rate is 14%.

- Sling procedures:
  - TOT- the success rate is close to 85%. Complications include obturator vessels and nerve injuries, adductor longus tendon injury, mesh complications
  - TVT- the success rate is close to 85%. Complications include retropubic space bleeding, bladder and urethral injuries, voiding problems, urinary retention, mesh erosion or exposure

Suburethral sling materials:
Synthetic materials
- Gore-Tex
- Marlex
- Silastic
- Mersilene (Dacron)
- Polypropylene (usually used)

Increased infection, rejection, erosion, urinary retention
- Native materials:
  - Giordano (1907) used gracilis muscle
  - Goebel (1910) used pyramidalis muscle
  - Price (1933) used fascia lata
  - Aldridge (1942), Millin, Studdiford used rectus abdominis fascia

Nowadays, autologous grafts from tensor fascia lata or rectus sheath are used as slings in TOT. We are harvesting autologous grafts by various minimal access or endoscopic methods and then doing TOTs with these prepared autologous grafts at our institute, SHIMIST, Sonepat with excellent results.

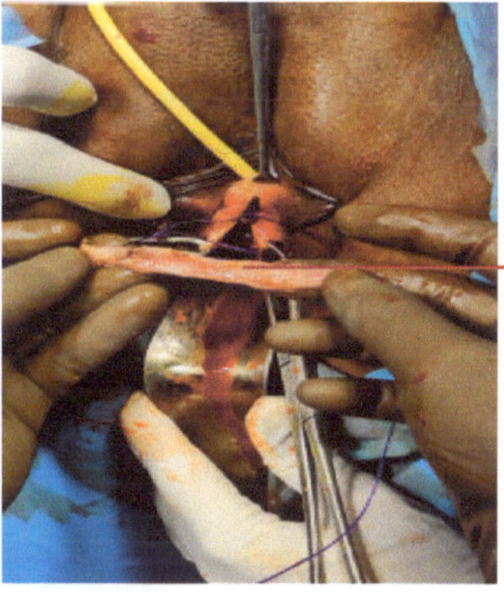

TFL graft harvested and used as sling in TOT

Complications:

- Hemorrhage (>200ml) and hematoma -2%.
- Voiding dysfunction-1.9%
- Erosion -0.5% to 1.3%
- Bladder perforation
- Others – Infection, Dyspareunia, bowel perforation, TVT tract fistula
- Hemorrhage and Hematoma
  - Observation
  - Local compression
  - Laparotomy if major vessel bleed.
- Voiding dysfunction and urinary retention

Causes:
- Overcorrection of urethral axis
- Inappropriately placed or excessively tightened tape.
- De novo detrusor inactivity
- Denervation due to excessive dissection

Signs and symptoms:
- Partial or complete urinary retention.
- Inability to void continuously.
- Slow stream with increased voiding time

Management:
- Serial dilatation with hegars dilator up to number 8 within a week of surgery.
- Redo surgery- in case of failure of urethral dilatation
  - Time -7-14 days.
  - Methods
    - Loosening the sling
    - Cut the sling in the middle and lyse it up to the inferior pubic ramus.
    - Urethrolysis- retropubic or vaginal
    - Success rates – 65 to 80%

Vaginal erosion:
- Observation with topical estrogens if asymptomatic with small erosions.
- Partial or complete tape excision and re-approximation of vaginal mucosa if symptomatic.

Urethral erosion
- Transvaginal excision of mesh and closure of urethrotomy
- Vascularized Martius fat pad graft.

Intravesical erosion – Very rare
- Usually an intraoperative complication
- Treatment – partial or complete excision of mesh with the reconstruction of the lower urinary tract.

Bladder perforation

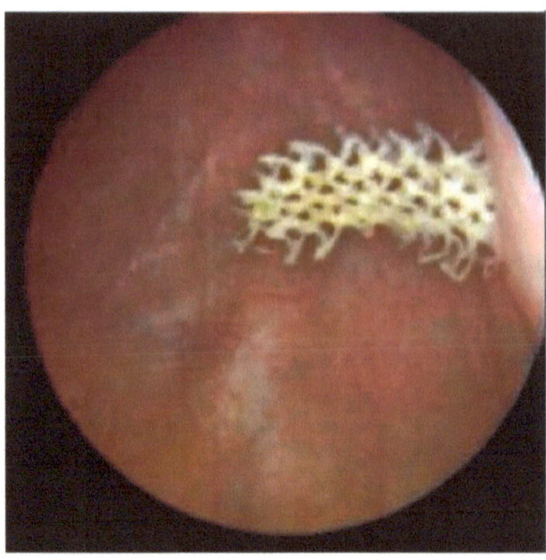

- Site
  - Left -1 to 3 o clock
  - right-9-11 o clock
- Treatment – Post-operative drainage – only if
- multiple perforations
- significant hematuria
- low perforations

The appropriate diagnosis and management of urinary incontinence amongst women is of utmost importance as it has a huge impact on women's social and personal lives. Proper history-taking, investigations and cause-specific treatment is the key. The management of urinary incontinence is huge and ever-evolving. Currently, autologous grafts harvesting mainly by endoscopic approach and using them in suburethral sling surgeries is a novel procedure under trial with excellent results.

MESOTHERAPY

Fahad Usman

Definition of Mesotherapy

- Mesotherapy treatment is a nonsurgical cosmetic solution aimed at diminishing problem areas in your body such as cellulite, excess weight, body contouring, and face/neck/intimate rejuvenation, just to name a few. It is administered via numerous injections containing various types of approved medicines, vitamins, and minerals.
- The content mixture of the injection varies by each unique case and specific area to be treated.
- Mesotherapy can also assist in reducing pain, and in replenishing hair loss in both men and women.

Techniques

- Intra-epidermal
- Papular
- Nappage
- Point by Point
- Meso perfusion
- Meso-Needling

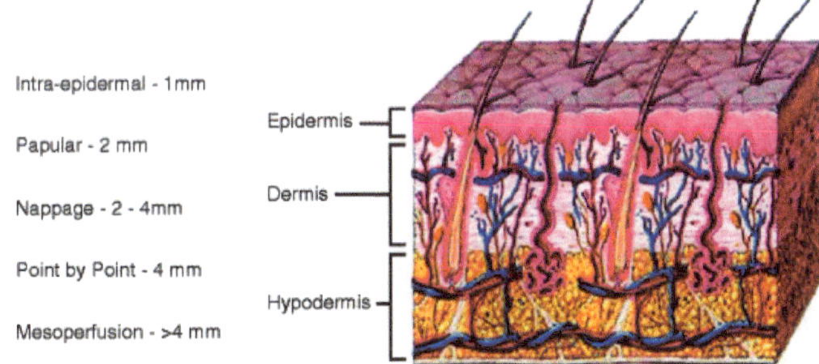

Figure 18: Mesotherapy Techniques [1]

INTRA-EPIDERMAL TECHNIQUE

- Multiple superficial injections into the epidermal level.
- <1mm depth "superficial nappage"
- Minimal or no Bleeding
- Minimal or no pain
- Cutaneous stimulation +++

- Needle: 30G x 13mm
- Bevel up. But only the bevel goes into the skin.

PAPULAR TECHNIQUE

- Intrabasal layer injection (junction of epidermis and dermis)
- Multiple Papules. 1-2mm depth.
- <0.1 ml per point
- Needle: 30G 4mm (or 12mm). Bevel up.
- Blanching of the skin to form a papule.
- Mostly for facial rejuvenation

NAPPAGE TECHNIQUE

- Multiplepricking technique 2-4 mm depth
- Needle: 30G 4mm.
- 2-4 injections per second. 2-4mm depth. 30 – 60°
- Constant unchanging pressure on the syringe piston
- Using a syringe or a mesotherapy gun

Over the whole of the face, neck, and back of the hands. Very superficial cutaneous micro-injections
- Small papules, barely visible, roughly 1cm apart.
- Most commonly used technique, for multiple indications.

POINT-BY-POINT TECHNIQUE

- Deep intradermic or hypodermic injections. 4-10mm depth.
- Needle: 4-13mm
- 0.5 to 2cm distance apart.
- Variable volume, might be >0.1 ml
- More Painful
- Subcutaneous injections in mesotherapy are used for injection lipolysis

MESOPERFUSION TECHNIQUE

- Deep hypodermic infusion
- Used for chronic pain
- 4-13mm depth.

Meso-Needling TECHNIQUE

- Devices: Dermapen or Dermaroller
- 0.5mm for the scalp & 0.5 to 1mm for the face

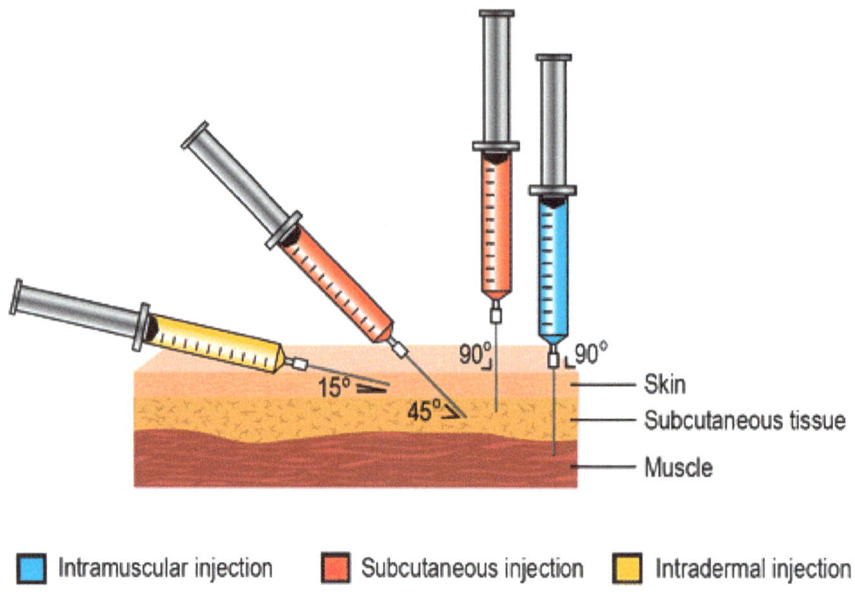

Figure 19: Angles for Injection [2]

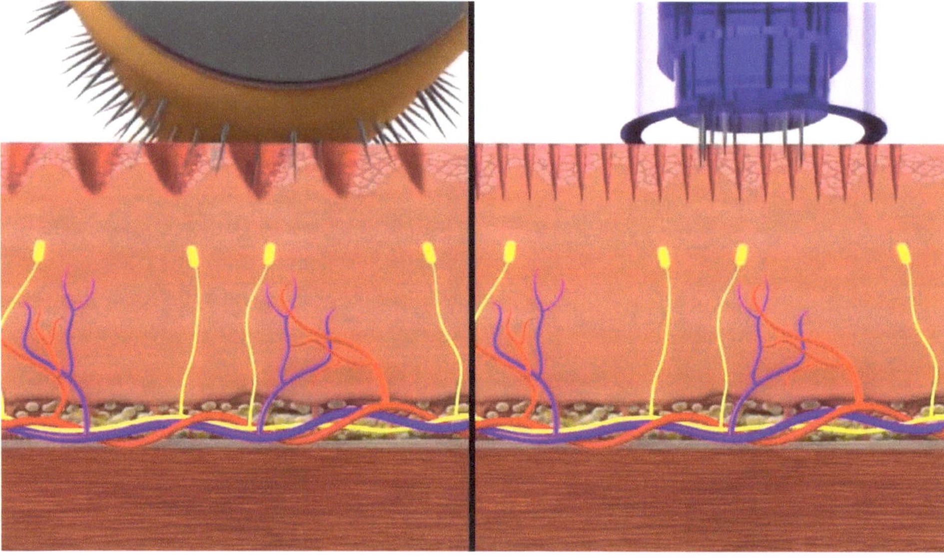

Figure 20: Meso-needling: Pen vs. Roller [3]

REFERENCES

1. https://link.springer.com/
   chapter/10.1007/978-3-642-21837-8_13
2. https://www.magonlinelibrary.com/doi/
   abs/10.12968/joan.2012.1.6.292
3. https://www.rmclinic.co.uk/4601-2/

STEM CELL AND AESTHETIC GYNECOLOGY

Fahad Usman

Stem Cell - Definition

A cell that can continuously divide and differentiate (develop) into various other kind(s) of cells/tissues.

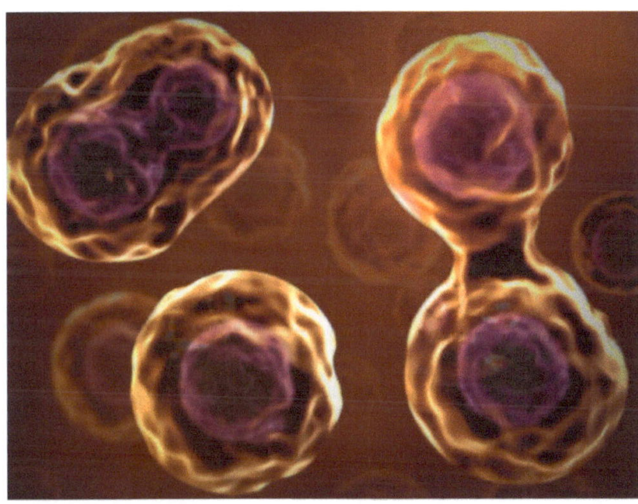

Figure 1: Cell Division [1]

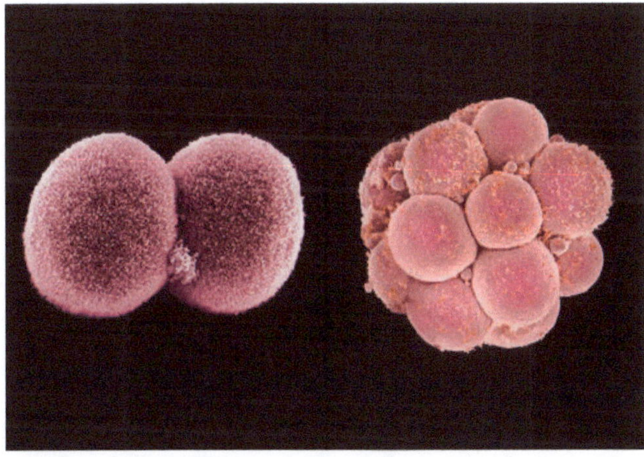

Figure 2: Human Embryonic Stem Cell [2]

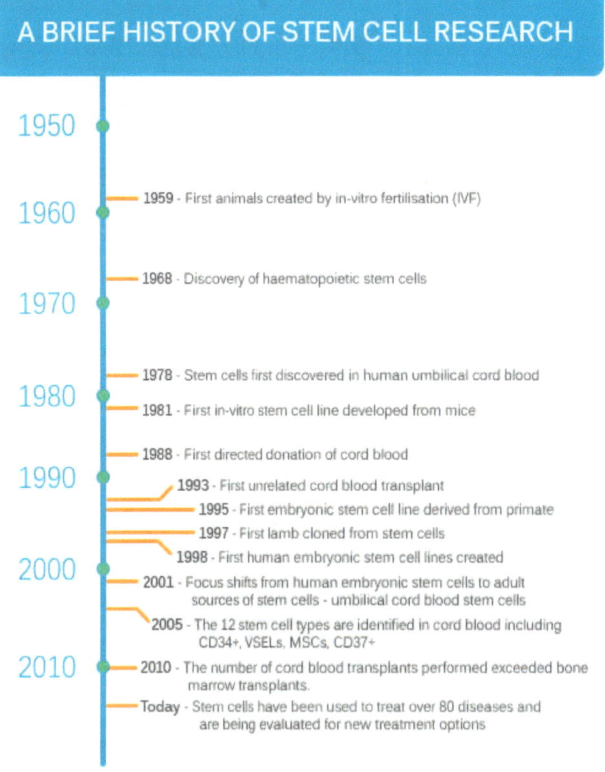

Figure 3: History of Stem Cells [3]

Characteristics of Stem Cells

- 'Blank cells' (unspecialized)
- Capable of dividing and renewing themselves for long periods (proliferation and renewal)
- Have the potential to give rise to specialized cell types (differentiation)

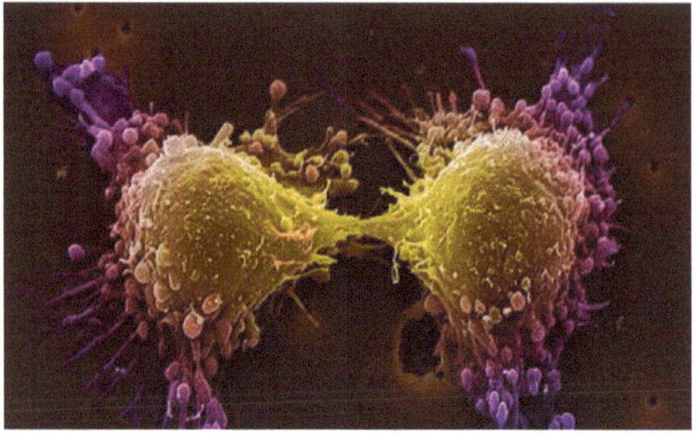

Figure 4: Coloured scanning electron micrograph of two prostate cancer cells in the final stage of cell division.

Types of Stem Cells

Stem cell type	Description	Examples
Totipotent	Each cell can develop into a new individual	Cells from early (1-3 days) embryos
Pluripotent	Cells can form any (over 200) cell types	Some cells of blastocyst (5 to 14 days)
Multipotent	Cells differentiated, but can form several other tissues	Fetal tissue, cord blood, and adult stem cells

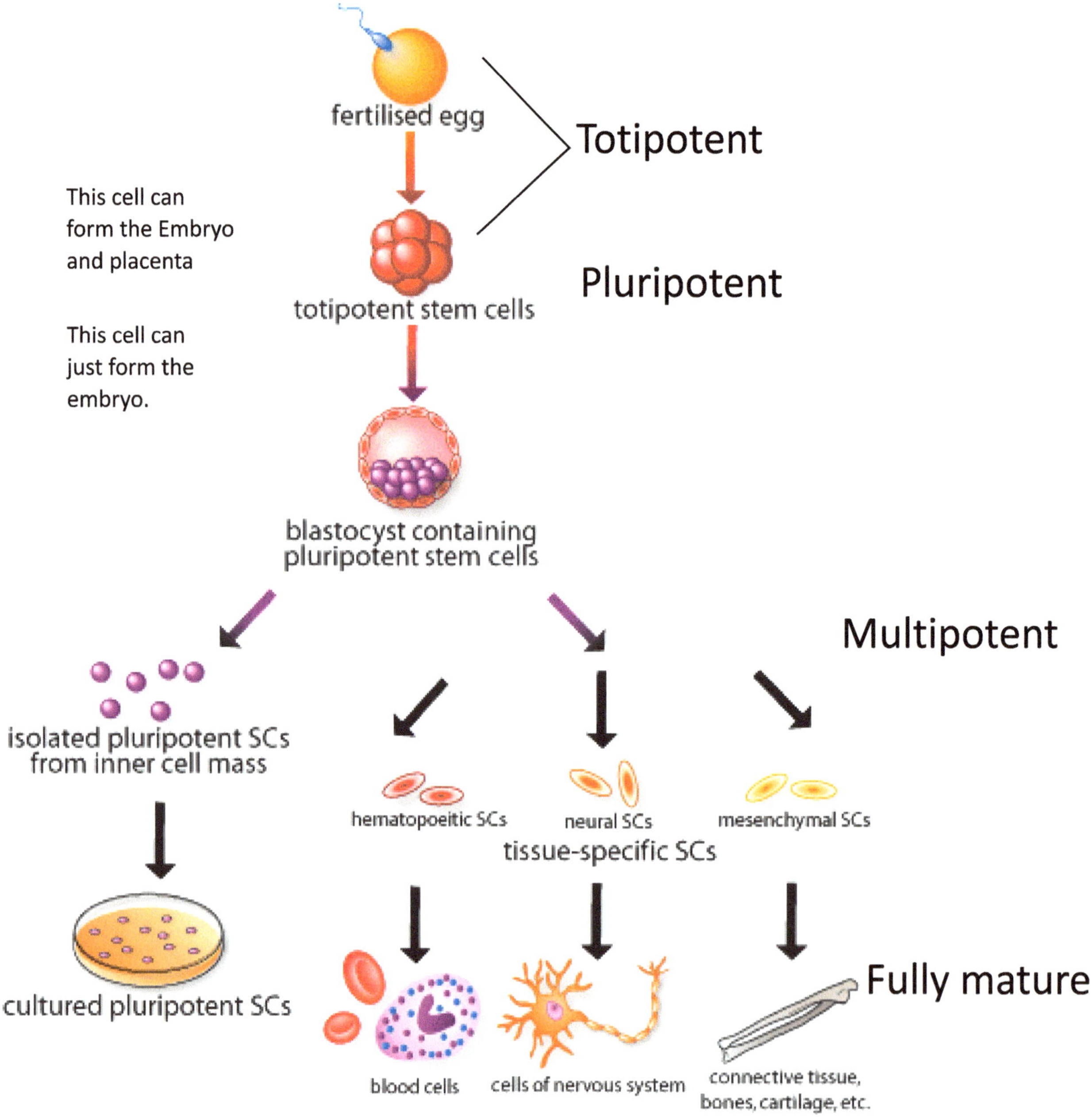

Figure 5: Development of Stem Cells

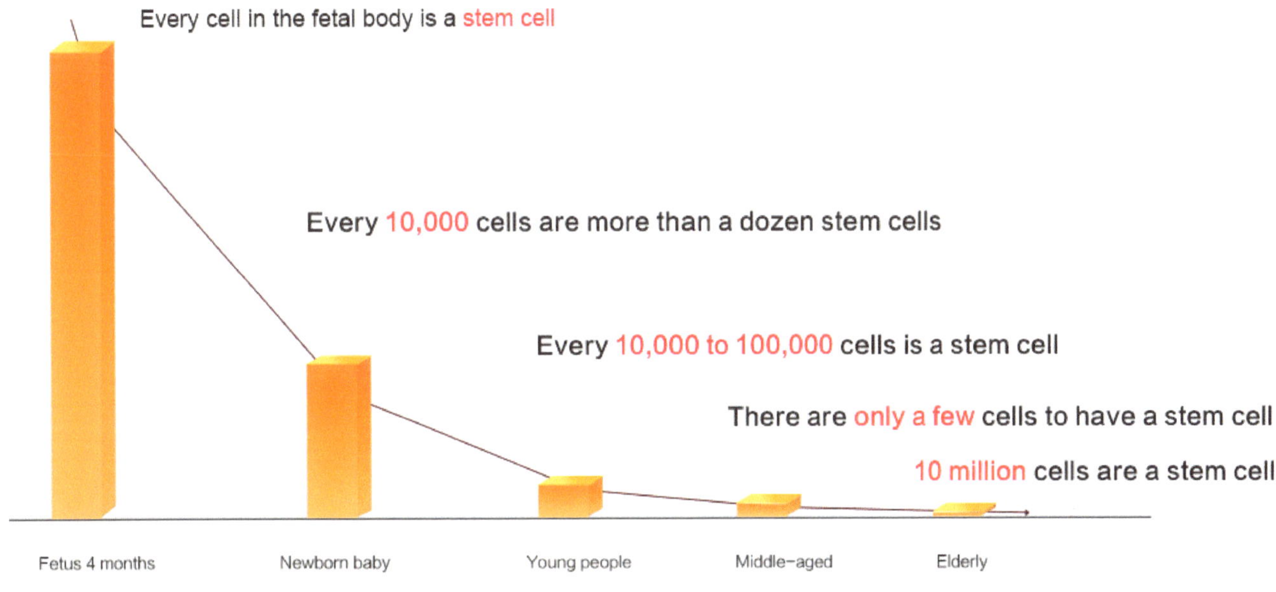

Figure 6: Age-wise Stem Cell Count

Bone Marrow

- Found in the spongy bone where blood cells form
- Used to replace damaged or destroyed bone marrow with healthy bone marrow stem cells.
- Treat patients diagnosed with leukemia, aplastic anemia, and lymphomas
- Need a greater histological immunocompatibility

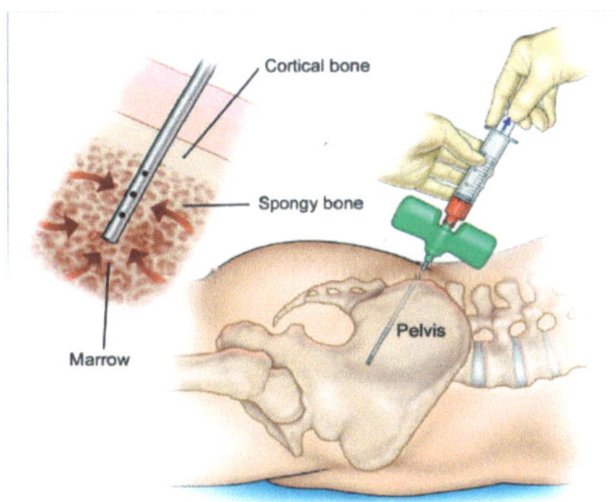

Figure 8: Isolation of Bone Marrow

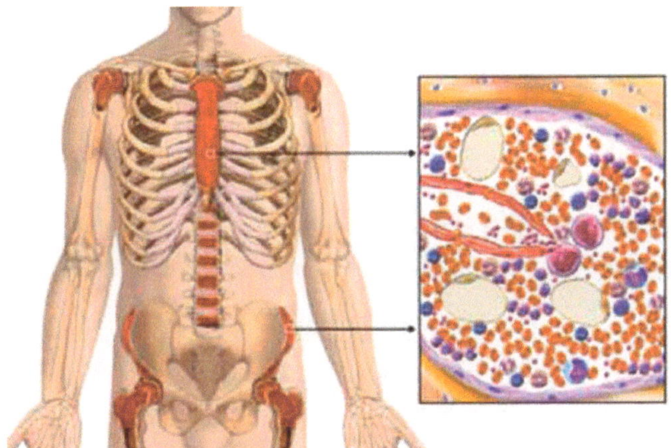

Figure 7: Bone Marrow

ADSC-Stromal Vascular Fraction (SVF)

SVF Composition

- Hematopoietic CD45 cells (9%)
- Monocytic CD13 cells (11%)
- Hematopoietic/ Connective Tissue CD 90 cells (29%)
- Endothelial progenitors CD31, CD105, CD146 cells (47%)
- Early lymphohematopoietic progenitors CD34/ CD133 (7%)
- The CFU-F assay was used to evaluate the frequency of mesenchymal progenitors in the SVF estimating a frequency of 1/4880, a value about 7 times greater than the reported data for bone marrow and comparable with the data reported for umbilical cord blood

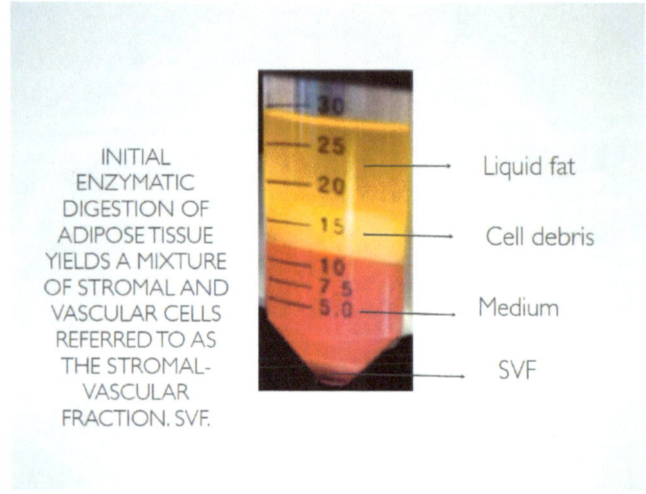

Figure 9: SVF Composition

Fate of Stem Cells After Implantation

- Disperse into the adjacent tissue and become smooth muscle, fibroblast, striated muscle, urothelium, blood vessel, fat, and hair follicle
- Differentiate into component cell types and integrate with the target tissue
- Secrete a plethora of growth factors
- Also attract the growth of blood vessels toward them – facilitate tissue formation

Use of Stem Cells in Functional Gynaecology

1. O-shot
2. P-shot
3. Peyronie's disease
4. Male genital enhancement
5. Intimate area rejuvenation
6. Labia majora augmentation
7. Premature Ovarian failure
8. Non-obstructive azoospermia
9. Endometriosis

Why IV-SVF for Anti-aging?

- Medicinal Signalling Cells (MSC) home to sites of inflammation and secrete immuno-modulatory and anti-inflammatory factors
- Inhibit cell surveillance
- Enhance proliferation and differentiation of endogenous progenitors
- Generalized repair

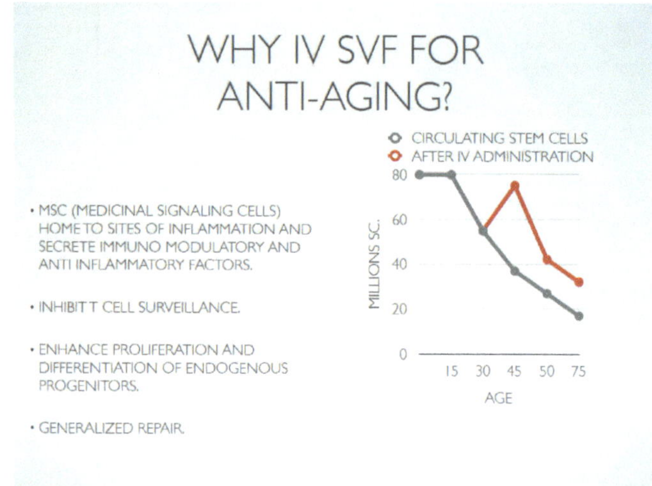

Figure 10: Increase in Stem Cells after IV treatment

Results of Anti-aging Stem Cell Treatment

- Youthful appearance with even skin tone, reduced age spots, fewer lines and wrinkles
- Reduced fatigue and tiredness
- Improved energy, stamina, and vitality
- Relief from aches, pains, and stiffness in joints
- A boost in libido, sexual prowess, and activity
- Healthy weight maintenance
- Greater muscle strength, reduced flabbiness
- Motivation to be active, exercise, and work
- Improved mood, happier and healthier outlook

REFERENCES

1. https://harvardsciencereview.org/2016/05/16/cellular-senescence-age-and-cancer/
2. Vascular & Endovascular Review 2018;1(1):17–21.
3. https://www.creative-biolabs.com/stem-cell-therapy/disease-specific-stem-cell-therapy-development.htm

FAT GRAFTING IN GYNECOLOGY

Salman Khan

Cosmetic gynecology covers a range of procedures aimed at enhancing the aesthetic appearance of the genital area. One specific application involves the use of fat grafting or fat transfer. This technique also known as lipofilling or autologous fat injection, involves taking fat from one part of the body (usually through liposuction) and injecting it into another part, the genital, Buttocks, breasts, face, etc.

In cosmetic gynecology, fat grafting is often used to rejuvenate and enhance the labia majora, which can lose volume and elasticity due to aging or other factors. By injecting a patient's fat into this area, it can restore volume, improve contour, and provide a more youthful appearance. It increases the thickness of the vaginal walls, rejuvenate the skin of the vulva, and restore genital volume. (23).

Over time, the labia majora suffer time-related insults including the loss of hyaluronic acid, collagen, and fat leading to noticeable rhytids and loss of volume; the resulting decrease in the majora to minora ratio causes the minora to look abnormally prominent. This subsequently can cause significant psychosocial impairment for a woman, who may inappropriately feel that her vulvovaginal area is 'abnormal' and she may thus suffer a decrease in sexual self-esteem.

An inherent component of fat grafting is liposuction, which is one of the most demanded procedures worldwide. Liposuction works by removing the excess fat surgically, resulting in improved contours in the desired areas. (10) There are a variety of liposuction techniques available, such as Suction-assisted, Power-assisted, Ultrasound-assisted assisted, or laser-assisted to aid fat removal.

Uses of Autologous Fat in Cosmetic Gynecology:

Adipose-derived stem cells (ADCs) are a rich source of stem cells that are widely distributed. Autologous fat transfer carries a very low chance of rejection. ADCs are a component of a complex mixture called the stromal vascular fraction (SVF), which also includes endothelial cells, extracellular matrix, and different immune cells.

Adipose-Derived Stem Cells

What is a stem cell? A basic working definition is that these cells have both a self-renewing capacity and the ability to produce daughter cells that have a more specialized function. (23) Human adipose tissue has emerged as an important source of stem cells. (24) Recently, we have discovered that fatty tissue has the highest percentage of adult stem cells of any tissue in the body, with as many as 5000 adipose-derived stem cells per gram of fat compared with 100 to 1000 stem cells per milliliter of bone marrow. In addition, one study showed that as many as 350,000 preadipocytes can be isolated from 1 g of adipose tissue.

These more primitive cells can clearly differentiate into adipose tissue, but recent studies have demonstrated the ability of adipose-derived stem cells to undergo multilineage differentiation, not just into fat but also into bone, cartilage, skeletal muscle, cardiac muscle, blood vessels, nerves, and skin Fully differentiated epidermis can form from adipose-derived stem cells in vitro, and we now have evidence that skin repair under normal physical conditions may involve stem cells.

Labia Majora Augmentation (Labia Puffing):

Labia Majora Augmentation is a procedure that aims at improving the aesthetic appearance of labia majora that are hypo-plastic or loose. This is achieved by Hyaluronic acid (HA) fillers and autologous fat grafting are common procedures. Autologous fat grafting can be sourced from various fatty areas, but typically from the thigh or inner knee, and is prepared using techniques such as labia puffing [14]. However, re-absorption of the graft must be considered to achieve the desired outcome. The surgeon's skill and anatomical knowledge are essential for a successful outcome. Nonetheless, caution must be exercised when using HA in this region to prevent complications such as granuloma formation. (12)

Volume Augmentation of the Mons Pubis and Labia Majora

Deflation of the mons pubis common with weight loss and hormonal changes may allow for posterior rotation and sagging of the labia majora. In the lithotomy position, the volume loss or paucity of fat appears as dents and puckers along the posterior one-third of the Majora. Fat transfer is the best option for augmenting both the mons pubis and the labia majora. It is best to inject the mons first to allow for elongation and elevation of the labia majora anteriorly. Next, the labia majora themselves are injected with fine cannulas (0.7-mm short blunt cannulas) using 1-cc syringes. Next, if there is a widening of the intervulvar commissure or cleft, grafting the superomedial portion of the labia majora may approximate the cleft, thus concealing the clitoral hood. Fat grafting of the mons and labia majora creates a youthful appearance in the standing mirror view.

G-spot Amplification:

Gräfenberg described the G-spot in 1950, which is positioned on the anterior vaginal wall midway between the cervix and pubic bone, 1-2 cm from the urethra, and is responsible for stimulating systematic orgasm as opposed to clitoral orgasm. (13) The scientific community, on the other hand, denies its existence. G-spot amplification is a minimally invasive procedure that involves injecting hyaluronic acid, PRP, collagen, silicone, or autologous fat into the bladder-vaginal septum to augment the protrusion of the G-spot into the vagina (3-5mm). Before the process, digital palpation is required to identify the correct location of the application. (14)

Under local anesthesia, G-spot augmentation temporarily enhances the size and sensitivity of the so-called G-spot for sensory reinforcement and stimulation with friction of the anterior vaginal wall during intercourse. As a result, higher frequency and intensity of vaginal orgasm are more likely. The results are not permanent and last between 5 to 9 months. Unfortunately, there is a dearth of scientific evidence to support the procedure's treatment of sexual dysfunction and safety. (15)

Lipofilling

To increase the thickness of the vaginal walls, rejuvenate the skin of the vulva, and restore genital volume, lipofilling, a technique involving the transfer of fat, is carried out. By grafting fat into the labial folds, this procedure thickens them, thereby shrinking the vaginal diameter [22].

Clinical Case

It is the case of a 39-year-old woman with a complaint of sexual dysfunction. When she was 23, she had her only child by vaginal delivery in Africa. An episiotomy was performed during the delivery; no obstetric forceps were used to extract the baby. No perineal immediate postpartum physiotherapy was performed.

The first sexual dysfunction symptoms started 7 years after birthdate when she resumed her sexual vaginal activity. Her symptoms dealt with vaginal laxity and included: flatus incontinence, an unpleasant feeling of a too-wide vagina, sexual dysfunction reported by her partner complaints of not feeling her vaginal walls, the overall patient's sexual dissatisfaction, and her specific conviction of not being able to reach orgasms. She did not notice any improvement in her symptoms after an intensive perineal physiotherapy treatment (40 sessions) that she started 7 years after birthdate.

Clinical examination showed a vaginal laxity with preserved vaginal tonicity, a retractile episiotomy scar, a slightly atrophic vaginal mucosa, and a pelvic floor muscle laxity with a diastasis of the anus elevators.

Treatment: During the intervention, sixteen milliliters of purified fat cells were injected into two linear anteroposterior tracts in the posterior vaginal wall and ten milliliters of the PRP-HA solution in the perineum focusing on the episiotomy scar.

Fat grafting to Labia Majora

The labia Majora (outside vaginal lips), like other parts of the body, aged and can become wrinkled and deflated. Aging, childbearing, menopause, and even weight reduction can all contribute to the loss of fatty tissue and elasticity in the labia. As the volume of the labia Majora decreases, it becomes less effective in protecting against friction and impact, resulting in pain during sexual intercourse. Furthermore, the labia minora (inner vaginal lips) may grow more visible, giving some women an unflattering appearance.

Fat grafting can be used to restore the appearance and function of a deflated labia Majora. Fat cells are extracted from the inner thigh, hips, or belly and injected into the labia Majora to revitalize and plump the area in this minimally invasive process.

- It produces more natural-looking results.
- It's an all-natural approach using your own body's fat – unlike filler injections, which your body may reject.
- The effects last longer than filler injections.
- Minimal downtime and recovery process.

Procedure Performed:

- Area for Harvesting
- Anesthesia / Tumescence Technique
- Fat harvesting (taking fat with cannula),
- Fat processing (processing the fat harvested),
- Fat transfer (injecting the fat into the tissue).

Areas for Harvesting

The abdominal area is the most preferred area for fat harvesting. However, it may not be easy to harvest abdominal fat in slim patients who do not have abdominal fat, or patients who have undergone abdominoplasty. In such cases, fat can also be harvested from the side of the abdomen, inner thigh, outer thigh, and mons pubis areas. The procedure performed to thin the mons pubis area is called 'mons pubis correction' or 'mons pubis reduction'. After a thinning process, the fat harvested is injected into the desired areas.

Tumescent Anesthesia

Tumescent local anesthesia is a type of local anesthesia that has been utilized for a variety of dermatological operations, including liposuction. It is a procedure that involves injecting a dilute local anesthetic solution into the subcutaneous tissue until it becomes hard and tense.

Tumescent technique, which permits liposuction totally by local anesthesia and with minimal surgical blood loss. (1) For infiltration local anesthesia, the conventional dosage of lidocaine is up to 4.5 mg/kg, and that with adrenaline is up to 7 mg/kg; however, in liposuction using tumescent anesthesia, the recommended maximum dose of lidocaine with adrenaline is up to 55 mg/kg. (2)

Harvesting

Current studies have not indicated increased viability from any one donor site, so harvesting sites are chosen for ease of accessibility and to improve the patient's body contours. (22) Through 3-mm incisions, a two-hole Coleman harvesting cannula with a blunt tip is attached

to a 10-ml Luer-Lok syringe. The cannula is pushed through the harvest site as the surgeon uses digital manipulation to pull back on the plunger of the syringe and create a gentle negative pressure. A combination of slight negative pressure and the curetting action of the cannula through the tissues allows parcels of fat to move through the cannula and Luer-Lok aperture into the barrel of the syringe. When filled, the syringe is disconnected from the cannula and replaced with a plug that seals the Luer-Lok end of the syringe. The plunger is removed from the syringe before it is placed into a centrifuge.

Fat Processing – Gravity / Centrifuge

Centrifugation separates the denser components from the less dense components to create layers. The upper level is the least dense and consists primarily of oil. The middle portion is fatty tissue. The lowest layer is blood, water, and any aqueous element (lidocaine). For sterility, a smaller centrifuge with a central rotor and sleeves that can be sterilized is preferred. The recommended centrifugation speed is 3000 rpm for 3 minutes. Larger centrifuges can create significantly more gravitational force at 3000 rpm than the smaller centrifuges commonly used in offices. After the oil layer is decanted, the Luer-Lok plug is removed to release the densest liquid layer. Absorbent material can be used to wick off any remaining oil. The refined fat is then transferred into a 1- or 3-ml Luer-Lok syringe

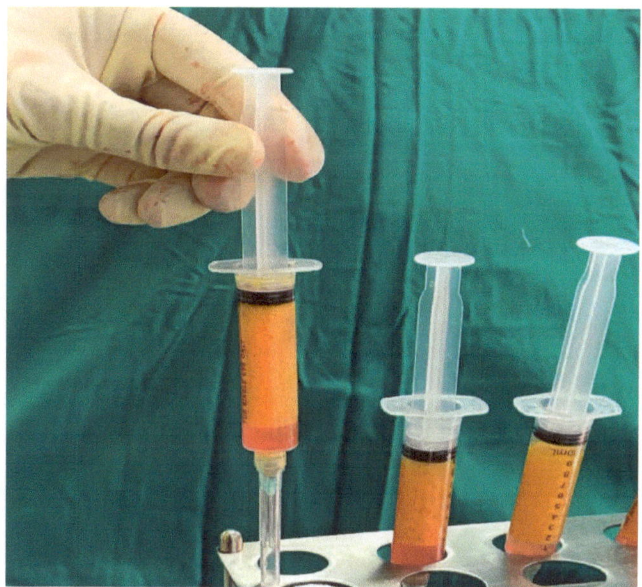

Figure 1: *10-ml Luer-Lok syringe*

Placement

The instruments used for the placement of fatty tissue are dramatically different from those used for harvesting: the placement cannulas are of a much smaller gauge, with only one hole at the distal end. Like the harvesting cannula, the proximal end of the infiltration cannula has a hub that will fit into a Luer-Lok syringe. For various situations in the face and body, cannulas with different tip shapes, diameters, lengths, and curves can be used. (22) The use of blunt cannulas allows placement of the fat parcels in a more stable, less traumatic manner. However, less blunt cannulas may give the surgeon more control for placement in the immediate sub-dermal plane, in fibrous tissue, and scars. A cannula with pointed or sharp elements can be used to free up adhesions. Through 2-mm incisions, the infiltration cannula is inserted and advanced through the recipient tissues into the appropriate plane. Fatty tissue should be injected only as the cannula is withdrawn—this, deposits the fatty tissue in the pathway of the retreating blunt cannula. As the cannula is withdrawn, the deposited fatty tissue parcels fall into the natural tissue planes as the host tissues collapse around them.

End Point

The amount of fat transported varies by situation. Fat absorption plays a crucial role in determining the endpoint or the amount of fat transported. 40-60% of fat is absorbed and the remaining survives to give the augmented appearance. Therefore, over correction by 50% is recommended.

REFERENCES

1. Barbara G, Facchin F, Buggio L, Alberico D, Frattaruolo MP, Kustermann A. Vaginal rejuvenation: current perspectives. Int J Womens Health. 2017; 9:513-519. doi: https://doi.org/10.2147/IJWH.S997002

2. Barbara G, Facchin F, Meschia M, Vercellini P. "The first cut is the deepest": a psychological, sexological, and gynecological perspective on female genital cosmetic surgery. Acta Obstet Gynecol Scand. 2015; 94(9):915-920. doi: https://doi.org/10.1111/aogs.126603

3. Halder GE, Iglesia CB, Rogers RG. Controversies in female genital cosmetic surgeries. Clin Obstet Gynecol. 2020; 63(2):277-288. Doi:

4. https://doi.org/10.1097/GRF.00000000000005194.

5. Mullerova J, Weiss P. Plastic surgery in gynecology: Factors affecting women's decision to undergo labiaplasty. Mind the risk of body dysmorphic disorder: A review. J Women Aging. 2018; 00(00):1-18. Doi:

6. https://doi.org/10.1080/08952841.2018.1529474 5.

7. Desai SA, Kroumpouzos G, Sadick N. Vaginal rejuvenation: From scalpel to wands. Int J Women's Dermatology. 2019; 5(2):79-84. Doi:

8. https://doi.org/10.1016/j.ijwd.2019.02.0036.

9. Wilkie G, Bartz D. Vaginal rejuvenation: a review of female genital cosmetic surgery. Obstet Gynecol Surv. 2018; 73(5):287-292. Doi:

10. https://doi.org/10.1097/OGX.00000000000005597.

11. Latif EZ, Diamond MP. Arriving at the diagnosis of female sexual dysfunction. Fertil Steril. 2013; 100(4):898-904. Doi: https://doi.org/10.1016/j.fertnstert.2013.08.0069.

12. Placik OJ, Devgan LL. Female genital and vaginal plastic surgery: An Overview. Plast Reconstr Surg. 2019; 144(2):284e-297e. Doi:

13. https://doi.org/10.1097/PRS.00000000000666010

14. Triana L, Robledo AM. Aesthetic surgery of female external genitalia. Aesthetic Surg J. 2015; 35(2):165-177. Doi:https://doi.org/10.1093/asj/sju020

15. Radman HM. Hypertrophy of the labia minora. Obstetrics and gynecology. 1976 Jul 1;48(1 Suppl):78S-9S.

16. Clerico C, Lari A, Mojallal A, Boucher F. Anatomy and aesthetics of the labia minora: the ideal vulva. Aesthetic plastic surgery. 2017 Jun;41:714-9.

17. Hodgkinson DJ, Hait G. Aesthetic vaginal labioplasty. Plastic and reconstructive surgery. 1984 Sep 1;74(3):414-6.

18. Alencar Felicio Y. Labial surgery. Aesthetic surgery journal. 2007 May 1;27(3):322-8.

19. Choi HY, Kim KT. A new method for aesthetic reduction of labia minora (the de-epithelialized reduction labioplasty). Plastic and reconstructive surgery. 2000 Jan 1;105(1):419-22.

20. Alter GJ. Aesthetic labia minora and clitoral hood reduction using extended central wedge resection. Plast Reconstr Surg. 2008;122:1780–1789. 16.

21. Alter GJ. Labia minora reconstruction using clitoral hood flaps, wedge excisions, and YV advancement flaps. Plastic and reconstructive surgery. 2011 Jun 1;127(6):2356-63.

22. Spyropoulos E, Christoforidis C, Borousas D, Mavrikos S, Bourounis M, Athanasiadis S. Augmentation phalloplasty surgery for penile dysmorphophobia in young adults: considerations regarding patient selection, outcome evaluation, and techniques applied. Eur Urol 2005 Jul;48(1):121e7. discussion 127e8.

23. Goodman MP. Female cosmetic genital surgery. Obstet Gynecol 2009 Jan;113(1):154e9.

24. Goodman MP, Placik OJ, Benson 3rd RH, et al. A large multicenter outcome study of female genital plastic surgery. J Sex Med 2010 Apr;7(4 Pt 1):1565e77.

25. Vogt PM, Herold C, Rennekampff HO. Autologous Fat Transplantation for Labia Majora Reconstruction. Aesthetic Plast Surg; 2011 Feb 27 [Epub ahead of print].

26. Klein A. Filler materials. In: Thorne CH, Bartlett SP, Beasley RW, Aston SJ, Gurtner GC, Spear SL, editors. Grabb & Smith's plastic surgery. 6th ed. New York City: Lippincott Williams & Wilkins; 2007. p. 468e74.

27. Sawhney CP, Banerjee TN, Chakravarti RN. Behavior of dermal fat transplants. Br J Plast Surg 1969 Apr;22(2):169e76.

28. Abu-Ghname A, Perdanasari AT, Reece EM. Principles and applications of fat grafting in plastic surgery. InSeminars in plastic surgery 2019 Aug (Vol. 33, No. 03, pp. 147-154). Thieme Medical Publishers.

29. Coldiron B, COLEMAN III WP, Cox SE, Jacob C, Lawrence N, Kaminer M, NARINS RS. ASDS guidelines of care for tumescent liposuction. Dermatologic Surgery. 2006 May;32(5):709-16.

SHOCKWAVE THERAPY

Nitesh Prajapat

CHAPTER

29

Extracorporeal Shockwave Therapy (ESWT) is an advanced treatment that uses acoustic shockwaves to break soft tissue calcifications, enhance collagen synthesis, release growth factors, and stimulate your body's healing process.

The therapy enhances blood circulation and accelerates healing.

The initial clinical application of ESWT technology was lithotripsy, a procedure that has been used since the 1980s to break kidney stones.

ESWT has undergone extensive clinical trials and is US FDA-approved.

INDICATIONS

- Lithotripsy for kidney stones and biliary calculi
- Tennis elbow
- Shoulder rotator cuff pain
- Achilles tendinitis
- Plantar fasciitis
- Bone healing and bone necrosis
- Nonhealing fractures
- Foot ulcers in diabetics
- Erectile dysfunction

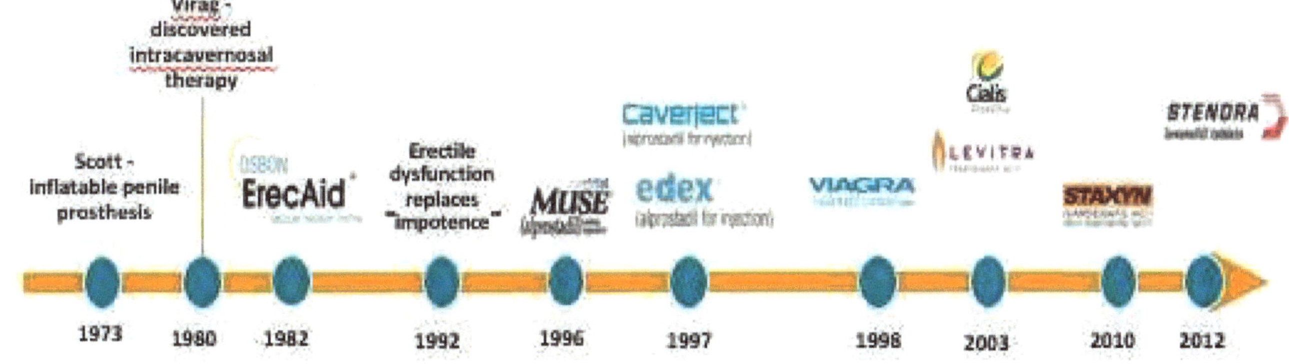

ED treatment algorithm (before 2018)

2018 AUA Erectile Dysfunction Guideline

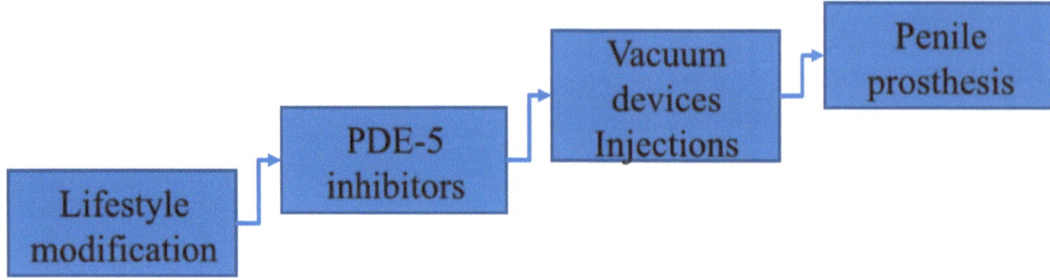

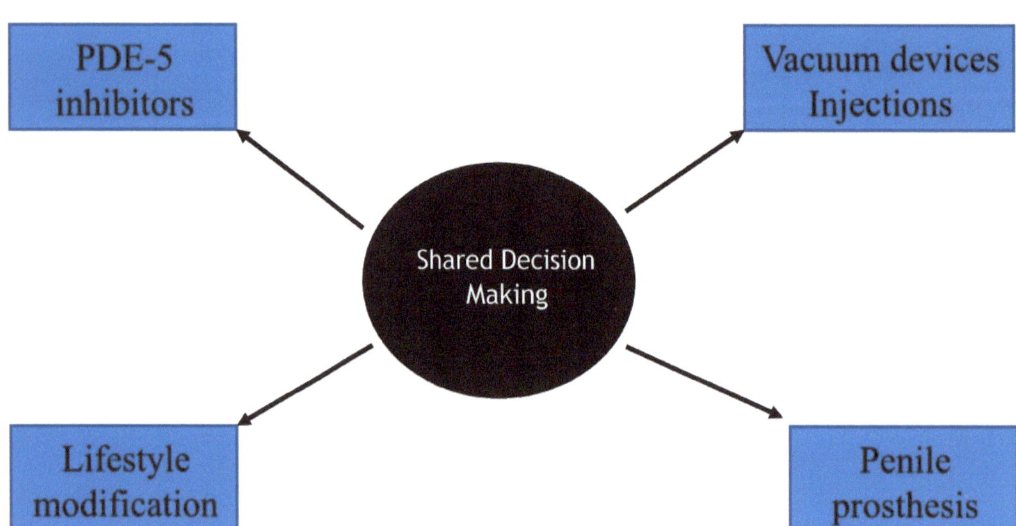

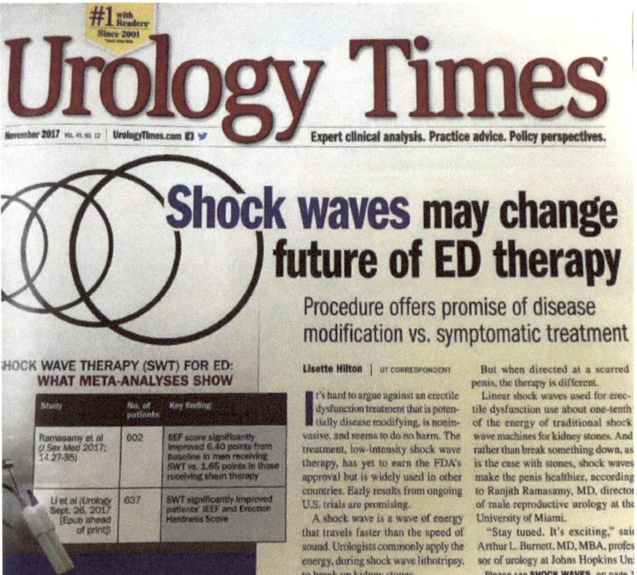

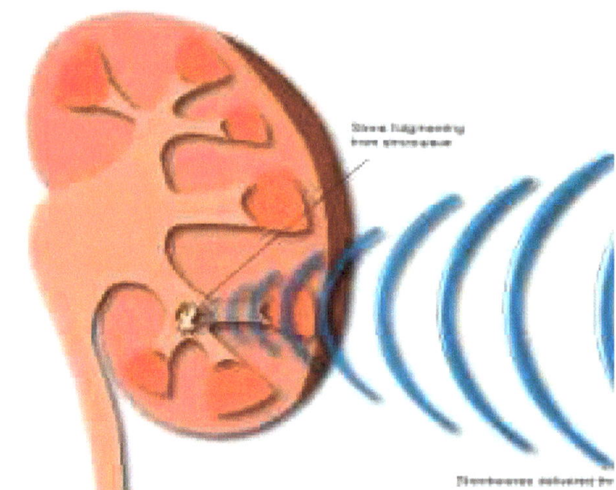

- Smaller focal volume
- Energy concentrated

ESWL vs. LI-SWT

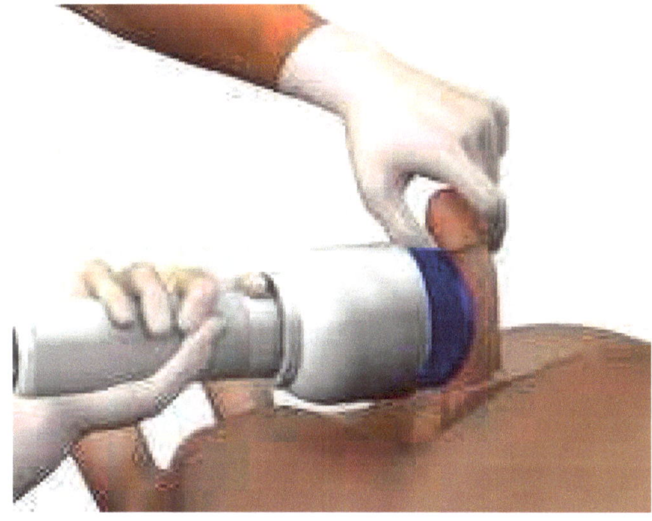

- Larger focal volume
- Energy spread greater area

Shockwave Therapy to Treat Other Medical Conditions

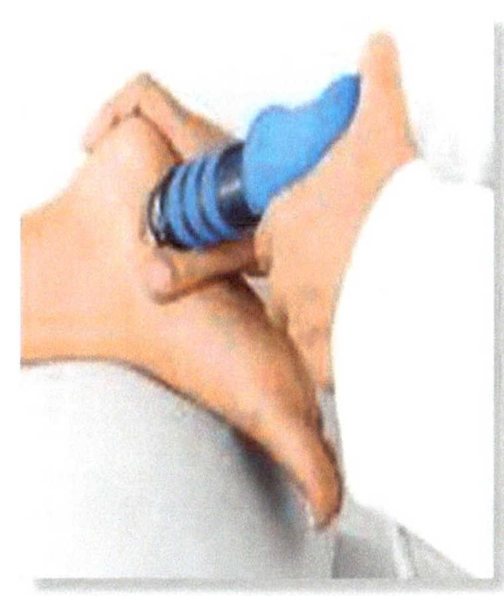

Plantar fasciitis

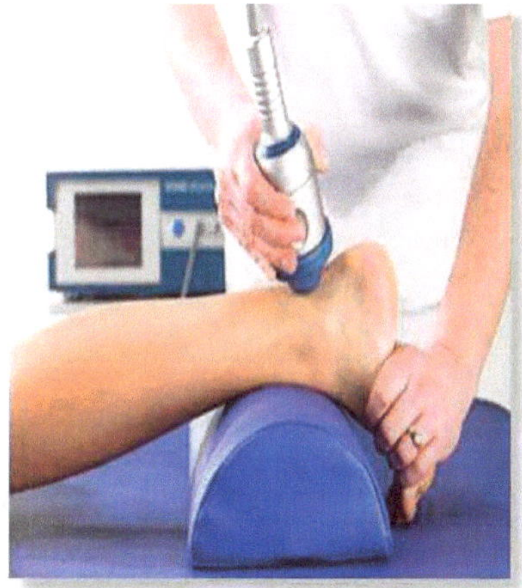

Achilles tendonitis

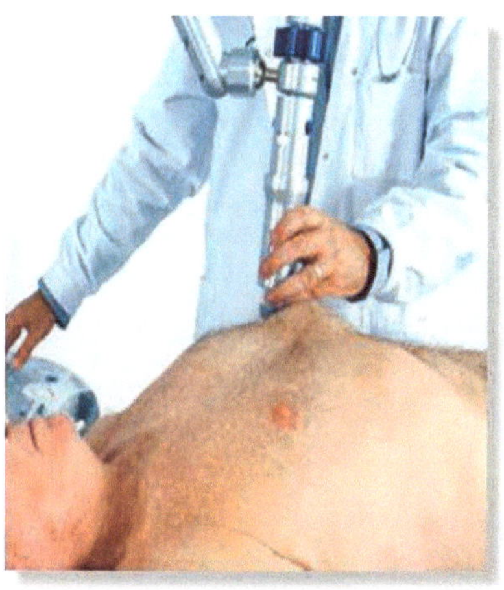

Myocardial revascularization

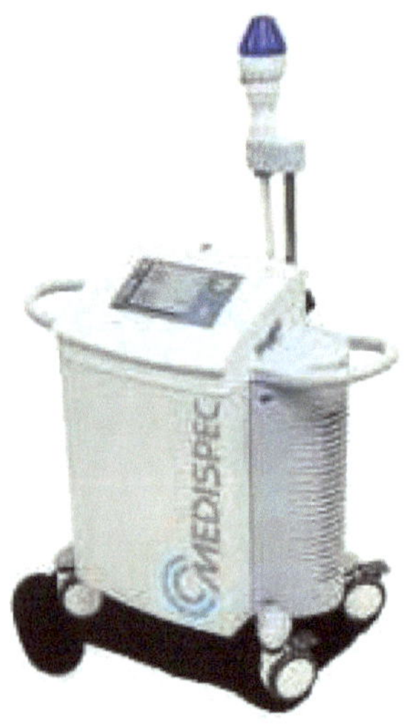

Several LI-ESWT Devices

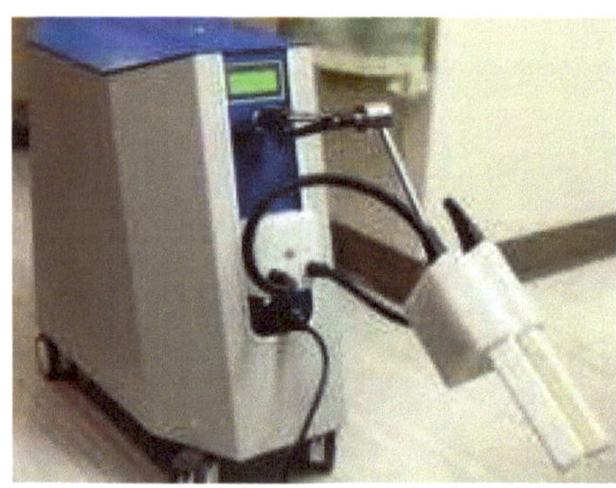

Direx (Israel) – MORENOVA

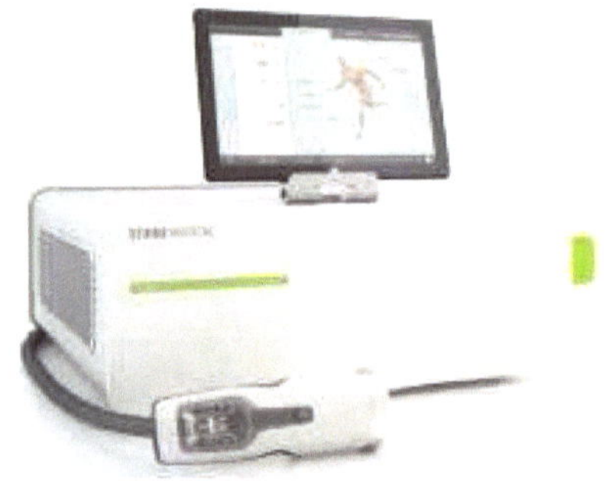

Medispec(Israel) – ED1000

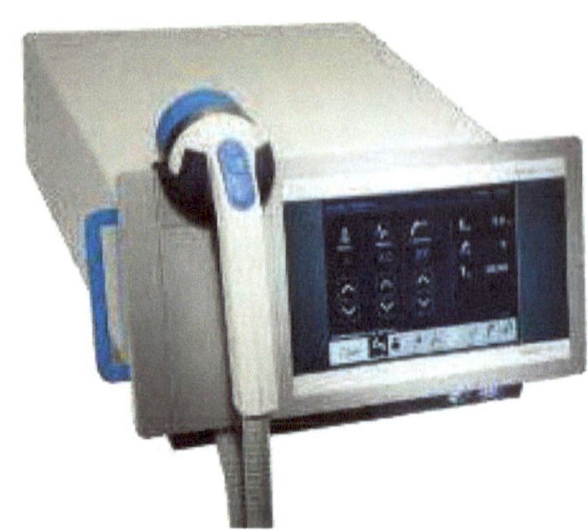

Dornier (France)- Aries 2

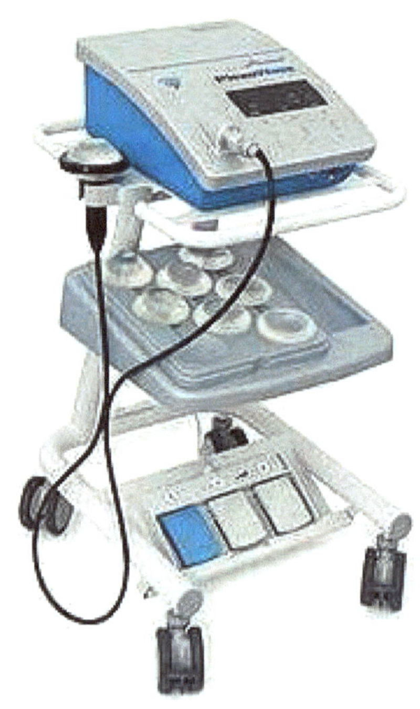

Stortz (Switzerland) - DUOLITH SD1 - FDA approved
Richard-Wolf GmbH (Germany) - PiezoWave2

SEXUAL MEDICINE REVIEWS

The Basic Physics of Waves, Soundwaves, and Shockwaves for Erectile Dysfunction

Jonathan Elliott Katz, MD,[1] Raul Ivan Clavijo, MD,[2] Paul Rizk, MD,[1] and Ranjith Ramasamy, MD[1]

Sex Med Rev 2020;8:100–105

- Shockwave: a disturbance that propagates through any medium (in this case liquid/tissue) at a speed faster than the speed of sound travels through that medium

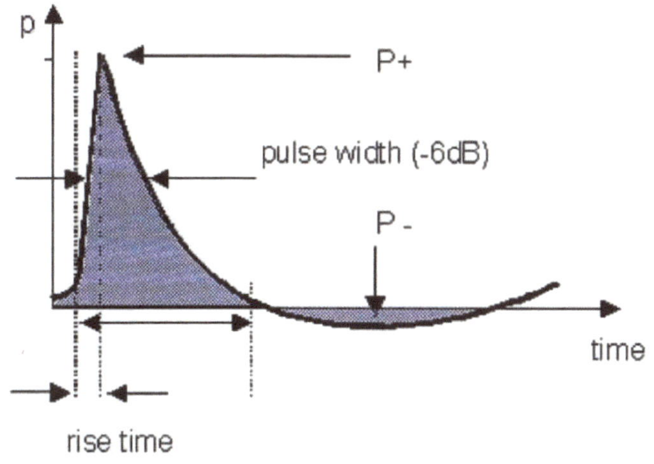

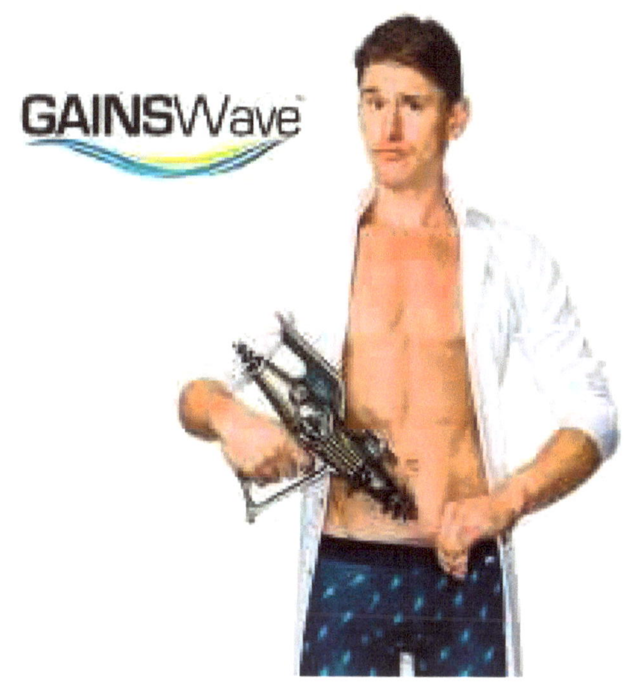

- Characterized by the rapid rise in pressure over a very short interval of time
- Energy density or energy flux density (EFD), is the amount of energy delivered to a specific area of tissue

$$EFD = [E\text{-}A] = [1\text{-}\rho c]\int p^2(t)\,dt$$

E = the energy of the shockwave p = pressure

A = area of the wave surface is A ρ = the density of the medium is

c = the propagation speed in the fluid t = time

Radial Shockwaves (Gainswave Technology)

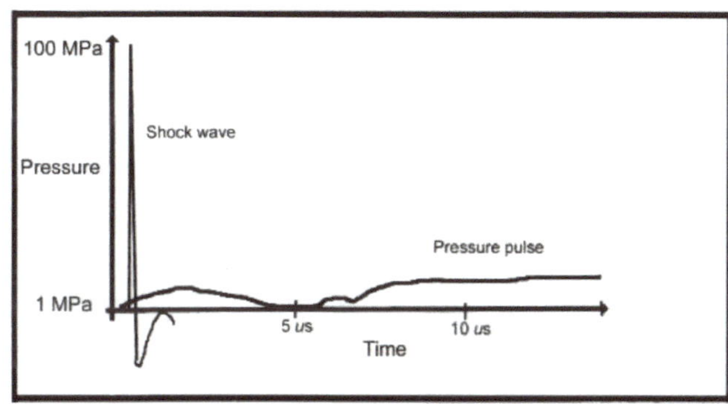

Focal vs Radial Shockwaves:

- maximum pressures are 100 times lower
- pulse durations are 1,000 times longer
- Corresponding lower EFD and depth of penetration
- Therefore, medical class 1 device (low-risk of harm to patient)

McClure, S., & Dorfmüller, C. (2003). Extracorporeal shock wave therapy: Theory and equipment. Clinical Techniques in Equine Practice, 2(4), 348–357. doi:10.1053/j.ctep.2004.04.008

SEXUAL MEDICINE REVIEWS

The Basic Physics of Waves, Soundwaves, and Shockwaves for Erectile Dysfunction

Jonathan Elliott Katz, MD,[1] Raul Ivan Clavijo, MD,[2] Paul Rizk, MD,[1] and Ranjith Ramasamy, MD[1]

Sex Med Rev 2020;8:100–105

While technically not a shock wave, **radial pressure devices** have also been marketed as shock wave devices in veterinary medicine. These machines work like a small jack hammer to transmit mechanical energy to the body. These devices have much lower energy and extremely limited penetration relative to true shock wave devices.

Parameter	Electro-hydraulic	Electro-magnetic	Piezo-electric	Radial Pressure
Peak Energy	Highest (E)	Moderate (1/3 E)	Low/Moderate (1/4 E)	Low (1/200 E)
Rise Time	Most rapid (T) Nanoseconds	Moderate 1,000 times T Microseconds	Moderate 1,000 times T Microseconds	Slow 1,000,000 times T Milliseconds
Focal Volume	Largest (V)	Small (1/15V)	Very Small (1/200V)	Not applicable: not focused
Total Energy	Highest (E)	Moderate (1/10 E)	Low (1/50 E)	Very Low (1/200 E)
Penetration Depth	Variable: Deepest (0 – 11cm)	Moderate (5cm)	Variable: Moderate (0 - 6cm)	Very shallow (< 1cm)

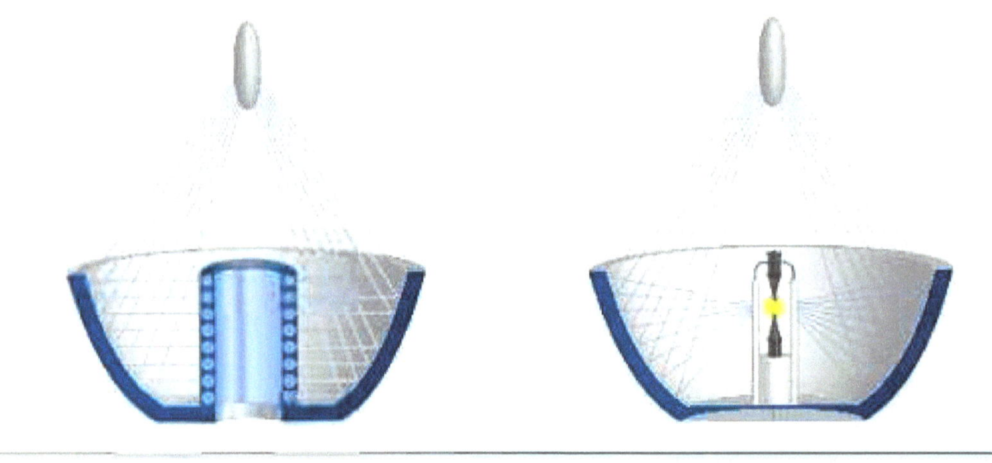

Cavernosal Tissue Response to Shockwaves

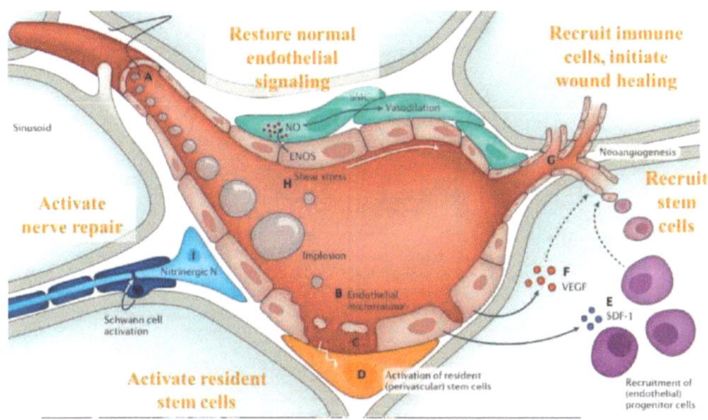

LiSWT for ED - Meta-Analysis of RCTs

- Meta-analysis of 7 randomized controlled trials using LiSWT for ED reporting IIEF-EF scores
  - 602 subjects
  - Age – 60y
  - Follow-up – 5 months
- Improvement in IIEF-EF score was 6.4 (Treat) vs. 1.6 (Sham)

Studies in this meta-analysis:

1. Kitrey ND, Gruenwald I, Appel B, et al. J Urol 2016.
2. Feldman R, Denes B, Appel B, et al. J Urol 2015.
3. Fojecki GT, Osther P. Poster ESSM 2015; København.
4. Srini VS, Reddy RK, Shultz T, et al. Can J Urol 2015.
5. Hatzichristou DG, Kalyvianakis DE. EAU, 2015, abstract 124.
6. Yee CH, Chan ESY, Hou S-M, et al. Int J Urol 2014.
7. Vardi Y, Appel B, Kilchevsky A, et al J Urol 2012.

LiSWT for ED - Meta-Analysis

- Meta-analysis of **7 randomized controlled trials** using LiSWT for ED reporting IIEF-EF scores
  - 833 subjects
  - Follow-up – 3-6 months
- Improvement in IIEF (mean difference: 2.00; 95% confidence interval [CI], 0.99– 3.00; p < 0.0001)
- Therapeutic efficacy at least 3 months
- Patients with mild-moderate ED had better therapeutic efficacy
  Studies in this meta-analysis:

1. Chitale S, Morsey M, Swift L, et al. BJU Int 2010.
2. Poulakis V, Skriapas K, de Vries R, et al. Asian J Androl 2006.

1. Zimmermann R, Cumpanas A, Miclea F, et al. Eur Urol 2009.
2. Srini VS, Reddy RK, Shultz T, et al. Can J Urol 2015.
3. Vardi Y, Appel B, Kilchevsky A, et al. J Urol 2012.
4. Yee CH,Chan ES,Hou SS, et al. Int J Urol 2014.
5. Olsen AB, Persiani M, Boie S, et al. Scand J Urol 2015.

Phase II Randomized, clinical Trial Evaluating 2 Schedules of **Low intensity shockwave theraoy for the treatment of erectile disfunction**

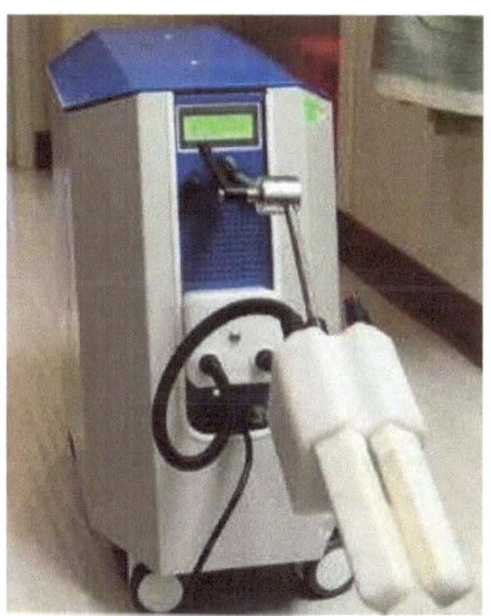

More Nova Shockwave Generator

- 80 men with ED (30-80 y/o)
- Baseline IIEF-EF: 11-25
- Randomized 1:1
  - Group A: 5 consecutive daily treatments of 720 shockwaves (N=45)
  - Group B: 6 treatments of 600 shockwaves qOD over 2 weeks (N=43)
- IIEF and EHS baseline and 1, 3 and 6 months

Phase II Randomized, clinical Trial Evaluating 2 Schedules of **Low intensity shockwave theraoy for the treatment of erectile disfunction**

Low -intensity

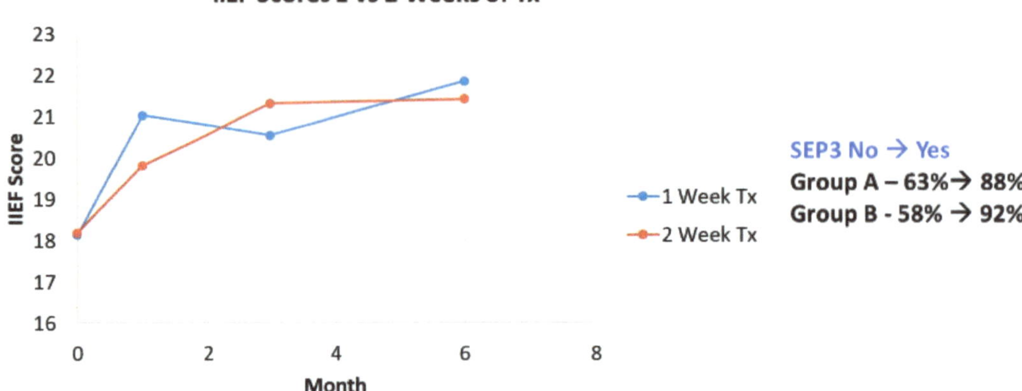

Group A: 720 shocks daily for 5 consecutive days
Group B: 600 shocks every other day for 6 days

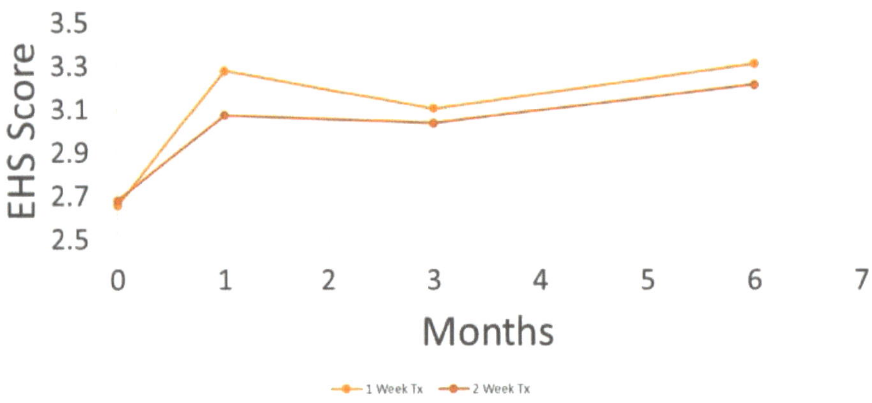

Treatment Group	MCID for IIEF at 6mo
1 week	66%
2 week	75%

ED treatment algorithm – SWT?

- Non-surgical ED treatment consists of PRN medications/ interventions.
- The goal of LI-ESWT is to restore spontaneous erection

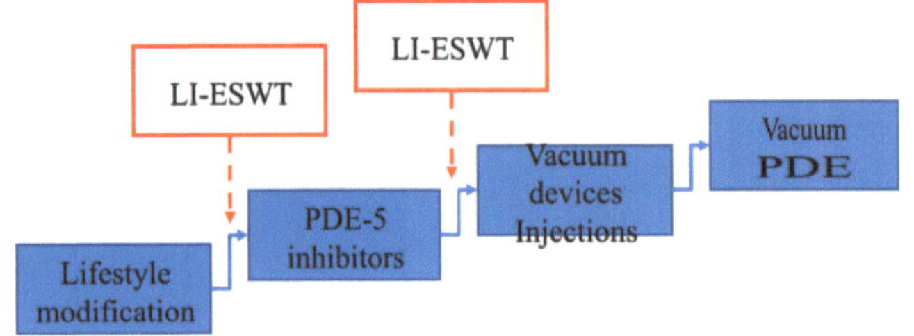

AUA ED Guidelines: Low-Intensity Shock Wave Therapy

- For men with ED, low-intensity extracorporeal shock wave therapy (ESWT) should be considered investigational. (Conditional Recommendation; Evidence Level: Grade C)
- Given the availability of other treatments that are less burdensome and known to be effective and the fact that ESWT is not FDA-approved, the Panel concludes that ESWT should only be used in investigational settings in the context of an institutional review board (IRB)-approved clinical trial.

SETTING UP COSMETIC GYNECOLOGY PRACTICE

Garima Srivastav

Aesthetic gynecology is the fastest-growing offshoot of gynecology.

There is an increasing number of patients becoming aware and demanding these procedures as well as more and more gynecologists inculcating cosmetic gynecology in their practice due to the easy learning curve, fewer complications, better patient compliance, and good results.

As the branch gains popularity, gynecologists, dermatologists, urogynecologists, plastic surgeons, and even general practitioners are now getting into the field.

Various training programs are being held for the same as by the Indian Association of Cosmetic Gynecology and, the American Board Of Aesthetic Gynecology to name a few. The author herself has trained 300 + doctors in India, Nepal, Dubai, Sharjah, Oman and Pakistan.

GOALS
- To balance the art, science, and business of aesthetic gynecology
- Keep the balance between medical and aesthetic patients

HOW TO SET UP YOUR PRACTICE
- Running a dedicated cosmetic gynecology practice.
- Building up pre-existing practice

LOCATION
Location is of paramount importance in establishing your practice. Your office should be visible and accessible to the general public. One should understand the demographics of patients in that particular location to be able to practice.

It should be easily approachable, safe, and close to major hospitals.

PHONE HANDLING
The person responsible for handling the front office and phone should be an expert salesperson and understand the basics of the subject.

They should be open in their way of speaking and not at all judgemental while handling patients.

WAITING AREA
The clinic should have a good aesthetic ambience too, with various banners and boards communicating various health issues that can be now addressed differently using technologies

CONSULTATION
The patient's concerns should be addressed. As a doctor, you must now not only learn to do the procedure but also be able to sell your skills to the patients.

A good patient hearing is the cornerstone of a good consultation in aesthetic gynecology.

PROCEDURE ROOM
It should be a minimum of 10* 12 feet to accommodate the procedure chair and various machines and utilities.

PROCEDURES
Before performing any procedure, the patient must understand the purpose, technique, results, and number of sittings and should have realistic expectations from the procedure.

A detailed informed consent should be signed by the patient.

TEAM
A good team is crucial for any practice. Documentation of the procedure, data collection, and post-procedure counseling are as important as the procedure itself.

MARKETING

Marketing is very crucial in the practice of aesthetic gynecology.

You should be an expert or hire a manager to do the same for you.

You should put yourself out there, be open to discussions on public platforms, and talk about newer modalities on your platform.

1. Start working on your social media.

   Make sure you put brochures, fliers, and videos talking about the various new technologies.
2. Be seen digitally, be on Google searches, and ads.
3. Arrange meetings with GPs, alternate medicine health practitioners, and colleagues.
4. Create and design a good web page.
5. Understanding awareness is the key.
6. Ask your patients to give reviews and put them on your profile.

WHAT NOT TO DO

- Do not start with a debt
  - This is the major cause of failure!!!
  - No profit is seen until the debt is paid back
  - Starts with injectable/Peels:
    - No inventory is needed
    - Shipped overnight
    - Get a laser later when practice going well and cash flow increases
    - Do not trust sales reps
    - Do not discuss fees with your patients/clients.

FINAL THOUGHT

- The cosmetic medical market has matured in the last 15 years, but the 5 areas above are not entirely tied to medicine, they're business strategies.

- You won't find "improving patient outcomes" here because those are simply table stakes.
- Patient Outcomes - You can't build a business marketing better patient outcomes.
- Outcomes are what the patient says they are.
- You can have a perfect outcome but if the patient's expectations are unrealistic
- The 'outcome' from the patient's point of view can still be negative.
- As cosmetic gynecology services are not always purely cosmetic but may have functional gynecology elements, many of these services overlap as in:

OBSTETRICS

PRP in C sec, episiotomy scars, tears, stretch marks, lax abdomen, pigmentation, body contouring, and weight loss.

GYNECOLOGY

Genitourinary Syndrome of Menopause, Aesthetic concerns in PCOD, vaginal laxity, labial deflation, hyperpigmentation, vaginal dryness, vaginal infection like BV and Candidiasis, and Lichen Sclerosis.

SEXUAL MEDICINE

FSD, Orgasm intensification shots, Clitoral hood reduction, vaginismus, vulvodynia, and dyspareunia.

Hence, every gynecologist can learn more about this new branch and can help improve the overall health care of our women.

Just like other branches, it may too take time to develop and be accepted over time.

Stay motivated! !

REFERENCES

1. Svenson, O. Acta Psychologica 47, 143–148 (1981).
2. Kruger, J. & Dunning, D. Journal of Personality and Social Psychology 77, 1121–34 (1999).
3. Gabriel, M. T., Critelli, J. W. & Ee, J. S. J. Pers. 62, 143–155 (1994).
4. Hoorens, V. & Harris, P. Psychology and Health 13, 451–466 (1998).
5. Alicke, M. D. & Govorun, O. in The Self in Social Judgment (eds Alicke, M. D., Dunning, D. A. & Krueger, J. I.) 85–106 (Psychology, 2005).
6. Cross, P. New Directions for Higher Education 17, 1–15 (1977).
7. Taylor, S. E. & Brown, J. D. Psychological Bulletin 103, 193S210 (1988).
8. Shedler, J. et al. American Psychologist 48, 1117–1131 (1993).
9. Colvin, C. R. & Block, J. Psychol. Bull. 116, 3–20 (1994).
10. Sharot, T. The Optimism Bias: A Tour of the Irrationally Positive Brain, New York: Pantheon Books (2011).
11. Johnson, D. D. P. & Fowler, J. H. Nature 477, 317–320 (2011).
12. Trivers, R. Deceit and SelfDeception: Fooling Yourself the Better to Fool Others. (Allen Lane, London, 2011).
13. Barber, B. M. & Odean T. Quarterly Journal of Economics 116, 261–292 (2001)
14. Johnson, D.D.P. 2004. Overconfidence and War: The Havoc and Glory of Positive Illusions. Cambridge: Harvard University Press (2004).
15. Enquist, M. & Leimar, O. J theor Biol 127, 187S205 (1987)

www.ingramcontent.com/pod-product-compliance
Lightning Source LLC
Chambersburg PA
CBHW041558110726
48005CB00002B/215